Handbook of Calf Health and Management

Handbook of Calf Health and Management

A Guide to Best Practice Care for Calves

Edited by Sophie Mahendran

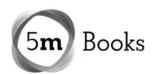

5m Books

First published 2021

Published by
5M Books Ltd,
Lings, Great Easton,
Essex CM6 2HH, UK
Tel: +44 (0) 330 1333 580
www.5mbooks.com

A Catalogue record for this book is available from the British Library

ISBN 9781789181340
eISBN 9781789181760
DOI 10.52517.9781789181760

Book layout by Servis Filmsetting Ltd, Stockport, Cheshire
Printed by by Ömür Printing & Binding, Istanbul, Turkey
Photos by the authors unless otherwise indicated

This book is dedicated to everyone who works tirelessly to ensure the safety, health and welfare of the calves in their care. While there are many jobs to juggle on farm, in the words of Ron Swanson: 'Never half-ass two things. Whole-ass one thing.'

Contents

Contributors

Editor

Sophie Mahendran, BVMedSci, BVMBVS (Hons), MSc, DipECBHM, MRCVS
Lecturer in Farm Animal Health and Welfare at the Royal Veterinary College, UK
Royal Veterinary College, Regional Veterinary Centre – South of England, Stinsford, UK
Business Centre, Kingston Maurward College, Dorchester

Authors

Benjamin Barber, BVetMed (Hons), MRCVS
Veterinary surgeon at Syncrgy Farm Health, UK

Dr Nicola Blackie, BSc, PhD
Lecturer in Production Animal Science at the Royal Veterinary College, UK

Dr Richard Booth, BVSc, PhD, BSc (Hons), MRCVS
Associate Professor in Veterinary Extension Services and Infectious Diseases of Cattle at the Royal Veterinary College, UK

Esme Moffett, BVMS, MRCVS
Veterinary surgeon at Synergy Farm Health, UK

Peter Plate, Dr med vet, MRCVS
Lecturer in Livestock Veterinary Extension Services at the Royal Veterinary College, UK

Tom Shardlow, BVSc, MRCVS
Veterinary surgeon at Synergy Farm Health, UK

Professor Claire Wathes, BSc, PhD, Dsc, FRASE, FRSB
Professor of Veterinary Reproduction at the Royal Veterinary College, UK

Preface

Ensuring the future of a dairy herd must start with the health and development of its youngstock – only then can a farm build strong foundations that will have long lasting positive results. However, calf health is often under-appreciated and can be overlooked in favour of the adult milking herd when deciding on herd priorities.

This book explains the reasons why successful calf rearing is vital, right from conception, all the way through to first service of heifers. It draws on the authors' wealth of knowledge and experience to provide both in-depth science and evidence-based reasoning for decision making in calf health. In addition to this, the authors have first-hand experience of rearing calves, and appreciate that it can be both one of the most rewarding and most frustrating jobs on a farm, often switching between the two on a daily basis!

This book offers some practical tips for both stockpeople to use during day-to-day rearing, as well as tips for vets who are dealing with youngstock herd health. It takes the reader through the important life stages of the calf in each chapter, highlighting common areas for improvement and outlining gold standard practice that we should aim for. Important information regarding legislation is also included for completeness, as well as descriptions of common diseases and health management procedures.

We hope you will find this book to be a useful guide in your future calf rearing enterprises.

Abbreviations

ACF	automatic calf feeder		FSH	follicle stimulating hormone
ACTH	adrenal corticotropic hormone		GH	growth hormone
ADG	average daily gain		IBK	infectious bovine keratoconjunctivitis
AFC	age at first calving		IBR	infectious bovine rhinotracheitis
AHDB	Agriculture and Horticulture Development Board		ICS	intercostal spaces
APHA	Animal and Plant Health Agency		LH	luteinising hormone
BAL	bronchoalveolar lavage		MDA	maternally derived antibodies
BCMS	British Cattle Movement Service		ME	metabolisable energy
BCS	body condition score		MIC	minimum inhibitory concentrations
BHV	bovine herpesvirus		ML	macrocyclic lactones
BRD	bovine respiratory disease		NPS	naso-pharyngeal swabs
BRSV	bovine respiratory syncytial virus		NSAID	non-steroidal anti-inflammatory drug
BVD	bovine viral diarrhoea		ORT	oral rehydration therapy
BVDV	bovine viral diarrhoea virus		PI	persistently infected
BW	bodyweight		PIR	parainfluenza virus
CE	calving ease		PLI	profitable lifetime index
CMR	calf milk replacer		PTA	predicted transmitting ability
CP	crude protein		RFID	radio-frequency identification
CPH	country parish holding		RFM	retained foetal membranes
DCAB	dietary cation-anion balance		ROC	receiver operator curves
DDD	defined daily doses		SARA	sub-acute ruminal acidosis
DLWG	daily live weight gain		SCC	somatic cell count
DM	dry matter		SNP	single nucleotide polymorphisms
ELISA	enzyme-linked immunosorbent assay		TCC	total coliform counts
			THI	Temperature–humidity index
FEC	faecal egg counts		TMR	total mixed ration
FPT	failure of passive transfer		TNZ	thermoneutral zone
			TPC	total plate count

Chapter 1

Pregnancy and the pre-partum environment

Claire Wathes and Sophie Mahendran

CHAPTER CONTENTS

Even prior to birth, the future of a calf is being defined by decisions made that lead to conception and development of the fetus. These include parent selection, the effect of genomics, methods of conception, the environmental and management factors affecting the dam (such as nutrition and heat stress). This chapter discusses the choices and impacts of the decisions made in this period, as well as briefly exploring some fertility issues, such as twinning and abortion.

BREEDING CHOICES

Producing and rearing good quality heifers represents the future of any dairy herd and this process begins at conception. Creating the right balance of selection traits in a breeding programme leads to greater sustainability and long-term profitability. Before breeding begins it is vital to establish the goals of the farm business over a number of years and plan ahead to achieve them. The farm business must consider carefully both how many and what type of animals will be required as replacements.

The advent of sexed semen and genomic testing have opened up more possibilities in terms of optimising the genetic potential for each herd. Any improvements made by this approach will remain with the herd over time, as opposed to management changes that improve the current performance. A detailed consideration of genetics is outside the scope of this book, so this section includes a brief summary of some of the key points.

> Within the UK, the Agriculture and Horticulture Development Board (AHDB) Dairy provides a series of comprehensive guides on genetics and breeding that explain the science behind genetic and genomic selection and their practical application in greater detail. The guides are freely available to download at www.dairy. ahdb.org.uk.

PARENT SELECTION

The majority of dairy herds breed their own replacement heifers using artificial insemination (AI). In the past, breeding decisions were made based on the known appearance and performance of the dams, while potential sires were assessed for a variety of traits based on the actual performance of their daughters. This information was used to derive their *predicted transmitting ability* (PTA). This is a measure used to express the genetic potential of an animal as a parent and which compares their individual values with an average genetic base for the population.

Genetic improvement depends on the desired traits being inherited by the offspring, with some traits being more heritable than others. Highly heritable traits are easier and quicker to improve through breeding. Milk production traits are highly heritable, with heritability values of 55% for milk yield and 68% for protein percentage. Other traits, including those for health and fertility, are

less heritable but consistent genetic progress can still be made through careful selection. Examples of these include susceptibility to mastitis (4%) and calf survival (5%).

GENOMIC SELECTION

The genome refers to the entire complement of the animal's genetic material. In cattle each cell contains approximately 22,000 genes made of deoxyribonucleic acid (DNA). Each gene contains a sequence of DNA building blocks, called nucleotides, which encode for the synthesis of a gene product. Minor differences in the structure of the genes between individuals may lead to alterations in which proteins are made and so affect how the cell performs.

The most common types of genetic variation are single nucleotide polymorphisms (SNPs). Each SNP represents substitution of a single nucleotide that occurs at a specific position in the genome (Figure 1.1).

This genetic variation ultimately affects the characteristics of the individual including productive capability, fertility, conformation and disease resilience. The actual performance is also

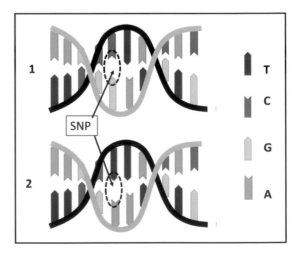

FIGURE 1.1 Comparison of the DNA sequences of two individuals at a specific position of the genome: in (1) there is a C nucleotide whereas in (2) there is a T nucleotide at this position.

influenced by the environment in which the animal is kept. Analysis of the genome provides information on the potential of each heifer (or their daughters in the case of bulls) to perform in different environments and farm types. In genomic selection, the PTAs are derived from DNA profiles based on genotype (rather than actual performance) and can be obtained from samples taken as soon as an individual is born (see Chapter 2). Testing young animals enables the farmer to take better informed decisions regarding whether to keep them as replacement females. Those heifers with less genetic potential can be sold (avoiding unnecessary rearing costs) or bred to a beef bull (producing higher value calves). By following this approach, the average genetic merit of the cows in the herd should improve over time as genetic changes are both cumulative and permanent.

How is genomic testing performed?

Tests can be based on either hair, tissue or blood samples. Tufts of hair samples (to total about 30–50 hairs) should be pulled (not cut) from a clean area, ensuring that the hair follicles are present. They should be placed immediately into a paper envelope or plastic bag, taking care to avoid any mixing between animals. Alternatively, tissue sampling ear tags can be utilised (see Chapter 2).

The results are then analysed to translate the genetic sequence into a genetic index. Other information can also be obtained, such as confirmation of parentage, level of inbreeding and the presence in the herd of harmful recessive genes. The two options are as follows.

- Low density chips are microarrays of microscopic spots containing specific DNA sequences (probes) attached to a solid surface. These provide a full range of trait information, as found in an AI bull catalogue, and are most reliable for breeds with large population sizes.
- High density chips provide information on extra traits such as polled or coat colour. They

are also recommended for females sired by a non-genomic tested stock bull or for heifers from less common dairy breeds.

Genomic tests for common breeds, such as Holsteins and Friesians, typically provide between 50% and 70% reliability as to the individual's genetic potential, depending on the trait. Other breeds currently have less information available, but this situation is steadily improving as more animals are tested. Some systems on offer can also provide information on crossbred animals.

Choice of dam

The first consideration is how many replacement heifers are required – this is established from calculating the replacement rate.

> The replacement rate is calculated by taking into account the culling rate plus expansion plans for the herd.
>
> A quick way to estimate this is to look at the average number of lactations in a herd. For example, a 200-cow herd with an average lactation number of 5 will need to replace ~20% (one-fifth) of the herd each year, therefore requiring ~40 replacement heifers per year.

Ideally, all the heifers which are being considered as replacements should be genomically tested so that the most informed choices can be made with respect to breeding decisions. The criteria used for selection will be farm specific, but it is important to maintain a good overall balance such as the traits included in the UK-based Profitable Lifetime Index (PLI), which selects for moderate-sized animals with good health traits and improved kilos of fat and protein in the milk. Good conformation, including that of the udder, is also important (Figure 1.2).

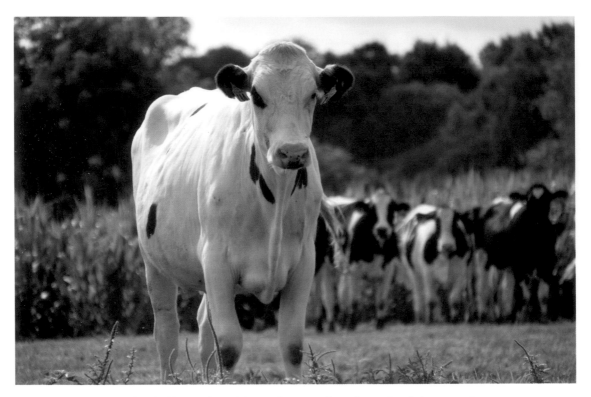

FIGURE 1.2 When selecting heifers to breed from, the overall conformation is important.

Choice of sire

Most farms will select a few bulls that fit their breeding strategy and milk contract (Figure 1.3). This may include an appropriate mix of dairy and beef, using both sexed and conventional semen. The reliability of the bull proof increases over time as actual information on daughter performance is added to data initially obtained from genomic testing to derive their PTA values. It is therefore prudent to include some proven sires in addition to using young genomic sires.

Trait selection

Traits for selection are divided into four broad categories: production traits, fitness traits, linear type traits and composite type. All are important, but only fitness traits directly related to rearing of heifers are considered here – calving ease and calf survival. Note that both the list of traits for which PTA values are calculated and their definitions vary between countries as sires are selected based on the most prevalent production systems and breeds. The definitions included here are for the UK.

Calving ease

This is a measure of the amount of assistance given at calving which is assumed to relate to calving ease. Calving ease (CE) indexes are expressed as 'per cent easy calvings' on a scale of –4% to +4% and are centred around a breed average of 0. Positive figures predict easier than average calvings and negative figures predict more difficult calvings. There are two CE indexes that together give a complete picture of a bull's calving performance.

- Direct calving ease (dCE%) predicts the ease with which a calf by that sire will be born.

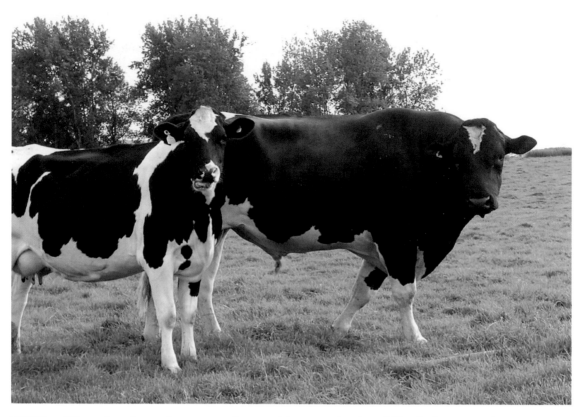

FIGURE 1.3 When choosing a sire, you need to consider several traits, picking bulls to complement each specific herd.

- Maternal calving ease (mCE%) predicts the ease with which a daughter of that sire will give birth.

It is important to select easy-calving sires for maiden heifers (dCE > 0.5%) to minimise the proportion of difficult calvings. However, birth weight, gestation length and cow stature are also heritable and all are influential at calving. dCE favours the birth of smaller calves, which may then develop into smaller cows and have more difficulty calving themselves. Conversely, mCE favours larger cows with a greater frame size, which is associated with larger calves. A bull with above-average mCE will therefore produce more difficult births in heifers, compared to a bull with below-average mCE, so it is important to consider both indices in the herd. dCE% is also more heritable than mCE% (7% versus 4%).

Calf survival

Calves of some sires are more likely to survive between birth and 10 months of age than those sired by other bulls. The typical range for calf survival PTAs is from –5% (poor) to +5% (excellent), which indicates a 10% difference in the probability of survival between the progeny of the worst and best bulls.

SEXED SEMEN

The first calves born using sexed semen straws were produced in 1999, and since then the technology has been constantly improving and its popularity steadily increasing. There are a number of benefits to its use in a dairy herd (1,2).

Benefits of using sexed semen

Easier calving: Avoids birth of bull calves with a higher risk of dystocia. This is particularly useful when breeding maiden heifers.

Genetic gains: Enables targeting the best heifers and cows in the herd to produce the herd replacements. It is then also possible to breed the less desirable cows with beef semen, so increasing the value of their calves. This increases the rate of genetic gain.

Avoids production of male dairy calves: Public perception on welfare is driving bans on exporting or killing unwanted male calves at birth.

Increase herd size: Increasing the production of replacement heifers within the herd facilitates herd expansion while avoiding the need to buy in replacements, which also improves biosecurity.

Income diversification: Can produce more breeding heifers than the farm requires, which can then be sold.

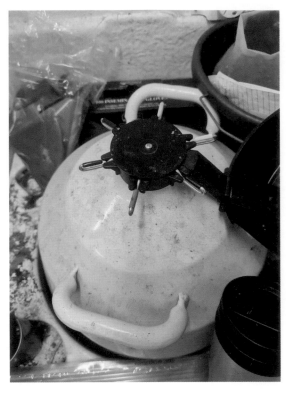

FIGURE 1.4 A flask containing semen straws being stored frozen on farm.

Fertility used to be lower in sexed semen compared to conventional semen straws, but new sorting techniques and higher numbers of sperm per straw have reduced this difference. However, management still needs to be excellent around breeding in order to achieve good conception rates, which can be maximised by the following.

- Using maiden heifers or cows with a good health history. Avoid heifers that are poorly grown or cows that have had mastitis, metritis/endometritis or lameness.
- Animals should receive a consistent diet, nutritionally balanced for energy, protein and minerals, and dietary changes avoided from 1 month before until 1 month after service.
- Good management pre-service is vital. Animals, particularly heifers, should be moved into small groups and handled quietly to reduce stress.
- Reliable heat detection is essential.

- Having good handling facilities available with a crush.
- Avoid breeding during times of heat stress.
- Handle the straws carefully, always with tweezers and never by hand. Taking straws out of the liquid nitrogen to check is best avoided, but if it is done then the time out of the liquid nitrogen must be minimised to less than 5 seconds (Figure 1.4).

EMBRYO TRANSFER

Embryo transfer is worth considering if a female in the herd has an exceptionally good genotype as it enables her to provide more replacements into the herd than would otherwise be possible. Details of the procedure are outside the scope of this book but, in brief, it involves treating the donor female with hormones that increase the number of ovarian follicles maturing at the same time. One option is then to collect the developing oocytes (eggs) from the follicles by aspiration, referred to as ovum pickup. The eggs are then transferred to a laboratory, fertilised and grown into 7-day-old embryos. Alternatively, the donor animal is inseminated and her reproductive tract is flushed out 6–8 days later to recover any embryos present. In either case, embryos are graded as to quality and those meeting the evaluation criteria can then be transferred into a recipient animal, which must have been synchronised to be at the same stage of the oestrous cycle. Good quality embryos can also be frozen and placed in storage for later use. This reduces conception rates slightly but storing frozen embryos means they can be used when most convenient on farm. The number of embryos recovered by either technique varies widely between individual animals. It is crucial to success that both donor and recipients are in optimum condition.

GENETIC DEFECTS

Several genetic defects can cause problems in dairy breeding. The advent of genomic testing has enabled geneticists to link more of these defects to individual genes or haplotypes (DNA sequences at specific locations on a chromosome that are transmitted together as a group). These conditions are most commonly caused by recessive genes, meaning the defect only appears when both the dam and the sire are carriers. Each parent has one normal and one faulty copy of the gene, referred to as being heterozygous. The genetic defect will then occur in about one in four of their offspring, which inherit both both copies of the faulty gene (and are said to be homozygous for that gene). The likelihood of both parents being carriers increases with the degree of inbreeding in the population. Most AI sires are now tested for known defective genes, although novel mutations may arise in future. Any sires found to be carriers can still be used in a breeding programme but they must be identified.

Depending on the type and severity of the defect, the affected offspring may die at an early stage of embryo development (apparent as reduced dam fertility), later in pregnancy or as a neonatal/young calf. Some common genetic defects include:

- **complex vertebral malformation**, which causes stillbirths or, more commonly, abortion or foetal reabsorption before 260 days of gestation
- **brachyspina**, which causes abortion and stillbirth associated with a shortened spinal cord, long legs and abnormal organs
- **Holstein cholesterol deficiency (HCD)**, which causes a lack of cholesterol in the animal's cells, usually leading to death within months of birth. Heterozygous animals (which inherit only one copy of the HCD gene) also have reduced levels of cholesterol and compromised health.

PREGNANCY

Conception and development of the placenta and fetus

Fertilisation takes place within the oviduct and involves a single sperm fusing with the egg membrane. The egg starts to divide, initially forming a ball of cells known as a morula, surrounded by the zona pellucida forming a protective layer around it. The morula moves from the oviduct into the uterus about 4–5 days after ovulation, and on around day 8 the embryo 'hatches' out of the zona pellucida. By this time the morula has hollowed out into a blastocyst with a fluid filled cavity enclosed by a single layer of trophoblast cells. The trophoblast later forms the external membrane of the placenta, becoming known as the chorion. The blastocyst also contains a group of cells called the inner cell mass, which will develop into the actual embryo. The trophoblast together with the inner cell mass are referred to as the conceptus (the products of conception) (Figure 1.5).

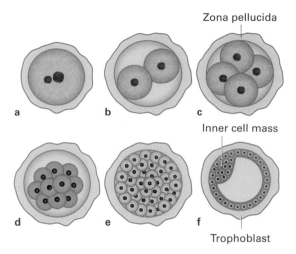

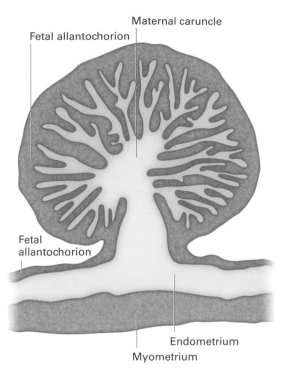

FIGURE 1.5 The formation of a blastocyst from a fertilised ovum. (a) Recently fertilised egg showing two pronuclei, one of which was derived from the successful spermatozoon; (b) cleavage divisions begin, yielding two cells; (c) four cell stage; (d) beginning of morula; (e) morula; (f) a cavity develops in the morula, forming a blastocyst. Throughout these early stages the conceptus is enclosed in the zona pellucida, but it will shortly hatch out of this and start to elongate.

FIGURE 1.6 The foetal allantochorion invaginates the maternal caruncle to form a convex placentome. This is where most of the nutrient, gas and waste exchange occurs between the foetal calf and its dam. The endometrium and myometrium together make up the uterine wall.

The conceptus continues to expand, and from around day 15 of pregnancy onwards, elongates dramatically to occupy the entire length of the uterine horn. From day 20 of pregnancy onwards, attachments start to form with the endometrium (the uterine lining). In ruminants, the endometrium already has a number of pre-formed attachment points called caruncles. As the trophoblast continues to expand within the uterus it progressively makes contact with each attachment point: projections known as villi then develop and penetrate into the caruncles. The villi form foetal cotyledons which together with the maternal caruncles become known as placentomes (Figure 1.6). Cattle therefore develop cotyledonary placentas, which each contain between 75 and 125 placentomes.

The inner cell mass also gives rise to three extra-embryonic membranes, which contribute to development of the placenta. The first to form is the yolk sac, which is a transient structure formed as an outgrowth of the primitive gut. The amnion is formed next as a complete sac around the embryo, which becomes filled with amniotic fluid and provides a protective 'pond' around the embryo. The amnion is the membrane that surrounds the calf at birth, when it may be referred to as the water bag (see Chapter 2). The third extra-embryonic membrane is the allantois. It expands to make contact with the external chorion, jointly forming a membrane called the allantochorion (or chorio-allantois), which becomes filled with allantoic fluid. The allantochorion is very well vascularised, with a network of blood vessels leading to and from the fetus via the umbilical cord, which traverses the amniotic cavity to act as the main transport system between the mother and fetus.

The growth of the placenta precedes that of the embryo/fetus, with most placental growth occurring in the first half of gestation, whereas the majority of foetal growth in terms of size and weight happens in the final third of pregnancy. The placenta is absolutely critical to foetal development as it provides the main route for the transfer of nutrients from the mother and for the disposal of waste products, such as urea and carbon dioxide. A study in beef and dairy cattle that examined the morphology of expelled placentas obtained immediately after calving both found highly significant relationships between the weight of the calf, the placental weight and the total cotyledonary surface area, confirming the importance of the placental surface available for nutrient transfer to the developing fetus (3).

Factors influencing foetal development

Throughout foetal development, growth occurs through cell proliferation together with differentiation of the individual cells into the many different cell types required to form a viable newborn animal. Each tissue experiences critical periods of rapid cell division when it is particularly vulnerable to damage (4). Growth requires an adequate supply of both nutrients and oxygen. The supply of nutrients to the fetus is through the placenta, so growth of the placenta is strongly linked to growth of the fetus. If the placenta does not reach a sufficient size in the first half of gestation then it will be unable to deliver sufficient nutrients in late pregnancy when the demand is greatest. It has been estimated that the uterine environment is responsible for about 60% of the variation in calf size at birth, with maternal and paternal genotype each contributing a further 20% of the variation (5).

Primiparous heifers

Most dairy heifers are bred for the first time at about 60% of their mature bodyweight and so conceive well before they are fully grown themselves (6). Studies in both teenage humans and adolescent sheep have shown that immature mothers who become pregnant preferentially partition nutrients towards their own continued growth at the expense of the developing fetus (7,8). Uterine size is also more restrictive during the first pregnancy. In a comparison of placental characteristics at birth in cattle, it was found that the average cotyledonary weight of a heifer's placenta was lower compared with placentas of cows, and they also had a smaller total cotyledonary surface area (9). Younger age in adolescent Holstein dams was, however, associated with a higher cotyledon number, suggesting some capacity for placental compensation (10). Despite this, age at first calving (AFC) does have a significant effect on birthweight, with calves born to Holstein heifers of <22 months of age averaging 2.75 kg less than those calving at over 22.5 months (3). Despite the growth restriction experienced *in utero,* calves born to primiparous dams are then capable of postnatal catch-up growth (11).

Multiparous cows

In subsequent pregnancies most multiparous cows are lactating and are likely to be close to peak lactation during early gestation. They are therefore partitioning a significant proportion of their feed intake towards the mammary gland for milk synthesis during a period that is critical for placental growth. Although the nutrient requirements of the embryo are low in early pregnancy, their metabolic activity is high and this represents a critical period when many organs start to develop (12). At the other end of pregnancy, the greatest accumulation of foetal mass occurs in the last 2 months of gestation (13) when cattle are often on restricted rations during the dry period. Studies have demonstrated that low birthweight calves are more likely to have older dams (lactations 3–6) with higher peak yields (>42 kg/day), producing calves that were on average 10 kg lighter and, unlike the offspring of primiparous heifers, they did not exhibit catch-up growth and so remained significantly lighter (11). Similarly, it has been found that the birth weight of the calves was reduced in offspring of multiparous Holstein cows with high cumulative milk production (>7200 kg) between conception and drying off (3).

EPIGENETICS

Factors affecting development of the fetus include not only its own genetic make-up and that of its dam, but also a range of other variables including dam age and size, foetal number, maternal nutrition (both before and during the pregnancy), maternal health and aspects of the external environment, such as temperature. All of these additional factors and their interactions affect not only size at birth, but more importantly how the calf develops into adulthood, including such key matters as productivity and longevity. This concept is known as developmental programming or epigenetics, and gave rise to an area of science referred to as the 'foetal origins of adult disease' (14).

Epigenetics looks at the observable characteristics (phenotype alterations) of an animal caused by different gene activity levels (whether individual genes are turned on or off in particular cells) but does not involve changes in an animal's DNA sequence. The differences in gene activity can be affected by the internal environment in which a fetus develops (the uterus), and also by the external environment in the first few weeks of a calf's life. Epigenetics helps to explain some of the paradigms about Nature versus Nurture. Subsequent exposure of the newborn calf to certain bioactive substances in the environment (including in milk and colostrum) can also cause epigenetic changes, leading to alterations in gene expression (15).

More basic genetics

Nearly every cell in the body contains all the same genetic information within its' DNA. However, only certain parts of this DNA sequence are utilised in different cell types due to the presence of specific transcription factors that regulate gene activation and protein production in a cell.

For example, the cells of the hair and the brain contain the same DNA, but different areas of the sequence are active, producing mature differentiated cells with very different functions.

A gene is a defined section of the DNA that codes for production of a specific protein (which is made up of a chain of amino acids). Each type of protein has a unique shape and chemical property that determines its function, for example, structural, chemical, immunological. Small changes to the DNA code for a protein (such as DNA methylation) will alter the protein's activity. The study of these changes is epigenetics.

Environmental factors that can affect gene expression in a calf including the health of the mother, and are summarised in Table 1.1.

TABLE 1.1 Examples of some of the environmental exposures that can affect a calf's epigenetics (16).

The mother's environment while pregnant	The calf's environment in the first few weeks of life
Maternal malnutrition, e.g. negative energy balance	Nutrition – extended feeding of colostrum
Foetal number	Infectious disease
High metabolic load, e.g. high milk production	Heat or cold stress
Raised body temperature, e.g. suffering an infectious disease	
Social stressors, e.g. changing management groups	
Maternal heat stress from a high environmental temperature in the summer	

Calves born to either undernourished dams, or high-yielding dairy cattle that have partitioned their energy into milk production rather than foetal growth, have altered gene expression to enable them to maximise the uptake and utilisation of nutrients in similar low nutrient environments (17). This may also happen in first calving heifers who are themselves still growing, and so have to partition their energy and protein intakes between their own body growth, and those of their calf. However, these epigenetic adaptations in the calf can become harmful if the calf then lives in a nutrient-rich environment, resulting in higher risks of developing obesity and insulin resistance characteristics (18).

HEAT STRESS

The changing global climate is resulting in an increased risk of heat stress during the summer months. The effect of heat stress has already been well studied in many hot countries, but now also needs to be considered in previously more temperate countries such as the UK.

> Heat/thermal stress is caused by an environment that results in an alteration in body temperature that is not entirely compensated for by the animal's thermoregulatory mechanisms or behavioural responses.
>
> Thermoregulatory responses include increased respiratory rate, panting and sweating.
>
> Behavioural responses include increased water intake, altered feed intake patterns (eating at cooler times of the day), decreased activity and movement, increased standing times and seeking shade.

When assessing environmental conditions, the temperature–humidity index (THI) is more informative than just temperature alone. Including a humidity assessment is important as this affects the ability of the body to lose heat by evaporation of moisture from the skin and respiratory tract. In people, the THI was originally designed to indicate the level of discomfort that would be felt – how hot and sweaty a particular environment would make you feel.

The upper threshold for cattle comfort is a THI of 72. Cows are able to tolerate much higher temperatures when the relative humidity is low as they can dissipate excessive heat more effectively by sweating. However, during hot and humid conditions, the cooling ability is compromised, and this has negative consequences for the cow and her fetus.

Heat stress in pregnant dry cows leads to reduced feed intake by the dam (19), as well as affecting the growth and physiology of the developing calf (20). Calves are born earlier with a gestation period shortened by ~4 days (21), and are born lighter and shorter, and experience higher morbidity and mortality rates. This can be due to depressed immune competence from compromised passive transfer from colostrum, along with altered energy metabolism (22, 23). Studies have also demonstrated long-term implications for the productivity of a calf born to a heat stressed dam, with dairy heifers going on to produce significantly less milk during their first lactation (24). The reason for this is thought to be that heat stress reduces blood flow to the uterus and placenta, so compromising the development of the calf through reduced delivery of oxygen and nutrients. This is amplified by heat stress during the dry period, as 60% of calf birth weight is gained during the last 2 months of gestation, with organs undergoing functional maturation in preparation for life outside the uterus (25).

Another effect of heat stress is a reduction in plasma levels of calcium and magnesium in pregnant cows, along with a reduction in colostrum levels of calcium, magnesium and phosphorus (26). These minerals are required for bone production in the calf, both in utero and after birth, so this process may be adversely affected by exposure of late gestation cows to heat stress.

Owing to these negative effects, keeping dry cows cool during the summer months is important. Measures to improve cooling include providing plenty of shade for cows to get out of direct sunlight, ample access to clean drinking water and, if housed, provision of fans in sheds to ensure air movement. In some countries, such as the southern USA, sprinkler cooling systems are used – something that may need to be considered as the climate changes elsewhere.

DAM NUTRITION AND BODY CONDITION

The effect of nutritional supply on foetal growth encompasses not only what the dam is actually being fed at different stages of pregnancy, but also her body condition, which affects the availability of additional nutrients through mobilisation of body tissue, in particular fat. In addition to the main building blocks of proteins, carbohydrates and fats, many micronutrients including vitamins and minerals are absolutely essential for foetal development. In cows the situation is further complicated by competition for nutrients within the dam – it used to be considered that the fetus acted somewhat like a parasite, drawing what it required from the host mother. In practice, however, the dam has significant control over the proportion of nutrients in her system that are made available to cross the placenta.

Undernutrition in early pregnancy leads to placental enlargement, thought to be an adaptation on the part of the fetus to try to extract more nutrients from the mother (27). Ill health during pregnancy can also lead to a short-term dramatic reduction in food intake, with the main organs affected being the foetal lungs and the morphology of the placentomes (28).

Care must be taken during the dry period to find a balance in the control of energy intakes in the dam to prevent excess weight gain, while ensuring a balance of micro- and macro-minerals is still provided. Mineral content is often lacking when the diet is based predominantly on grass or with low-quality forage. The pre-partum diet of the cow has been linked to the occurrence of anaemia in newborn calves due to poor iron transfer from the dam. This is exacerbated in primiparous heifers by their own requirement for iron due to their continued growth, as well as that of their fetus. Research indicates that during periods of heat stress and restricted feed intakes in late gestation, calves are born with decreased levels of haemoglobin and a reduced haematocrit level (26). The resultant calf anaemia can reduce growth rates and adversely affect health and mortality levels. Vitamin E is another colostral component that varies depending on dam supplementation, and can help with the calf's development of cellular immunity (29).

During the transition period (from 3 weeks prior to calving), the dam's diet needs to include volatile fatty acids (VFAs) to help prepare the digestive tract for the transition back onto a milking cow ration, as well providing an increase in energy to compensate for a reduction in dry matter (DM) intake that occurs around calving (Figure 1.7). As well as correct energy levels, ensuring adequate metabolisable protein levels in dry cow rations is important, with the recommendation being for 12% of dry matter intake being crude protein (CP) (30). Arginine (an amino acid) is also known to increase placental blood flow, which is beneficial for calf development (31). Calves born from dams that were fed inadequate protein have higher mortality rates (32).

A good diet in the dam also helps to ensure that she produces good quality colostrum. Although maternal feed protein levels do not directly affect immunoglobulin levels in the colostrum, they do impact other colostrum constituents that can affect absorption by the calf's intestines (33). The fat content of colostrum is also important as it supplies a large amount of energy to support metabolism and thermoregulation in the newborn calf (34) (see Chapter 3).

Ensuring an appropriate body condition score (BCS) for the calving cow of between 2.5 to 3 is vital. It has been shown that optimal maternal BCS during gestation improves their daughter's fertility in terms of non-return rate and number

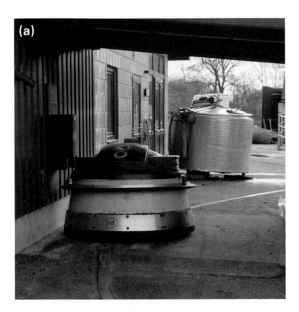

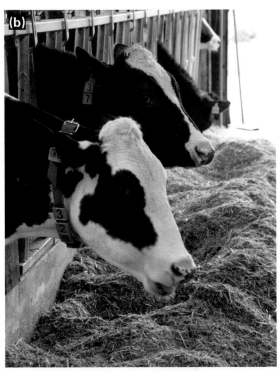

FIGURE 1.7 (a) Use of robotic feed pushers can help ensure cows fed in an alley system have frequent stimuli to feed throughout the day. (b) Image of dry cows with ample access to a total mixed ration (TMR) feed.

of inseminations per conception (31). Fat cows have a much higher occurrence of dystocia during calving, as do cows that have a large change in body condition during the dry period, and this increases the risk of mortality in the calf. Over conditioned cows (BCS > 3.5) are also at an increased risk of developing milk fever (35) – see section below for more detail.

One cause of fat cows at calving is an extended dry period. The energy requirements of a non-lactating cow are relatively low, and so it is common for dry cows to gain excess weight, especially if out at grass. Aiming for accurate calving dates and a dry period of ~8 weeks is best. Some studies have assessed the effect of short dry periods (<30 days), and have found that it can help maintain a more stable BCS and is beneficial for cows with long milking persistency (36). However, it must be noted that the colostrum quality in these cows may be poorer. Estimated DM intakes for the early dry period are approximately 13 kg/day, and for the close-up period the figure is about 11 kg/day for a 650 kg cow (32).

Summary

- In addition to genotype, the environment in the uterus has a significant influence on the development of the calf.
- Inappropriate nutrition at any stage of pregnancy can have permanent effects on subsequent performance and prevent animals from reaching their genetic potential.
- Different organs develop at different stages of pregnancy, but such key aspects as fertility, production capacity, size and immunity can all be influenced.
- Both long-term undernutrition and short-term changes (e.g. following heat stress, or infection) are significant.

Take home message – getting the diet right at all times during pregnancy is important not just for current milk production but for lifetime impacts on the offspring.

Hypocalcaemia

Hypocalcaemia (commonly referred to as milk fever or parturient paresis) is a condition of the dam that occurs around the time of parturition following a massive increase in calcium requirements for colostrogenesis and milk production. While a lack of maternal calcium may not directly affect the calf, hypocalcaemia at the time of calving can lead to a delay in stage 2 labour (foetal expulsion). Calcium is required for muscular contractions, with low levels causing ataxia and decreased uterine and abdominal contractions during labour (37). This can delay or prevent the cow from being able to calve herself, with this extended calving duration increasing the risk of mortality in the calf.

Controlling milk fever in the dam can be achieved through several methods, with all of them focused on the transition period approximately 3 weeks prior to calving. Feeding either a low calcium diet, placing calcium binders in the ration (38), or feeding a ration that manipulates the dietary cation–anion balance (DCAB) can be effective at controlling this metabolic disease. Grass is generally high in calcium, so should be avoided if possible during this period (Figure 1.8). Transition diets may focus on artificially lowering calcium levels in the dams' body, so encouraging her natural homeostatic mechanisms to increase calcium release from her bone stores. The DCAB diet helps to upregulate these same calcium release mechanisms by manipulation of the blood pH level. In addition, making sure the dry cow ration contains sufficient magnesium is important, with addition of 50 g/cow of magnesium chloride to the water being beneficial.

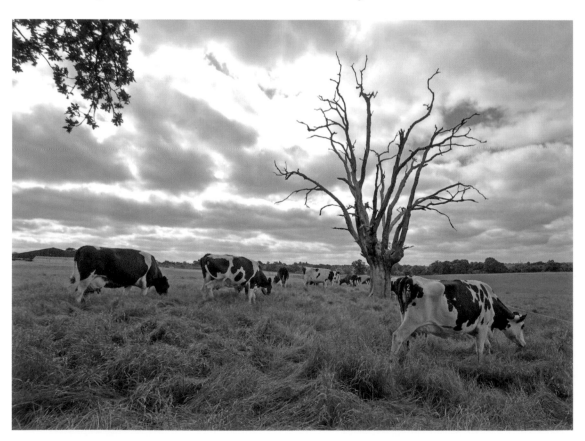

FIGURE 1.8 Grazing transition cows on high grass diets can lead to high calcium intakes and problems with calcium mobilisation around parturition. Picture courtesy of N. Blackie.

DCAB diets for prevention of hypocalcaemia

DCAB diets are low in potassium and sodium (cations), and contain additional chloride and sulphur (anions). This helps to produce a metabolic acidosis to lower the blood pH level in the cow (a low DCAB). This has the effect of enhancing tissue responsiveness to parathyroid hormone (PTH), which stimulates calcium mobilisation from the bones and increases intestinal absorption of calcium, and upregulates osteoclasts in the bone, which mobilises calcium from bone reserves. This diet also increases the loss of calcium through the kidneys into the urine. The overall effect is to upregulate the cow's ability to increase her calcium levels, helping to ensure that she can cope with the large increase in demand at calving.

The level of a DCAB diet is expressed as a positive or negative value based on the charges of the anions and cations. A partial DCAB diet will reduce the DCAB to 0 mEq/kg DM, whereas a full DCAB diet will give a value of −100 to −150 mEq/kg DM.

Checking the pH level of urine (should be pH < 8.2) can help monitor whether DCAB diets are being effective.

A failure to regulate calcium metabolism in the periparturient cow can lead to clinical milk fever, with a recumbent cow that requires intravenous (IV) calcium treatment (Figure 1.9).

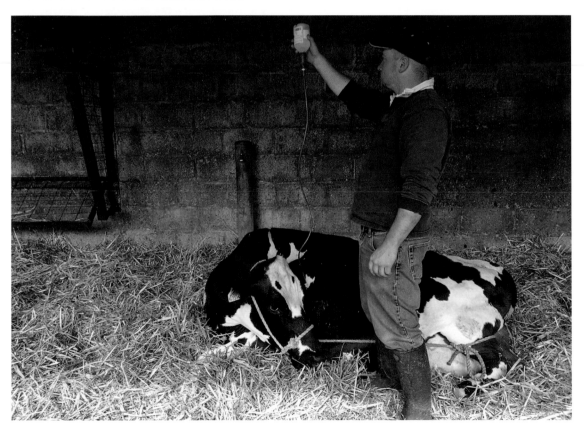

FIGURE 1.9 Treatment of a cow with milk fever by intravenous calcium administration. The cow is restrained by a halter tied to her back leg to prevent her from rising.

TWINNING

Twinning occurs in ~3–5% of pregnancies in dairy herds, but in less than 1% in most beef herds (39). The twins may be either monozygotic (formed from one fertilised egg, which splits into two identical halves during early embryonic development, resulting in genetically and physically identical twins) or dizygotic (formed following a double ovulation, so each involves a different egg and sperm, meaning they are completely different and may be of either sex). Monozygotic twins are much less common than dizygotic twins, with one study reporting that they represented only about 5% of the total in a Holstein population (40). In either case, the pregnancy is more likely to fail.

Twin fetuses are growth restricted and have much higher neonatal mortality, with one large-scale study reporting one or both calves as dead in 28% of twin calving events compared with 7% for singleton births (41). Those twins that survive do not remain stunted and do not appear to suffer adverse health consequences as adults. Each twin initially grows its own placenta but the number of available attachment points in the uterus as a whole remains unchanged so that each has fewer placentomes. These are, however, able to grow larger in compensation so the total placental weight is higher in twins even though the weight of placenta per fetus remains lower. The nutrient supply from the mother is also likely to become rate limiting. The size difference of twins in comparison with singleton calves becomes most apparent in the last two months of gestation, coincident with the time of maximal foetal growth.

Apart from pregnancy losses and neonatal mortality, another major concern in cattle carrying dizygotic twins is the birth of freemartins. In about one-half of such pregnancies one twin will be male and the other female. The extra-embryonic membranes of the two placentae fuse where they come into contact at about 6 weeks of gestation (Figure 1.10). This allows exchange of blood, cells and hormones between the two fetuses. If these are

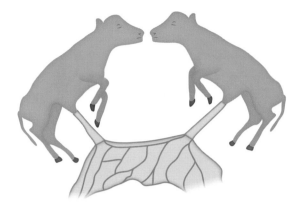

FIGURE 1.10 Diagram showing twin fetuses attached via their umbilical cords to a fused placenta.

of opposite sex, then the condition causes infertility in 90% of the female calves.

The reason for the problem is that the development of testes in the male fetus occurs earlier in pregnancy than the development of ovaries in the female. The testes produce a hormone called anti-Müllerian hormone, which inhibits the development of the female reproductive tract (42). At birth the external vulvar region of the female calf usually looks fairly normal but the calf may have an enlarged clitoris and large tufts of vulvar hair. The reproductive tract will also be blind ended, with the ovaries failing to develop correctly and remaining very small. The absence of follicles leads to an inability to produce oestrogen. The 'ovaries' may instead produce the male hormones testosterone and androstenedione, which affect the developing nervous system. In some individuals this leads to more aggressive behaviour and heifers born as freemartins do not themselves come into oestrus but may instead be more inclined to seek out other animals on heat. When mixed sex twins are born it should therefore be assumed that the female will be infertile. In some cases, however, one twin may abort at an earlier stage of gestation (but after the developmental damage was done), so the female may appear as a singleton at birth. These may then be reared as a potential herd replacement and not identified until the breeding period, when they fail to conceive. One study that genotyped infertile female heifers reported that about one-quarter of those failing to conceive tested positive to a Y chromosome-specific primer developed for embryo sexing (43).

A number of factors have been associated with the twinning rate in the Holstein population. These include parity, with the rate estimated at 1.2% for nulliparous compared to 5.8% for multiparous cows (41). Heritability for conceiving twins is low, estimated at <0.1 (39). The main reason that the twinning rate is thought to be higher in dairy than beef breeds is associated with the level of milk production. It was suggested that greater blood flow to the liver increases steroid metabolism in high producing cows, so reducing circulating concentrations of oestradiol and allowing two follicles to proceed to ovulation (44).

ABORTION

The normal gestation length of a cow is about 285 days, but this can be influenced by the sire, the breed and it also tends to be shorter if the cow is carrying twins or is heat stressed. Bovine abortion is defined as expulsion of a dead fetus after 42 days and before 260 days of gestation (Figure 1.11). The majority of abortions are sporadic rather than epizootic. Abortion rates should be <5% within a herd, but can reach 10% and it is often challenging to determine the cause. Aborted fetuses may be autolytic due to death some days/weeks before they are expelled and in over one-half of the cases submitted for diagnosis no infectious agents are identified (45). Nevertheless, abortions may be indicative of an underlying disease or management issue in the herd and some infectious agents causing abortion are zoonotic. It is therefore important to keep good records of when they occur and to investigate possible causes thoroughly.

In addition to the loss of the fetus, an abortion often has adverse effects on the fate of the dam. Depending on the stage of gestation when it occurs, the cow may either need to be rebred (so increasing her calving interval) or she may start the

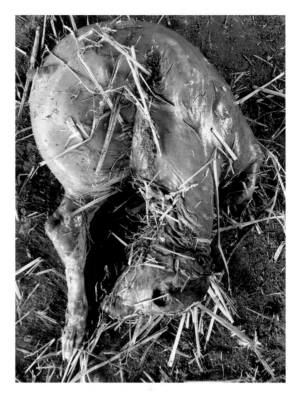

FIGURE 1.11 An aborted cattle fetus.

next lactation prematurely. In one large study of Holstein heifers, 4.8% aborted and this increased their risk of leaving the herd without completing a first lactation by an odds ratio of 2.7, with one-third of the affected animals dying or being culled within 50 days from calving (46).

The many causes of abortion are generally subdivided into infectious (bacterial, viral, protozoan and fungal pathogens (Table 1.2)) or non-infectious causes. Maternal infections during pregnancy may impact foetal development directly by crossing the placenta or indirectly by causing placentitis. The outcome of an infection is highly dependent on the stage of pregnancy when the initial infection occurs. Other infectious diseases that cause the dam to become pyrexic (have a high fever, e.g. mastitis, pneumonia), hypoxic (e.g. severe anaemia) or endotoxaemic can also cause abortion. Non-infectious causes include environmental factors such as extreme temperatures, genetic abnormalities in the fetus

TABLE 1.2 Infectious causes of foetal death and abortion in cattle

Bacterial	Viral	Protozoan	Fungal
Arcanobacterium pyogenes[a]	Akabane virus[b]	*Anaplasma marginale*[b]	*Aspergillus* spp.
Brucella abortus[a]	Aino virus[b]	*Neospora caninum*	*Mortierella wolfii*
Campylobacter spp.[a]	Bluetongue virus[b]	*Tritrichomonas foetus*	*Mucor* spp.
Chlamydophila spp.[a]	Bovine herpesvirus 1		
Coxiella burnetti[a]	Bovine parvovirus		
Histophilus somnus	Bovine viral diarrhoea virus		
Leptospira spp.[a]	Epizootic bovine abortion[b]		
Listeria monocytogens[a]	Epizootic haemorrhagic disease virus[b]		
Salmonella spp.[a]	Lumpy skin disease[b]		
Ureaplasma spp.[a]	Rift Valley fever[a,b]		
	Schmallenberg virus[b]		

Source: Information from (45,48,49).
Notes: [a]Zoonotic disease; [b]diseases which have arthropod vectors.

and ingestion of toxic agents by the dam such as nitrates and mycotoxins.

Climate change associated with changes in host or vector distribution and increased global marketing of cattle have both contributed to some of the diseases which can cause abortion reaching new countries. For example, the distribution of Rift Valley fever and Bluetongue disease are both currently being influenced by climate change. New diseases such as Schmallenberg virus emerged for the first time in Europe in 2011 (47).

Bovine viral diarrhoea virus

Bovine viral diarrhoea virus (BVDV) is a pestivirus belonging to the family *Flaviviridae* and is classified by sequence differences as type 1 or 2 (BVDV-1 or -2). It exists as either cytopathogenic (cp) or non-cytopathogenic (ncp) biotypes, with the ncp biotype causing the majority of field losses (50). BVDV infection is generally via the oronasal route but direct transmission to the reproductive tract via semen or embryo transfer is also possible (51) and can cause abortion in cattle. An estimated 7% of foetal deaths are attributed to BVDV (52), but vaccination of cows reduces the abortion rate compared with unvaccinated cohorts (53). The outcome of infection is highly dependent on the time of foetal

infection. If the fetus becomes infected before it develops immune competence (prior to gestation day 120) then the virus may cause early embryonic death, later abortion or birth of an immunotolerant calf that is persistently infected (PI) (51). The PI calf can continuously shed virus from all secretions and is therefore a major source of infection within a herd. BVDV-aborted fetuses may be fresh, autolysed or mummified (54) and many different foetal lesions have been described in association with a BVDV infection (55).

Bovine herpesvirus 1

Bovine herpesvirus 1 (BoHV1) is a member of the *Herpesviridae* family. Following initial infection, the body is usually unable to eliminate the virus completely so it is able to remain in an inactive, latent state in neural tissue and macrophages. It can then be reactivated in times of stress or following a subsequent disease challenge. BoHV-1 causes infectious bovine rhinotracheitis (IBR), an acute and highly contagious inflammation of the upper respiratory tract which is endemic in many parts of the world. It can also cause conjunctivitis and encephalitis and is recognised as an important cause of abortion (56). A meta-analysis of over 7500 animals showed that pregnant cattle vaccinated against BoHV-1 had an overall decrease of abortion risk of 60% (53). Abortions may occur from about 2 weeks to 2 months after catching IBR (57), with aborted fetuses usually showing a degree of autolysis.

Neospora caninum

Neospora caninum is a protozoan parasite that can cause abortion early in the second trimester. Infected cows are asymptomatic but can abort repeatedly. Dogs are the definitive hosts, with cows ingesting sporulated oocysts in feed, water or soil contaminated with dog faeces. These give rise to tachyzoites which are transmitted through the placenta to infect the fetus. Calves born carrying the parasite are also capable of vertical transmission to their offspring when they start to breed themselves (58). One study reported an incidence of 7.2% seropositivity of dairy heifers on 18 UK farms (59). The seropositive animals were more likely to experience foetal loss or abortion in both their first and second pregnancies, with odds ratios of 5.8 and 7.0, respectively. Perinatal mortality was also increased about fourfold in seropositive heifers at both their first and second calving.

Leptospira spp.

Leptospira spp. are zoonotic spirochetes which that are transmitted through contact with infected urine, milk or placental fluid, transplacentally or venereally (45). Approximately 75% of UK cattle have been exposed to *L. hardjo*, for which they are the maintenance host; after infection they may harbour the bacteria in their kidneys for months, excreting leptospires in their urine and so acting as a reservoir of infection for other cattle. Infection in pregnant animals can result in abortions, foetal death, premature births and the birth of weak and/or low-weight calves. Abortion usually occurs 3–12 weeks following infection with most abortions occurring during the last three months of pregnancy. The disease may also cause subfertility and early embryonic death, so compromising reproductive efficiency (60).

Campylobacter spp.

The members of the genus *Campylobacter* are gram-negative epsilon bacteria. The most significant pathogenic taxa in cattle are *C. fetus* and *C. jejuni*.

C. fetus subsp. *fetus* colonises the gastrointestinal tract and is usually associated with horizontally transmitted abortion in cattle, whereas *C. fetus* subsp. *venerealis* is restricted to the genital tract and is the primary cause of venereally transmitted infectious infertility and embryonic mortality. *C. jejuni* is mainly associated with abortion outbreaks in sheep but can cause sporadic abortions in cattle (61).

Brucella abortus

Brucella abortus is a zoonotic, gram-negative coccobacillus, transmitted via ingestion of fetus, placenta, uterine discharge or materials contaminated by these products. Abortions generally occur after the fifth month of gestation. Brucellosis is a notifiable disease in the UK, so potential cases must be reported to the UK Government Animal and Plant Health Agency (APHA). The country has been officially free of Brucellosis since 1991, although sporadic cases have been reported since.

Listeria monocytogens

Listeria monocytogens is a zoonotic, gram-positive coccobacillus, transmitted through ingestion of spoiled feed or feed contaminated with infected fetus, placenta or uterine discharge. Abortion generally occurs in the last trimester. Infected cows can show clinical signs of fever, weight loss, endometritis and retained foetal membranes (45).

Schmallenberg virus

Schmallenberg virus (SBV) is a novel virus which belongs to the Simbu serogroup of the genus *Orthobunyavirus* (47). SBV is transmitted by *Culicoides* midges and affects both domestic and wild ruminants. The clinical signs of disease in adult cows are quite mild and include fever, a drop in milk yield and diarrhoea (62). SBV can both persist in and cross the placenta to replicate in the fetus. Depending on the time of exposure, this may result in abortion or severe congenital malformations causing dystocia and birth of non-viable calves. A case control study on Swiss dairy farms found that the abortion rate increased from 3.7% to 6.5% in the years before and after the infection emerged (63).

Bluetongue virus

An *Orbivirus* virus, bluetongue virus (BTV) infects both domestic and wild ruminants, with its geographical distribution primarily dependent on the distribution of *Culicoides* midges (64). Many serotypes of BTV exist, including the BTV-8 strain which is currently circulating in Europe (65). The virus can cross the placenta, and infection before 70 days of gestation usually leads to death *in utero* and absorption or abortion of the conceptus. Fetuses infected between 70 and 130 days develop fatal malformations of the central nervous system and are usually aborted, but may survive to term but with congenital malformations in newborn calves (66, 67).

Mycotic pathogens

Mycotic abortions can be caused by various moulds and yeasts of which *Aspergillus fumigatus* is the most common pathogen. Disease usually occurs when animals are housed indoors and fed poorly prepared hay or grass silage, so is more prevalent in the winter months. The fungal pathogens enter the respiratory or gastrointestinal tract and then gain access to the systemic circulation and spread to the placentomes, causing placentitis. Abortion generally occurs between 6 and 8 months of gestation (45).

Good practice in cases of abortion

- Establish a closed herd policy where possible, with good biosecurity. If not possible, buy in stock from a herd with accredited health status.
- Screen and isolate bought in animals for abortive agents such as IBR, bovine viral diarrhoea (BVD), leptospirosis and neosporosis.
- Record all abortions (date, cow, stage of gestation, veterinary findings).
- In the UK, report cases to APHA.
- Undertake a disease investigation if the annual incidence of abortion in your herd exceeds 4% or if several occur in a short space of time.
- Isolate animals which have aborted and dispose safely of the fetus and placenta.
- Avoid any contact of the potentially infected material with pregnant women or dogs.

PREMATURE CALVES AND GROWTH RETARDATION

Premature calves are typically defined as being born <265 days of gestation, and display signs such as a low birth weight, small frame, a short silky hair coat, floppy ears due to poor cartilage development, incomplete eruption of incisors, laxity of the joints and tendons and a domed forehead (68) (Figure 1.12). These calves may suffer from a poor ability to regulate their body temperature so are prone to becoming cold, and may also have gastrointestinal dysfunction with a reduced ability to digest and absorb nutrients, which impacts colostral passive transfer. Premature calves may also suffer from a lack of lung surfactant production (a mixture of lipids and proteins which reduces the

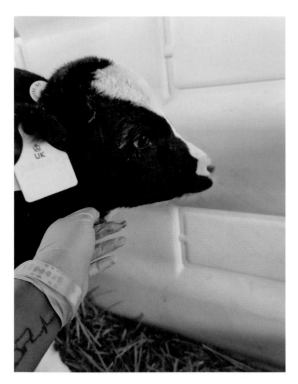

FIGURE 1.12 A premature calf with a domed forehead.

surface tension and increases their gas exchange ability), resulting in respiratory distress syndrome (69).

Some calves may experience a reduction in their growth and development while in the uterus of the dam, despite being born at a normal gestation length – this is referred to as intra-uterine growth retardation or dysmaturity. This is thought to occur due to placental insufficiency in a cow trying to support twins, or as a result of placentitis caused by either an infectious or inflammatory assault on the dam.

The viability and survival of these calves depends on the level of underdevelopment of internal organs, but they will all be at a higher risk of developing respiratory and enteric infections, as well as self-trauma caused by calves struggling to sit and stand. These calves will require extra supportive nursing and TLC to improve chances of survival, and if this is not possible, euthanasia must be considered.

REFERENCES

1. Seidel GE. Update on sexed semen technology in cattle. Animal 2014;8(suppl. 1):160–4.
2. Holden SA, Butler ST. Review: Applications and benefits of sexed semen in dairy and beef herds. Animal 2018;12(s1):s97–s103.
3. Kamal MM, Van Eetvelde M, Depreester E, Hostens M, Vandaele L, Opsomer G. Age at calving in heifers and level of milk production during gestation in cows are associated with the birth size of Holstein calves. J Dairy Sci 2014 Sep 1;97(9):5448–58.
4. Widdowson EM, McCance RA. A review: New thoughts on growth. Pediatr Res 1975;9(3):154–6.
5. Penrose LS. Data on the genetics of birth weight. Ann Eugen 1952 May;16(4):378–81.
6. Margerison J, Downey N. Guidelines for optimal dairy heifer rearing and herd performance. In: Garnsworthy PC (ed.) Calf and heifer rearing: principles of rearing the modern dairy heifer from calf to calving. Nottingham University Press 2005. p. 307–38.
7. Frisancho AR, Matos J, Leonard WR, Yaroch LA. Developmental and nutritional determinants of pregnancy outcome among teenagers. Am J Phys Anthropol 1985;66(3):247–61.
8. Wallace JM, Aitken RP, Milne JS, Hay WW. Nutritionally mediated placental growth restriction in the growing adolescent: Consequences for the Fetus. Biol Reprod 2004 Oct 1;71(4):1055–62.
9. Van Eetvelde M, Kamal MM, Hostens M, Vandaele L, Fiems LO, Opsomer G. Evidence for placental compensation in cattle. Animal 2016 Aug 1;10(8):1342–50.
10. Kamal MM, Van Eetvelde M, Vandaele L, Opsomer G. Environmental and maternal factors associated with gross placental morphology in dairy cattle. Reprod Domest Anim 2017;52(2):251–6. Available from: http://doi.wiley.com/10.1111/rda.12887.
11. Swali A, Wathes DC. Influence of primiparity on size at birth, growth, the somatotrophic axis and fertility in dairy heifers. Anim Reprod Sci 2007 Nov;102(1–2):122–36.
12. Robinson JJ, Sinclair KD, McEvoy TG. Nutritional effects on foetal growth. Anim Sci 1999;68(2):315–31.
13. Prior RL, Laster DB. Development of the bovine fetus. J Anim Sci 1979;48(6):1546–53.

14. Barker DJP. Fetal origins of coronary heart disease. BMJ 1995 Jul 15;311(6998):171–4.

15. Bagnell CA, Steinetz BG, Bartol FF. Milk-borne relaxin and the lactocrine hypothesis for maternal programming of neonatal tissues. Ann N Y Acad Sci 2009 Apr 1;1160(1):152–7.

16. Koch C, Hammon HM. Epigenetics – programming starts at insemination! In: European Calf Conference. Berlin; 2019. p. 25–7.

17. Schoonmaker J. Effect of maternal nutrition on calf health and growth. In: TriState Dairy Nutrition Conference; 2013. p. 63–80.

18. McMillen IC, Adams MB, Ross JT, Coulter CL, Simonetta G, Owens JA, et al. Fetal growth restriction: Adaptations and consequences. Reproduction 2001;122(2):195–204.

19. Tao S, Dahl GE, Laporta J, Bernard JK, Orellana Rivas RM, Marins TN. Physiology Symposium: Effects of heat stress during late gestation on the dam and its calf. J Anim Sci. 2019 Apr 29;97(5):2245–57.

20. Monteiro APA, Guo JR, Weng XS, Ahmed BM, Hayen MJ, Dahl GE, et al. Effect of maternal heat stress during the dry period on growth and metabolism of calves. J Dairy Sci 2016 May 1;99(5):3896–907.

21. Tao S, Thompson IM, Monteiro APA, Hayen MJ, Young LJ, Dahl GE. Effect of cooling heat-stressed dairy cows during the dry period on insulin response. J Dairy Sci 2012 Sep 1;95(9):5035–46.

22. Monteiro APA, Tao S, Thompson IMT, Dahl GE. In utero heat stress decreases calf survival and performance through the first lactation. J Dairy Sci 2016 Oct 1;99(10):8443–50.

23. Tao S, Dahl GE. Invited review: Heat stress effects during late gestation on dry cows and their calves. J Dairy Sci 2013;96(7):4079–93.

24. Dahl GE, Tao S, Monteiro APA. Effects of late-gestation heat stress on immunity and performance of calves. J Dairy Sci 2016 Apr 1;99(4):3193–8.

25. Sangild PT, Schmidt M, Jacobsen H, Fowden AL, Forhead A, Avery B, Greve T. Blood chemistry, nutrient metabolism, and organ weights in fetal and newborn calves derived from in vitro-produced bovine embryos. Biol Reprod 2000;62(6):1495–504.

26. Kume S, Toharmat T, Kobayashi N. Effect of restricted feed intake of dams and heat stress on mineral status of newborn calves. J Dairy Sci 1998 Jun 1;81(6):1581–90.

27. Mccrabb GJ, Egan AR, Hosking BJ. Maternal undernutrition during mid-pregnancy in sheep: Variable effects on placental growth. J Agric Sci 1992;118(1):127–32.

28. McMullen S, Osgerby JC, Milne JS, Wallace JM, Wathes DC. The effects of acute nutrient restriction in the mid-gestational ewe on maternal and fetal nutrient status, the expression of placental growth factors and fetal growth. Placenta 2005 Jan;26(1):25–33.

29. Nemec M, Butler G, Hidiroglou M, Farnworth ER, Nielsen K. Effect of supplementing gilts' diets with different levels of vitamin E and different fats on the humoral and cellular immunity of gilts and their progeny1. J Anim Sci 1994 Mar 1; 72(3):665–76.

30. National Research Council. Nutrient requirements of dairy cattle. 7th ed. Washington, DC: National Academies Press; 2001.

31. Flynn NE, Meininger CJ, Haynes TE, Wu G. The metabolic basis of arginine nutrition and pharmacotherapy. Biomed Pharmacother 2002 Nov 1;56(9):427–38.

32. Quigley JD, Drewry JJ. Nutrient and immunity transfer from cow to calf pre- and postcalving. J Dairy Sci 1998;81(10):2779–90.

33. Hough RL, McCarthy FD, Kent HD, Eversole DE, Wahlberg ML. Influence of nutritional restriction during late gestation on production measures and passive immunity in beef cattle. J Anim Sci 1990 Sep;68(9):2622–7.

34. Le Dividich J, Herpin P, Rosario-Ludovino RM. Utilization of colostral energy by the newborn pig. J Anim Sci 1994;72(8):2082–9.

35. Heuer C, Schukken YH, Dobbelaar P. Postpartum body condition score and results from the first test day milk as predictors of disease, fertility, yield, and culling in commercial dairy herds. J Dairy Sci 1999 Feb 1;82(2):295–304.

36. Shoshani E, Rozen S, Doekes JJ. Effect of a short dry period on milk yield and content, colostrum quality, fertility, and metabolic status of Holstein cows. J Dairy Sci 2014 May 1;97(5):2909–22.

37. DeGaris PJ, Lean IJ. Milk fever in dairy cows: A review of pathophysiology and control principles. Vet J 2008 Apr 1;176(1):58–69.

38. Thilsing-Hansen T, Jørgensen RJ, Enemark JMD, Larsen T. The effect of zeolite a supplementation in

the dry period on periparturient calcium, phosphorus, and magnesium homeostasis. J Dairy Sci 2002 Jul;85(7):1855–62.

39. Wakchaure R, Ganguly S. Twinning in cattle: A review. ARC Journal of Gynecology and Obstetrics 2016;1(4):1–3.

40. Silva del Río N, Kirkpatrick BW, Fricke PM. Observed frequency of monozygotic twinning in Holstein dairy cattle. Theriogenology 2006 Sep 15;66(5):1292–9.

41. Silva del Río NS, Stewart S, Rapnicki P, Chang YM, Fricke PM. An observational analysis of twin births, calf sex ratio, and calf mortality in Holstein dairy cattle. J Dairy Sci 2007 Mar 1;90(3):1255–64.

42. Vigier B, Tran D, Legeai L, Bézard J, Josso N. Origin of anti-Mullerian hormone in bovine freemartin fetuses. J Reprod Fertil 1984;70(2):473–9.

43. McDaneld TG, Kuehn LA, Thomas MG, Snelling WM, Sonstegard TS, Matukumalli LK, et al. Y are you not pregnant: Identification of Y chromosome segments in female cattle with decreased reproductive efficiency. J Anim Sci 2012 Jul;90(7):2142–51.

44. Wiltbank MC, Fricke PM, Sangsritavong S, Sartori R, Ginther OJ. Mechanisms that prevent and produce double ovulations in dairy cattle. J Dairy Sci 2000 Dec 1;83(12):2998–3007.

45. Givens MD, Marley MSD. Infectious causes of embryonic and fetal mortality. Theriogenology 2008 Aug 1;70(3):270–85.

46. Bach A. Rumin nutr symposium: Optimising performance of the offspring: Nourishing and managing the dam and postnatal calf for optimal lactation, reproduction, and immunity. J Anim Sci. 2012 Jun;90(6):1835–45.

47. Fischer M, Hoffmann B, Goller KV, Höper D, Wernike K, Beer M. A mutation "hot spot" in the Schmallenberg virus M segment. J Gen Virol 2013 Jun 1;94(6):1161–7.

48. Ali H, Ali AA, Atta MS, Cepica A. Common, emerging, vector-borne and infrequent abortogenic virus infections of cattle. Transbound Emerg Dis 2012;59(1):11–25.

49. McDaniel CJ, Cardwell DM, Moeller RB, Gray GC. Humans and cattle: A review of bovine zoonoses. Vector Borne Zoonotic Dis 2014;14(1):1–19.

50. Ridpath JF. BVDV genotypes and biotypes: Practical implications for diagnosis and control. Biologicals 2003;31(2):127–31.

51. Lanyon SR, Hill FI, Reichel MP, Brownlie J. Bovine viral diarrhoea: Pathogenesis and diagnosis. Vet J 2014;199(2):201–9.

52. Rüfenacht J, Schaller P, Audigé L, Knutti B, Küpfer U, Peterhans E. The effect of infection with bovine viral diarrhea virus on the fertility of Swiss dairy cattle. Theriogenology 2001 Jul 15;56(2):199–210.

53. Newcomer BW, Walz PH, Givens MD, Wilson AE. Efficacy of bovine viral diarrhea virus vaccination to prevent reproductive disease: A meta-analysis. Theriogenology 2015 Feb 1;83(3):360–365.e1.

54. Anderson VM, Bartlett JW, Fox NC, Fisniku L, Miller DH. Detecting treatment effects on brain atrophy in relapsing remitting multiple sclerosis: Sample size estimates. J Neurol 2007 Nov 25;254(11):1588–94.

55. Grooms DL. Reproductive losses caused by bovine viral diarrhea virus and leptospirosis. Theriogenology 2006;66(3):624–8.

56. Ackermann M, Engels M. Pro and contra IBR-eradication. In: Vet Microbiol 2006;113(3–4):293–302.

57. Muylkens B, Thiry J, Kirten P, Schynts F, Thiry E. Bovine herpesvirus 1 infection and infectious bovine rhinotracheitis. Vet Res 2007;38(2):181–209.

58. Williams DJL, Hartley CS, Björkman C, Trees AJ. Endogenous and exogenous transplacental transmission of Neospora caninum – How the route of transmission impacts on epidemiology and control of disease. Parasitology 2009;136(14):1895–900.

59. Brickell JS, McGowan MM, Wathes DC. Association between Neospora caninum seropositivity and perinatal mortality in dairy heifers at first calving. Vet Rec 2010 Jul 17;167(3):82–5.

60. Loureiro AP, Lilenbaum W. Genital bovine leptospirosis: A new look for an old disease. Theriogenology 2020;141:41–7.

61. Sahin O, Yaeger M, Wu Z, Zhang Q. Campylobacter-Associated diseases in animals. Annu Rev Anim Biosci 2017 Feb 8;5(1):21–42.

62. Wernike K, Hoffmann B, Beer M. Schmallenberg virus. Dev Biol (Basel) 2013;135:175–82.

63. Wüthrich M, Lechner I, Aebi M, Vögtlin A, Posthaus H, Schüpbach-Regula G, Meylan M. A case-control study to estimate the effects of acute clinical infection with the Schmallenberg virus on milk yield, fertility and veterinary costs in Swiss dairy herds. Prev Vet Med 2016 Apr 1;126:54–65.

64. Carpenter S, Wilson A, Mellor PS. Culicoides and the emergence of bluetongue virus in northern Europe. Trends Microbiol 2009;17(4):172–8.

65. Wilson A, Mellor P. Bluetongue in Europe: Vectors, epidemiology and climate change. Parasitol Res 2008;103(suppl. 1):S69–77.

66. MacLachlan NJ, Conley AJ, Kennedy PC. Bluetongue and equine viral arteritis viruses as models of virus-induced fetal injury and abortion. Anim Reprod Sci 2000;60–61:643–51.

67. Osburn BI. The impact of bluetongue virus on reproduction. Comp Immunol Microbiol Infect Dis 1994 Aug 1;17(3–4):189–96.

68. Palmer J. Prematurity, dysmaturity, postmaturity. In: Proceedings of the IVECCS VI; 1998. p. 722–3.

69. Karapinar T, Dabak M. Treatment of premature calves with clinically diagnosed respiratory distress syndrome. J Vet Intern Med 2008 Mar 1; 22(2):462–6.

Chapter 2

Calving

Sophie Mahendran and Claire Wathes

CHAPTER CONTENTS

The start of a calf's life can pave the way for its success or otherwise. This chapter details the normal changes in the dam around calving, the natural physical processes involved in delivering the calf both with and without assistance, along with information on things that can go wrong and how to assist.

THE CALVING PEN

The type of calving pen that a farm has will vary depending on farm scale, thus management strategies need to be adopted that suit available space.

The ideal grouping of cows will include a far-off dry cow group, a close-up dry cow group (fed a transition diet for 3 weeks pre-calving), and ideally a separate calving area (sometimes referred to as a maternity pen).

Movements of cows between social groups is a stressful event involving re-establishment of social hierarchy and the exhibition of negative behaviours, such as displacement from feeding areas, that have adverse impacts on a cow's feed intake at this critical time. Ideally group changes should only be made once a week and the moving of individual animals avoided (ideally pairs or small groups should be moved together).

The Welfare of Farmed Animals (England) Regulations 2000

Where calving cows are kept in any roofed accommodation they shall have access at all times to a well-drained and bedded lying area. They shall be kept in a pen or yard which is of such size as to permit a person to attend the cows, and it shall be separate from livestock other than calving cows.

Calving pens MUST NOT be used as sick cow pens, as this creates a highly contaminated environment with increased risks of spreading disease to vulnerable animals.

Group calving pens should have at least 15 m² of space per cow, and be designed so that there is enough accommodation for 140% of the average monthly calvings on a farm. Individual calving pens should provide at least 25 m².

In smaller units, the close-up and actual calving pen may be the same area, but this is not ideal due to the difficulty in maintaining adequate calving pen hygiene. The calving pen must be kept clean in order to minimise the risk of introducing infections to both the dam (mastitis and metritis), and the calf (diarrhoea pathogens and infectious diseases such as Johne's disease). Daily bedding with ample straw is vital, and regular cleaning out of the pen every 3–4 weeks is needed to keep bacterial loads as low as possible (Figure 2.1). Additionally, placentas and wet areas from calving fluids should be removed as often as possible. Substrates other than straw can be used for a calving pen (sand or sawdust), but they do not offer the same levels of comfort, and require more frequent cleaning out to avoid pooling of residues on the surface of the bedding.

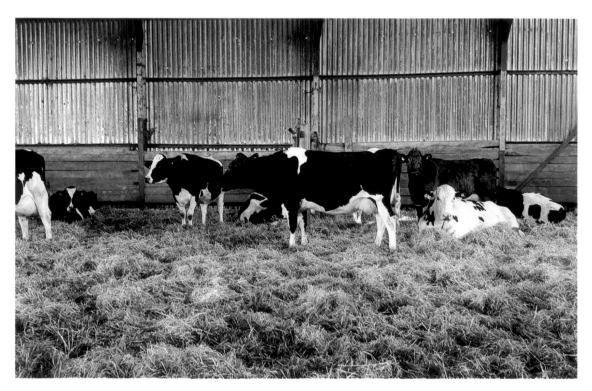

FIGURE 2.1 A group calving pen showing high stocking levels and poor straw hygiene.

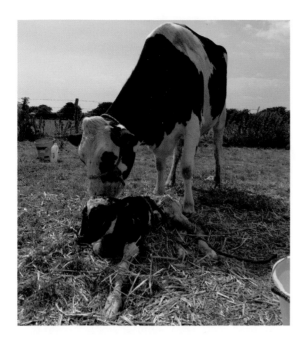

FIGURE 2.2 Outdoor calving in favourable weather conditions may be used, but high levels of hygiene must be maintained.

Calving pens can be either group or individual pens, but whatever the design, they should offer an area of quiet comfort with minimal cow disturbance. Calving outdoors in the UK is possible, but care must be taken to restrict grass intakes to prevent calcium imbalances, and to provide shelter from both heavy rain and also from the sun to prevent heat stress (Figure 2.2).

Group pens offer the simplest calving pen design, removing the stress of needing to move cows at the correct time prior to calving. Research has also demonstrated that cows tend to have a shorter duration of calving when in a group calving pen compared to individual calving pens (1). Many cows will choose to give birth in the corner of a pen as it is slightly more sheltered, so providing as many corners or hiding places as possible can enable cows to find a place to calve that makes them feel secure. Research has shown that cows who experience a prolonged calving period will seek additional isolation (2).

One problem with group pens is that as a cow approaches parturition, she can become attracted to amniotic fluids, afterbirth and new calves of other cows. This may cause confusion as to who has delivered, as expectant cows may try to mother freshly delivered neonates as their own.

Larger herds may be able to run an all-in, all-out calving pen system, where cows remain as a stable group, and are only moved into the milking herd once all the animals have calved. This reduces stressful group changes, but only works when there are enough animals calving in a short space of time, and the calving pen has access to either the parlour or a mobile milking device.

Individual calving pens offer the ability to fully clean the area between cows, as well as mimicking the natural behaviour of a calving cow isolating herself from her herd mates. However, moving a cow into an individual pen must be timed carefully to avoid disturbance of the calving process (see 'Management of the cow during delivery' below).

When calving heifers on farms that have a separate milking heifer group, it is a good idea to also have a separate heifer calving group. If heifers are to enter a milking group with multiparous cows, it is a helpful to let heifers become acclimatised to their new companions in the dry period. It is also best to transfer heifers into the dry cow group 8 weeks prior to calving – this allows for social acclimatisation as well as exposure to herd pathogens that will help improve colostrum quality.

HORMONAL CONTROL OF LATE PREGNANCY AND PARTURITION

During late pregnancy the calf and associated foetal membranes and fluid occupy an increasing amount of space within the abdominal cavity. The fetus becomes stressed and releases a peptide called adrenal corticotropic hormone (ACTH) from its pituitary gland, which triggers the onset of calving by initiating a synchronised cascade of events within the dam. First, the muscular layer of the uterus, known as the myometrium, needs to be activated and to start uterine contractions.

TABLE 2.1 Summary of key hormones which are important during calving.

Hormone	Source	Main function
Adrenal corticotropic hormone (ACTH)	Foetal pituitary gland	Release initiates calving cascade
Cortisol	Foetal adrenal gland	Causes changes in hormone production within the placenta
Progesterone	Ovary (corpus luteum)	Keeps the uterus quiescent during pregnancy, so progesterone concentrations need to fall before calving can progress
Oestradiol	Placenta	Promotes development of oxytocin receptors in the uterus, relaxation of the cervix and pelvic ligaments, and secretion of mucus by the cervix and vagina
Prostaglandin F2α	Placenta and endometrium	Causes regression of the corpus luteum (so progesterone levels fall), and stimulates uterine contractions
Prostaglandin E2	Placenta	Promotes dilation of the cervix and rupture of the foetal membranes
Oxytocin	Cow's pituitary gland	Stimulates uterine contractions

Second, the cervix must dilate sufficiently to allow the calf to pass through. In addition, the reproductive tract starts to secrete mucus which provides lubrication to help the calf pass easily through the birth canal. The key hormones involved in driving these processes are listed in Table 2.1.

SIGNS OF CALVING

The most reliable signs indicating that a cow will calve within the next 24 hours are relaxation of the pelvic ligaments combined with prominent distension of the udder. Rectal and vaginal temperatures are also between 0.4–0.6°C and 0.6–0.7°C lower than normal on the day of calving compared with 2 days earlier, but care needs to be taken as there are also normal diurnal variations. The DM intake is also reduced on the day of calving, so cows fitted with rumination collars or boluses should show a drop in feed and water intake, along with a reduction in rumination. Other signs that calving is approaching include a raised tail and mucus may be seen hanging from the vulva. The cow will often become restless, and may kick at her abdomen, bellow and detach herself from the rest of the herd.

She may also have increased periods of lateral recumbency and changes in position, probably due to abdominal discomfort.

There are currently several types of devices on the market to aid calving detection. These all involve a sensor which needs to be placed on the cow (Figure 2.3). This transmits a radio wave signal to a receiver that analyses the data; when the threshold is reached a voice and/or text message is sent to the farmer's mobile phone (3). These can all be helpful in providing warning of the impending calving when regular supervision

---

Available technology to detect onset of calving

1 Inclinometers/accelerometers which can detect a raised tail head.
2 Pressure sensors attached to abdominal belts which monitor uterine contractions.
3 Vaginal probes detecting a decrease in vaginal temperature and expulsion of the allantochorion.
4 Devices placed in the vagina or on the vulvar lips that detect calf expulsion.

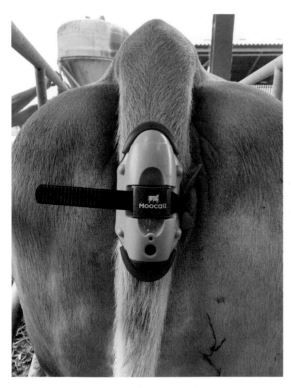

FIGURE 2.3 A Moocall device on the tail of a cow that can detect the onset of calving by the position of the cows' tail. Picture courtesy of N. Blackie.

of the calving pen is difficult. So far, however, they have only been tested on relatively small numbers of animals and none are 100% accurate under field conditions. They are also unable to identify cows with dystocia.

MANAGEMENT OF THE COW DURING DELIVERY

Placing cows into individual pens to calve is best for hygiene considerations, but the timing needs to be optimal. Although a cow will usually choose to separate herself from the herd when she goes into labour, separation from herd mates too soon can be stressful.

Research has shown that cows should not be moved once late Stage 1 or Stage 2 of labour has begun (signs of abdominal contractions or mucus is seen outside the vulva), as this can delay progress through Stage 2 of labour (4). This is due to activation of neural mechanisms which inhibit oxytocin release and myometrial contractility (5), increasing the still birth rate. Movement to individual calving pens should therefore be between 24 hours before calving to the early onset of Stage 1 labour, when there are signs of a raised tail head and a tense enlarged udder (6). Farms that have constant supervision of the calving pen may choose to move cows 'just in time', once Stage 2 of labour is well under way and the feet and head of a calf are showing. The effect this has on the progression of labour is unknown, but seems to work well in larger herds.

THE NORMAL CALVING PROCESS

The calving process is divided into three stages.

- Stage 1 – Initiation of uterine contractions and preparation of the birth canal.
- Stage 2 – Passage of the calf through the birth canal.
- Stage 3 – Expulsion of the placenta.

Stage 1 – Initiation of uterine contractions and preparation of the birth canal

During this stage contractions of the uterus begin at a rate of 12–24 contractions per hour. This helps to reposition the calf into the normal delivery position (anterior/forward presentation with the front legs extended out) (Figure 2.4). The contractions push the calf against the internal os of the cervix, which helps to initiate the dilation process, aided by breakdown of the collagenous tissue. There is also relaxation of the pelvic ligaments. Stage 1 usually takes between 4 and 24 hours, tending to be shorter in multiparous cows.

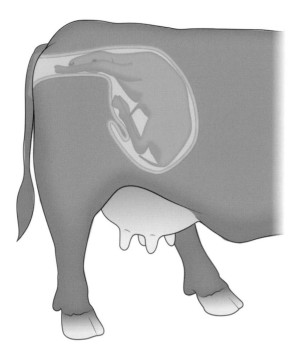

FIGURE 2.4 The normal position of a calf in the uterus just prior to delivery.

Stage 2 – Passage of the calf through the birth canal

The cow usually lies in lateral recumbency and will have strong myometrial contractions, increasing in frequency to around 48 per hour (7). These are accompanied by abdominal contractions (straining). As pressure of the calf against the cervix increases, this stimulates the Ferguson reflex – a neural pathway to the brain triggering the increased release of oxytocin, which in turn increases the force of the myometrial contractions. The allantochorion usually ruptures, with the escape of fluid through the vulva (Figure 2.5).

The amniotic sac (waterbag) protruding from the vulva is another sign that the calf has entered the birth canal. This should not be ruptured manually as the pressure helps to dilate the cervix and also protects the foetal head as it passes through the birth canal (8). The pressure of the calf's feet and head may, however, cause the amniotic sac to rupture, with the release of the amniotic fluid

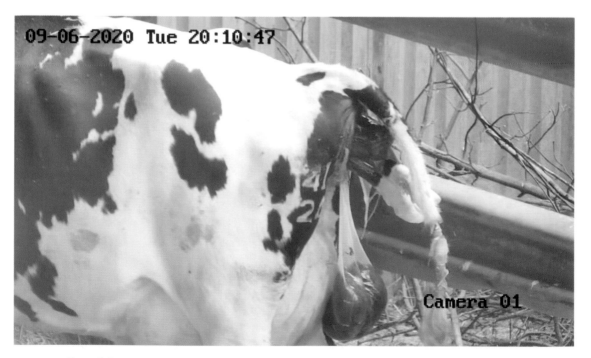

FIGURE 2.5 Part of the water bag is still intact and can be seen hanging from the vulva as the head and front legs pass out of the birth canal.

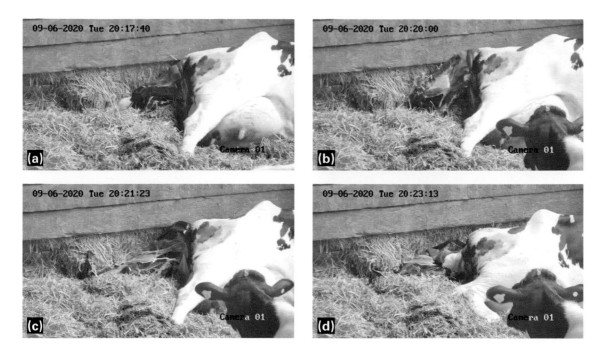

FIGURE 2.6 A series of photos showing the progression of a normal stage 2 labour over a 5 minute period.

adding to the lubrication. The calf's feet and head, then the shoulders, body and finally hips and back legs (when in a normal anterior position) should then appear (Figure 2.6).

While the calf is actually in the birth canal it will become hypoxic (short of oxygen), as it no longer continues to receive an adequate supply of oxygen from the placenta. The umbilical cord usually breaks as the calf is born. This stage normally takes up to 1 hour in multiparous cows, and up to 3 hours in primiparous heifers.

Stage 3 – Expulsion of the placenta

The abdominal contractions stop after the calf is born but the myometrial contractions continue and help to dislodge the foetal component of the placenta from the maternal caruncles. Rupture of the umbilical cord causes a sudden decrease in blood flow through the cotyledonary villi in the foetal cotyledons, causing them to collapse, and this helps the foetal and maternal components

of the placentomes to separate (Figure 2.7). This process should be complete by 6–12 hours after delivery of the calf, with about two-thirds of cows taking less than 6 hours (9). Definitions of retained placenta vary but are usually said to occur when passage takes longer than 12 to 24 hours.

Myometrial contractions continue for several days after giving birth, stimulated by oxytocin release during suckling or milking. This is important to push the lochia containing blood, mucus and remaining placental tissue out of the uterus and to start to return it to its non-pregnant size. Uterine involution mostly occurs in the 2 weeks after calving and should be complete within 4–5 weeks (10).

DYSTOCIA

Dystocia is when there is an abnormal or difficult calving, and this can happen for multiple reasons (Table 2.2).

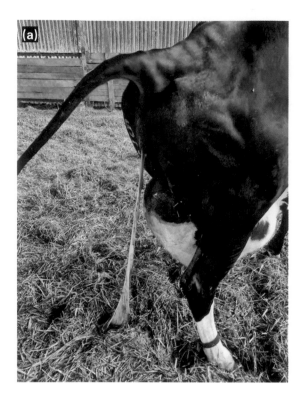

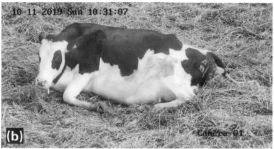

FIGURE 2.8 Use of CCTV in the calving pen allows close monitoring of calving animals.

FIGURE 2.7 The placenta can be seen hanging from the vulva immediately after delivery of the fetus, but should be expelled within 6 hours.

WHEN TO INTERVENE/ASSIST A CALVING

Careful monitoring of the calving pen is vital. Larger herds are able to employ staff to do this on a 24 hour basis, but smaller herds will have to rely on periodic monitoring. Installation of a camera in the calving pen can be very helpful, with Wi-Fi enabled devices allowing monitoring via mobile phones by multiple people (Figure 2.8). Ideally, a calving pen should be checked at least every 2 hours to avoid missing animals that may need assistance.

Making the decision to assist with a calving will vary slightly between a multiparous cow and a primiparous heifer, with Stage 2 labour taking up to 3 hours in heifers. A good rule of thumb is to intervene when the feet of the fetus have been visible for 2 hours ('two feet–two hours' rule) without any signs of significant progression (11). It is normal for the greatest delay in the passage of the calf to occur once the muzzle and forehead have emerged, but the eyes are not yet visible.

The decision to assist a calving is motivated by wanting to reduce the likelihood of a stillbirth, but intervening too early may lead to injuries to the birth canal due to insufficient dilation, an increased risk of stillbirth (1), and poor technique and hygiene causing iatrogenic trauma and increased risk of infections.

Prior to assisting with a calving, you need appropriate facilities that allow stress-free restraint, and are safe if the cow becomes recumbent. Simple systems can make use of a swinging gate, held closed by string or rope that is easily released if the cow lies down (Figure 2.9). This can be a very effective method, and does not take up any additional room in the calving pen when not in use. Additionally, special gates can be purchased that have removable bars for carrying out veterinary procedures, such as caesarean sections.

Calving gates are another way, and these have locking head yokes down to the floor so that if the cow becomes recumbent, they will not be strangled and can be quickly released.

In addition, provision of good lighting is essential as many assisted calvings will happen at night.

TABLE 2.2 Causes of dystocia in the cow, with summaries of identification and correction.

Problem	Description	How to tell this is occurring	Methods of correction
Maternofoetal disproportion	Either due to a very large sized calf (more common with beef breeds) or a small pelvis size in the dam (mostly seen in young heifers).	Presentation of a large pair of feet at the vulva, with crossing of the forelimbs demonstrating the shoulders are being forced together in the pelvis. Failure of progression of stage 2 labour after appearance of the feet.	If delivery through the birth canal is not possible, veterinary assistance for a caesarean section, or if the calf is dead, a fetotomy, will be required.
Incomplete cervical dilation	May occur due to environmental stressors, or if calving occurs pre-term.	An internal examination by insertion of a clean, gloved hand with plenty of lubrication through the vagina will allow palpation of only a partly dilated cervix – a clear taught ring will be palpable, not large enough for a calf to pass through.	Manual stretching of the cervix by insertion of both hands into the cervix and gentle outward pressure over a period of 10–20 minutes may produce sufficient dilation. If dilation is not possible, delivery via caesarean section will be required.
Malposition/ presentation of the calf	This is any position other than an anterior presentation with both front feet and head extended forwards. A posterior position is associated with 5× higher risk for dystocia and stillbirth. There may also be legs flexed back at various joints, or lateral deviation of the head. Reasons for occurrence of malpresentations are unclear, but may include oversized calves that are unable to move position in the uterus, or twins.	Unproductive straining during stage 2 labour. Internal examination by insertion of a clean, gloved hand with plenty of lubrication through the vagina will determine if a malpresentation is occurring. Check that both feet belong to either the front or back legs, by assessing the flexion of the joints. In front legs, the fetlocks and knee bend in the same direction, but in the back legs, the fetlock and hock bend in opposite directions.	Gentle repositioning of the calf can be conducted, with limbs and the head being straightened out. Care must be taken to use lots of lubrication, and covering of the feet and nose with the hand to protect the uterine wall from trauma is important. Retropulsing the calf to give more room for manipulation can be useful. When correction of position is proving difficult (no change achieved after ~10 minutes), veterinary assistance should be sought.
Malformation of the calf	This is when the calf has not developed in a normal way, which may lead to it being unable to pass through	Unproductive straining during stage 2 labour. Internal examination by insertion of a clean, gloved hand with plenty	If the calf is unable to pass through the birth canal, veterinary assistance for a caesarean section, or if the

TABLE 2.2 (Continued)

Problem	Description	How to tell this is occurring	Methods of correction
	the birth canal. This can happen due to infectious diseases, e.g. bluetongue.	of lubrication through the vagina, and careful palpation of the calf will allow identification of abnormalities.	calf is dead, a fetotomy, will be required.
Twinning	The position of the twin calves may prevent them from aligning in the birth canal normally. Mortality in twin calves is ~3× higher than singles.	Unproductive straining during stage 2 labour. Twins are often presented abnormally in the birth canal, so on internal examination it may just feel like an abnormal presentation. However, after delivery of one calf, an internal exam should be done to check for the presence of another calf.	Prior to assisted delivery of a calf, checking that both feet and the head of the calf in the birth canal belong to the same calf is important – this is done by carefully tracing the limbs back to the thorax. Twin calves may try and enter the birth canal at the same time, causing an obstruction.
Uterine inertia	May be caused by hypocalcaemia (milk fever) or a pre-term calving. It can also occur when a calving cow is disturbed during late stage 1, or during a prolonged labour, or with twins.	Lack of progression from stage 1 of labour. Internal examination by insertion of a clean, gloved hand with plenty of lubrication through the vagina, and careful palpation will reveal a calf and birth canal with no obvious abnormalities, but there is a failure of progression of delivery.	Correction of underlying metabolic condition such as hypocalcaemia will help re-establish uterine contractions. However, the cow will usually require assistance to calve, with the use of calving aids to provide gentle traction on the calf to remove it.
Uterine torsion	May be caused by excessive foetal movement, as the calf lies within one uterine horn, and can swing over, causing a twist in the cervix and an inability for the calf to pass through the birth canal.	Unproductive straining during stage 2 labour. Internal examination by insertion of a clean, gloved hand with plenty of lubrication through the vagina, and careful palpation of the cervix will indicate a corkscrew feeling to the cervix, which is often not fully dilated.	Establishing the direction of the torsion is important (many twist counter clockwise). Veterinary assistance is generally required for these cows, with various methods of correction including grasping the calf per vaginum and manually flipping the calf back over, or placing the cow in lateral recumbency and rolling her over whilst stabilising the calf in place by either holding it internally, or placing a board over the cow.

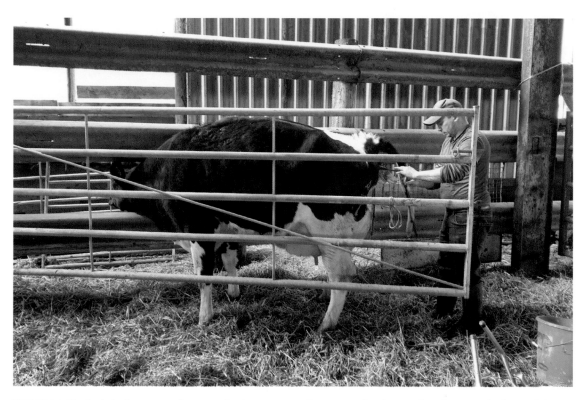

FIGURE 2.9 Restraint of a cow using a swinging gate to allow examination and assistance during calving.

Pre-prepared calving kit

- Container to transport warm water for washing – ideally ~20 L so that excess can also be given to the cow to drink after calving
- A clean bucket
- Rectal gloves
- Plenty of lubrication (powdered lubricant can be helpful as this is sometimes easier to introduce into the birth canal than liquid lubricant and the use of a pressurised sprayer may also be helpful to help introduce lubricant into the uterus)
- Paper towels
- Three calving ropes – two for the feet (ideally different colours), and one for the head
- A Vink calving jack
- A drug box with a non-steroidal anti-inflammatory drug (NSAID), oxytocin, antibiotics (e.g. amoxicillin) and a range of needles and syringes
- A calf resuscitator +/– Doxapram to stimulate breathing.

Once the cow is safely restrained, an internal examination can commence. The vaginal area should be wiped clean to remove any faecal contamination, and the assistant's arms washed and rectal gloves applied to help maintain cleanliness.

If the amnion or foetal legs are already present outside of the vulva, and they feel dry and cold, the cow has been calving at least 30 to 60 minutes. If the tongue of the calf is swollen and discoloured, this indicates that the calf has been stuck at the vulva for at least 3 hours.

Lots of lubrication should be used on the assistant's hand and arm, with the introduction of

TABLE 2.3 Summary of the malpositions of a calf.

Anterior (forward) malpresentation	Posterior (backwards) malpresentation
Transverse presentation – either the back of the calf or all four legs of the calf are presented at the entry to the cow's pelvis.	
Forelimb flexion (uni- or bilateral) at the knee or shoulder	Unilateral hindlimb flexion at the hock or hip
Lateral deviation of the head (often occurs when calf is dead)	Breech position – bilateral hindlimb flexion, with only a tail palpable on internal examination

lubricant into the birth canal and uterus being of great benefit if calving has been occurring for more than a couple of hours. The cervix should be assessed for how dilated it is, and if a band of tension is palpated, manual dilation should be attempted prior to trying to deliver the calf.

Thorough palpation of the calf should be done to determine which limbs are present, check that they are in a normal position (along with the head), and to check they both belong to the same calf. This is done by tracing your hand down along the limbs to the body of the calf, and moving across to check that the other limb presented is connected to the same body. The viability of the calf can also be assessed – this is done by pinching the interdigital or lingual areas, or checking for a swallowing or anal reflex (12).

If a malpresentation is detected, this must be corrected prior to attempted delivery of the calf. If the forelimbs are presented, they should be extended straight out so that the nose of the calf is approximately halfway up the length of the metatarsal bones, otherwise the elbows will still be bent and could catch on the lip of the pelvis. Calves presenting in a posterior position (backwards) must be delivered in this orientation, and these are easily identified when the hooves point upwards. However, in this position, reduced dilation of the cervix is more likely, so manual dilation may be necessary. Assisted delivery of a posterior calf should not be attempted before the hocks are able to be visualised outside of the vulva, as this indicates that the birth canal is sufficiently dilated for passage of the calf.

If a malpresentation is detected, but the cow is straining forcibly, veterinary assistance should be sought in order to provide both a sacrococcygeal epidural (~5 mL of procaine injected into the most cranial moving intervertebral joint) and the use of a β2 agonist (e.g. clenbuterol), which is a smooth muscle relaxant that aids manipulation of the calf without causing damage to the uterus. In addition,

Casting a cow using Reuff's method

- This process requires at least two people, and a large, deeply bedded pen for the cow to lie down in.
- A long rope ~10 m is needed.
- Place the rope around the cow's neck and secure with a bowline knot so that it does not tighten when pulled.
- Pass the rope around the cow so that the rope passes across the withers and behind the front legs. Pass the long end of the rope underneath the section at the withers to form a half-hitch loop near the withers.
- Repeat this process to pass the rope around the cow so that it sits in front of the udder and tuber coxae, passing the long end of the rope underneath the section that is along the back to form another half-hitch.
- Tighten the rope, making sure the half-hitches are positioned just left of midline along the back of the cow.
- Stand behind and to the left of the cow, and pull on the rope to cause her legs to buckle, so she becomes recumbent.

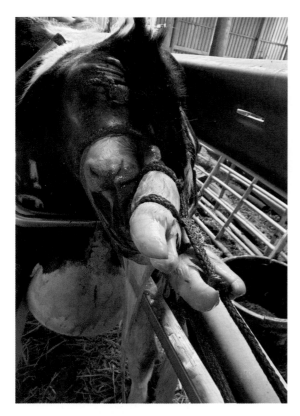

FIGURE 2.10 Signs of a large calf due to crossing of the front feet indicating pressure at the shoulders of the calf.

NSAID pain relief should be given to all cows that have an assisted delivery, with unassisted deliveries also benefiting from this treatment.

If the feet look very large, this may indicate a calf that will be unable to fit through the pelvic canal (Figure 2.10). Another sign of this is when the front legs are crossed over, indicating that the shoulders are being tightly compressed within the cow's pelvis, and may require veterinary assistance for a caesarean section. If the calf feels quite tight within the pelvic canal (very little room to move your hand around it), casting of the cow onto her left side may be of benefit (Figure 2.11). This can be achieved using a long rope, following Reuff's method. Being in left lateral recumbency helps to maximise the space within the birth canal and relieves pressure from the rumen.

Once the position and size of the calf have been assessed, calving ropes should be placed on both of the legs – a double throw should be placed, with one half-hitch above the fetlock and one below, thus spreading the tension placed on the limb and reducing the risk of injury, such as dislocation and fracture, to the calf's leg (Figure 2.12). Ideally, the knots should be placed on the dorsal (top) aspect

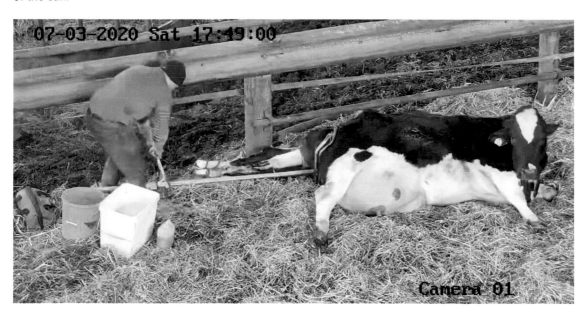

FIGURE 2.11 Calving assistance through the use of a calving aid, with the cow in left lateral recumbency to minimise compression by the uterus.

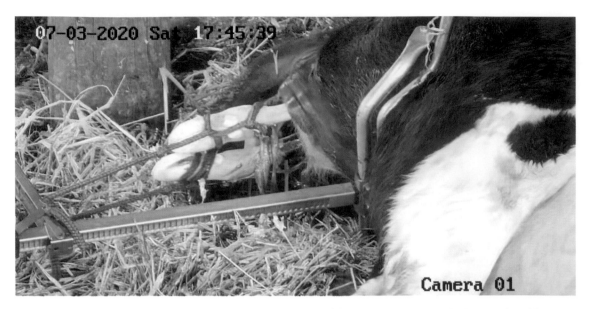

FIGURE 2.12 Calving ropes applied to the front feet of the calf. The blue rope is applied correctly with a half-hitch on the proximal and distal aspect of the fetlock. The red rope has slipped down distal to the fetlock, increasing pressure on the calf limb.

of the leg to give the best alignment. A head rope can also be of benefit in most cases, with the easiest method of application being to place one longer rope behind the cranium and tucked underneath both ears. Each end of the head rope is then used to apply pressure. This method can be easier to use successfully (and with less risk of trauma to the calf) than a loop of rope being passed behind the head, and through the mouth of the calf.

Use of a calving aid (often referred to as a jack) can be of great benefit, but must be used with great care as excess force can cause trauma to both the dam and calf. Combined abdominal and uterine contractions from the cow can produce up to 75 kg of force on the calf (13), with this reduced by up to 30% if the cow remains standing rather than in lateral recumbency. One man pulling on the calving ropes alone is able to produce an additional 75 kg of traction, with this being the maximum amount of pressure that is recommended before the risk of causing trauma becomes too high (14). A calving aid is capable of producing 400 kg of traction on a calf, and this must never be used to forcibly extract a calf from a cow.

The type of jack used is important, with a Vink calving jack with a ratchet design being the most suitable. The rump frame helps to keep the jack in place, and the ratchet mechanism allows alternate traction on each leg, which helps to slowly advance the calf through the birth canal.

The key to calving a cow is to be patient. Trying to rush a calving will only result in injury to the cow and/or calf. Once the ropes are in place, the calving aid can be used to apply traction in a steady and controlled manner. It can be useful to have an additional person handling the calving aid so that one hand can remain within the birth canal, assessing how tight the calf is and whether there is enough room for the calf to pass through. Pressure should only be applied to the calf when the dam has a contraction, and be released when the contraction ends by allowing the pole of the calving aid to be lifted upwards to allow the ropes to slacken, enabling optimal foetal circulation and oxygenation.

When delivering the first half of the calf, it is best to keep the angle of the calving aid straight/horizontal to avoid too much pressure on the calf's ribs,

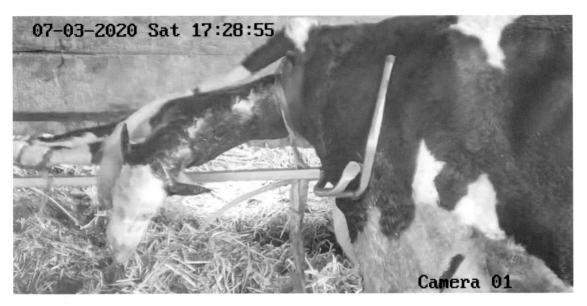

07-03-2020 Sat 17:28:55

Camera 01

FIGURE 2.13 Rotating of the calf once the thorax has been delivered can ensure the calf hips are lined up with the widest part of the cow hips.

risking severe bruising and fractures. This is especially important in posterior presentation, where a straight horizontal or even raised upward angle is required. Other injuries that can be caused by a tight vaginal delivery include a ruptured liver, intracranial haemorrhage, vertebral fractures and head and tongue oedema. Once the thorax of the calf has been delivered, the calving aid can be angled down slightly to mimic the natural arc that a calf would take. Rotation of the calf along its axis by 45° at this point can also be of benefit, ensuring that the hips of the calf enter the cow's pelvis aligned to its widest diameter. This can be achieved by applying traction in an upwards direction to only the lower leg.

If delivering a calf in posterior position, it is important once the calf's hips are engaged in the birth canal and traction is applied that the calf is delivered within approximately 5 minutes. This is because the umbilical cord becomes compressed, preventing oxygenation of the calf, which leads to anoxia that will be fatal if the calf is not delivered and able to breathe.

In some cases (often beef breeds), calves may become hip locked, meaning that the hips of the calf become stuck within the pelvis of the cow.

This is more likely to occur if the passage of the cranial end of the calf has been very tight, and is one of the main reasons that electing for a caesarean section for large calves is much safer. Once a calf becomes hip locked, attempts may be made to rotate the calf by 45° so that it is aligned with the widest diameter of the dam's pelvis (Figure 2.13). Plenty of lubrication should also be introduced. If the cow is recumbent, getting her to stand up can be helpful as this will change the position of the calf within the pelvis as well. If the calf is not able to be delivered, either a caesarean section or a fetotomy will have to be performed, with the forequarters of the calf removed, and the pelvis split in half to allow removal.

If a cow is carrying twins and delivers the first calf naturally, it may take her up to 1 hour to deliver the second calf herself. However, it is not uncommon for at least one of the twins to exhibit malpresentation, so careful monitoring is required. If the first twin requires assistance to be delivered, the second twin should also be delivered immediately due to the higher risk of the cow developing uterine inertia or damage to the umbilical cord of the remaining calf.

Caesarean section

It is beyond the scope of this book to fully describe the procedure for carrying out a caesarean section on a cow, but Figure 2.14 presents a series of photographs demonstrating the normal surgical procedure. The decision to carry out a caesarean is based on assessment of the cause of the dystocia, but this decision should be made early to provide the highest chance of a live calf being delivered.

After application of pain relief, antibiotics, a smooth muscle relaxant and local anaesthetic (via a paravertebral block, inverted L block or line block), the area is surgically prepared via clipping and scrubbing. A sharp incision ~30 cm long is then made through the skin in the left paralumbar fossa, following by use of either the scalpel or surgical scissors to cut through the muscle layers and peritoneum. Once in the abdomen, the position of the calf is identified by palpation, with the aim being to identify a limb that can be used to help exteriorise the uterus prior to an incision being made. The calf's legs can then be exteriorised through the hole in the uterus, and passed to an assistant who can help to lift the calf out of the cow. The assistant will then need to ensure the calf is ok (as detailed in 'Post-partum care of the calf' immediately below).

POST-PARTUM CARE OF THE CALF

During an unassisted delivery, the dam may remain recumbent for several minutes, before rising to sniff and lick her new calf. If a calving is assisted, it can be helpful to bring the calf around to the front of the cow, to allow her to begin this process (Figure 2.15).

As well as drying the calf off, licking stimulates improved breathing, circulation and activity of the calf. The vitality and vigour of the calf can be assessed by observations of its behaviour (Table 2.4) (15). Cattle are prey animals, so their instinct should be to stand up as quickly as possible after birth in case of the need to run from predators (Figure 2.16).

If the dam shows no interest in the calf, it is important to dry the calf off to prevent it from losing excess body heat. This can be done by rubbing with straw or a towel, and placing the calf underneath an infrared heater.

During parturition the calf is in a state of stress, and so releases catecholamines such as epinephrine (adrenaline) into its body (16). These are important for stimulating absorption of fluid from the calf's lungs in order for them to breathe and function properly. If a calf is born in a posterior presentation, it may be beneficial to raise them up by their back legs to encourage drainage of fluid from the upper respiratory tract, however, this must only be for ~10 seconds, and swinging of the calf in this position is unnecessary. The best way to encourage breathing and full inflation of the lungs is to sit the calf up in sternal recumbency, so allowing full expansion of both lungs – leaving the calf on its side means that the lower lung is compressed (17). Vigorous rubbing of the thorax with straw is beneficial to stimulate the absorption of fluid from the lungs, and the initiation of steady breathing. Additional stimulation can be applied by poking straw up the nostril of the calf to stimulate the nasal receptors, or hypothermal stimulation by pouring cold water down the calf's ear to induce gasping (12). If the calf is slow to establish rhythmical breathing, doxapram may be used (2–5 mL sublingually), which is a respiratory stimulant to increase the rate and depth of breathing.

If a calf fails to establish thoracic breathing by ~1 minute after birth, or is exhibiting gasping, use of a respirator can be of benefit. These are similar to an Ambu bag used in human medicine, with a compressor to push air into the lungs. They can also be reversed to allow sucking of mucus out of the upper respiratory tract. The respiratory tract should be cleared first prior to administration of air, and when this is done, it is of benefit to occlude the oesophagus to prevent pushing air into the rumen (18).

During an assisted delivery, or a prolonged natural delivery, the calf can be starved of oxygen and become hypoxic and acidotic (12). Normal blood pH for a calf is pH 7.2, with calves suffering

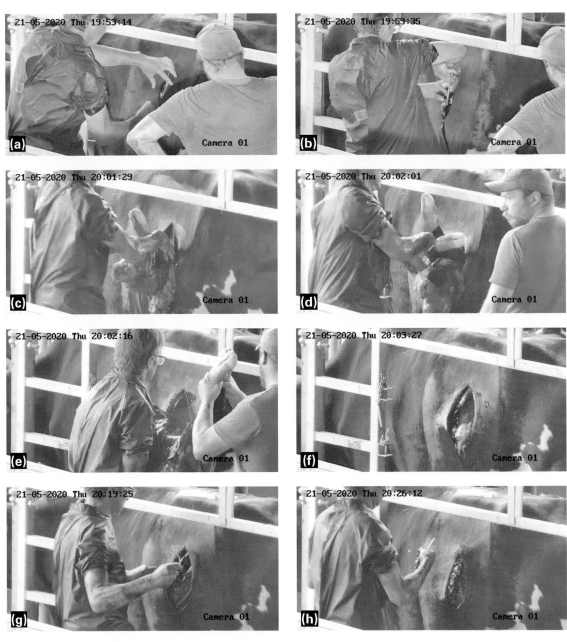

FIGURE 2.14 A series of images illustrating the process of a caesarean section. After application of local anaesthetic, and surgical preparation of the site, an incision is made through the skin, muscular layers and into the peritoneum. The uterus is then identified, and a limb of the calf identified and manoeuvred out of the incision in the abdominal wall. The uterus is then incised, and the calf removed. The uterus is closed by one or two layers of an inverting suture pattern, and the muscle layers and skin closed.

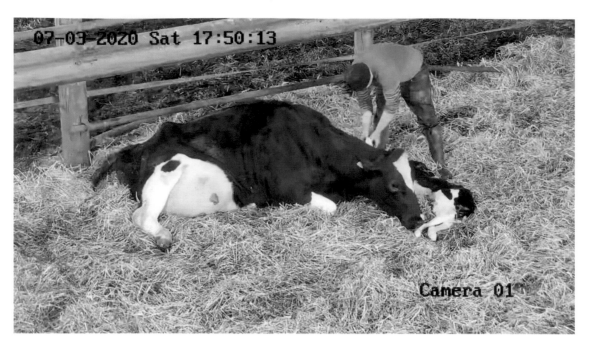

FIGURE 2.15 Moving the calf around to the front of the cow after delivery can allow the dam to start licking and stimulating the calf.

TABLE 2.4 Key milestones in the early life of a calf.

Behaviour	Time after birth
Lifting its head	3 minutes
Sitting in sternal recumbency	10 minutes
Attempting to stand up	20–30 minutes
Standing spontaneously and attempting to suckle	60–90 minutes

from severe acidosis having a pH of below 7.0. These calves will have reduced vigour and are slower to stand, but the most reliable indicator is having a reduced suck reflex. Severely acidotic calves (indicated by an inability to raise their heads) have a much higher risk of postnatal mortality, and will benefit from administration of intravenous (IV) bicarbonate solutions to raise their blood pH level. Preparations of 8.4% bicarbonate solutions are available, with 60 mL given intravenously working well in the authors' experience.

As mentioned, being born is a stressful and painful process for a calf, and so the provision of NSAIDs for pain relief to the calf can significantly improve welfare and calf vigour for up to 48 hours after delivery (19). This will also improve the suckling attempts made by the calf, and their feeding vigour in the first few days of life.

During stage 2 of labour, the umbilical cord of the calf ruptures and the vessels and urachus retract up into the calf's abdomen. Disinfection of the navel must be done as soon as possible after birth, both to prevent the tracking of infection up into the abdomen, but also to promote drying and healing of the area. Many stockpeople use 10% iodine in a dip cup. Alternatively, spraying of the navel can be used, but care must be taken to ensure full coverage (Figure 2.17). Chlorhexidine based products are also available, but should not contain alcohol.

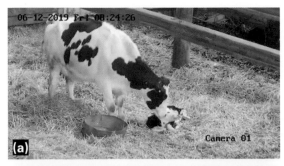

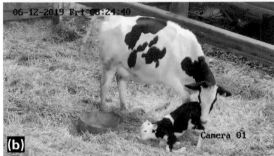

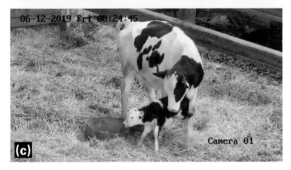

FIGURE 2.16 Three sequential images taken over 20 seconds show the calf rising from sternal recumbency to standing, watched carefully by the dam.

The final part involved in care of the neonate is colostrum management, which is covered in detail in Chapter 3.

POST-PARTUM CARE OF THE COW

Once a calf has been delivered, a final internal examination should be conducted to ensure that a twin calf is not present, and also to check for any tears to the reproductive tract or excessive bleeding from ruptured blood vessels. If the cow

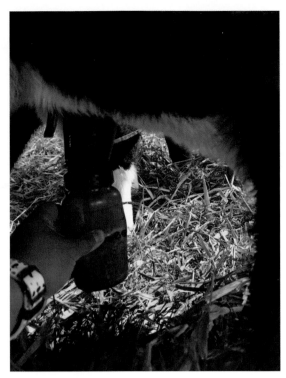

FIGURE 2.17 Application of 10% iodine to the navel via a teat dip cup.

is recumbent, she should be given some time to spontaneously rise to her feet, but if she does not do this within 20 minutes of delivery, she should be encouraged to stand (Figure 2.18).

Provision of highly palatable feed and also warm water to drink encourages feed intakes in the dam. The addition of calcium supplements to the drinking water can be of benefit to prevent milk fever. If a calving was assisted, thorough washing and disinfection of all equipment is important to prevent introduction of dirt and contamination to the next cow they are used on.

Retained foetal membranes (RFM)

Separation of the foetal component of the placenta is regulated by hormonal changes which cause breakdown of the linkages between the foetal and maternal components of the placentomes, together with activation of a maternal immune response

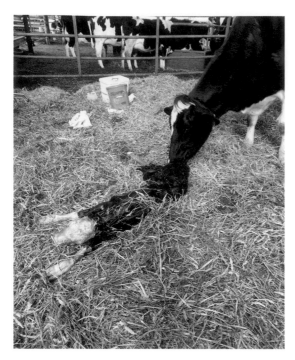

FIGURE 2.18 Cows that experience an uncomplicated calving should get back to their feet within a couple of minutes, and start licking and cleaning their calf.

against the foetal membranes. Sometimes the placenta does not detach itself from the uterus and remains hanging out of the vulva. The underlying mechanisms causing this separation failure remain uncertain, but there is good agreement that RFM results in considerable economic loss as it adversely affects the subsequent performance of the cow due to decreased milk production, a longer interval to first oestrus, lower conception rates and a higher risk of metritis, ketosis and mastitis (9). The reported incidence of RFM varies between studies/herds from 4–24% (29). Risk factors for RFM include premature delivery caused by infection or pharmacological induction, twin births, dystocia, Caesarean section, dietary deficiencies in antioxidants (Vitamin E, selenium, and β-carotene), infectious agents such as BVDV, and immunosuppression (9). Manual removal of a retained placenta should be strongly discouraged as it damages the uterine lining, resulting in more severe uterine infections and reduced fertility.

Medications used around the calving period

Corticosteroids

These may be used to induce calving due to a medical condition in the dam, for example, if a heifer has been bred too early, so is too small herself, or if she is in calf to a large beef bull. It is no longer considered ethically acceptable to induce cows in block calving herds in order to complete the calving season.

The most common method is a single injection of synthetic glucocorticoid such as dexamethasone, betamethasone or flumethasone. This mimics the rise in cortisol normally induced by foetal ACTH, and can be used from about day 255 of gestation onwards (30). Calves are born within 22–190 hours after treatment, taking longer when treatment is given 14 days compared with 5 days before the estimated due date. Calving is often more difficult than usual and there is a significantly increased risk of retained placenta. The incidence of RFM is worse if short as opposed to long acting formulations of corticosteroids are used, and may be as high as 93% (31).

Oxytocin

This is available to treat cows with RFM. Oxytocin is a very powerful hormone and it is important to remember that in a physiological situation it is released from the pituitary gland in small pulses, usually of short duration, with each pulse driving a uterine contraction. If too much is given as a single injection this can cause excessive contraction, and downregulation of subsequent responsiveness. No controlled studies are available to indicate any benefits of pre-calving treatment for uterine inertia. A number of studies have, however, concluded that oxytocin does not benefit cows with RFM (9, 32), or improve involution rates and health of the reproductive tract in normally calving cows (33).

Prostaglandins

Both PGF2α and its synthetic analogues have been used to induce calving. This should not be attempted until at least 270 days gestation and is again accompanied by an increased risk of retained placenta. Post-partum administration of prosta-glandin analogues is not useful in promoting the expulsion of the placenta in a cow with RFM (9, 32) or uterine involution in normal cows (33).

Non-steroidal anti-inflammatory drugs

NSAIDs act by inhibiting the synthesis of pros-taglandins, which are an essential element of the calving cascade. They should not therefore be administered before the calf is born. Although heavily pregnant animals may show signs of dis-comfort, use of the NSAID flunixin meglumine has been associated with increased risks of stillbirth (34). Another NSAID, meloxicam, administered prior to calving did not benefit symptoms of dys-tocia, but demonstrated a modest increase in sub-sequent milk yield (35). Other studies investigating the effects of treatment with NSAIDs on milk yield have, however, produced inconsistent results (35).

Antibiotics

If there has been significant manipulation of the calf within the uterus, the likelihood of contami-nation and dirt being introduced into the uterus is high, so coverage of the dam with antimicro-bials is recommended, for example, a beta-lactam based antimicrobial.

Relaxin

Relaxin is a peptide hormone which plays a key role in the birth process of many mammalian species as it causes relaxation of the pelvic ligaments and cervical dilatation. During evolution cows have lost the gene which makes relaxin, although they still retain the ability to respond to it (36). Although not currently available, it is possible that synthetic relaxin might prove a useful aid in future to treat animals with dystocia.

Separation of cow and calf

One a calf has been delivered, consideration of the appropriate timing for separation of calf and dam will be farm dependent. The bond between calf and dam develops slowly after calving, beginning with licking of the calf (37). Some time together is thought to be beneficial for both animals, such as allowing the cow to lick the calf to provide drying and stimulation. However early separation within a couple of hours is thought to minimise the distress response for both the cow and calf compared to separation at a couple of days old (38).

Possibly the most important consideration for early separation of dam and calf is to prevent infec-tious disease transmission (39). On a herd level, Johne's disease is significantly linked to calf expo-sure of contaminated faeces from infected cows in the calving pen. The likelihood of contact with other pathogens shed by adult cows such as *E. coli*, rota and coronavirus is also increased by delayed cow–calf separation. To minimise this risk, snatch calving techniques may be used if there are suf-ficient staff available on the farm. This method removes the calf from the calving pen immediately upon delivery, but requires constant supervision of the calving pen.

One method of reducing the likelihood of calf exposure to infectious pathogens is to use a cuddle box. This is a modern concept in perinatal calf care, with the aim being to remove the calf from the potentially harmful and contaminated environ-ment of the calving pen, while still allowing the dam access to the calf for her to lick, dry and clean off. The cuddle box is literally a box to place the calf inside, and can either be inside or outside of the calving pen. The cuddle box is kept completely clean, with fresh straw for each calf and thorough cleaning and disinfection between calves. You can also place feed and water for the cow in the same area as the box, so encouraging her to consume as soon after calving as possible – feed with a dam's own amniotic fluid on it will encourage the cow to eat it. Some designs of cuddle box come complete with a locking head yoke design for the cow, allowing restraint for milking. This allows harvesting and feeding of fresh colostrum from the dam, and the presence of the calf helps to keep the cow calm and quiet while she is milked.

Regardless of how long the calf is left with the dam, it needs to be transported to the calf housing using clean equipment. This might include a wheelbarrow, or for longer distances a transport box or trailer.

An alternative to complete separation of dam and calf are restricted suckling systems. These are more common on smaller farms, and can take two forms: only separating the cow and calf during milking time to allow the cow to be fully milked out; or only allowing the calf access for a set period each day for suckling. These systems have been shown to improve natural behavioural development in the calf (40), as well as having a positive impact on udder health in the dam (41).

Perinatal mortality

Perinatal mortality is usually defined to include both stillbirth of a full term (≥260 days gestation) calf, and mortality within the first 24 hours of life. It is calculated by dividing the number of dead calves at 24 hours after birth by the total number of calves born during the period under investigation. A number of studies have monitored rates of perinatal mortality and consistently found average values of around 6–10% (20–23). Under good management conditions perinatal mortality can be maintained below 5%, but this is rarely achieved in practice. A mortality rate >5% (per year and herd) is, however, often used by veterinarians as an investigation threshold.

The figures are often poorly monitored on farm and the reasons for mortality are rarely diagnosed at farm level, even when free post-mortem examinations have been offered. High calf mortality rates have economic costs due to the lost value of the calf, disposal costs, loss of genetic gain for the herd and possible increased costs needed for replacements. The mortality rate is also increasingly being used by external organisations as a key welfare indicator. Farms should therefore adopt a robust recording system to know precisely what their perinatal mortality rate really is. Establishing the main causes is then an essential step towards putting appropriate measures in place to reduce future risks.

Without a thorough post-mortem it is not always clear if a calf died before calving, during calving or within 24 hours after birth, and farmers tend to overestimate the numbers dead before parturition begins (24). A number of risk factors have been identified, of which the main ones are summarised in Table 2.5. In practice it is often not possible to

TABLE 2.5 Summary of main risk factors for calf perinatal mortality.

Factor	Increased risk rate	Comment
Assisted calving	4-fold	This includes dystocia, trauma to calf and prolonged calving. The risk of mortality is much increased, although assistance explains less than one-half of overall deaths.
Dam age	2-fold	The rate is approximately double for primiparous compared with multiparous dams. It is related to disproportion between calf size and dam size with a more restrictive birth canal in primiparous cows. The risk increases if age at first calving is <22 months.
Twins	3-4-fold	Twins are at higher risk, potentially caused by a prolonged or more difficult calving.

Calf size	3-fold	Very large calves are at greater risk. This is related to the sire, in particular breeds, but there is also variation within breeds which interacts with the risk of dystocia.
Calf sex	1–1.4 fold	In some studies, the risk increased slightly for male compared with female calves. This is probably related to calf size because male calves weigh more at birth and calf birth weight is a better predictor of perinatal mortality than gender.
Disease		Investigations of some herds, particularly those with high mortality rates, have found evidence of disease associated with a variety of pathogens including *Coxiella burnetii*, bovine viral diarrhoea virus, pathogenic *Leptospira* spp., *Neospora caninum*, *Chlamydia abortus*, *Streptococcus* spp. and *Escherichia coli*.
Farm size		Some, but not all, studies have reported increased mortality rates in larger herds. This is likely confounded by the staff time available for supervision at calving.
Calving location		Some studies have found increased risks associated with calving at pasture, calving in small pens compared with larger yards, and calving in tie stalls compared with loose housing. These effects are, however, hard to separate from effects of supervision.
Calving supervision		Both the frequency of observations, particularly overnight and at weekends, and the skills and training of the farm staff are influential. The farm policy for the timing of intervention during stage 2 labour is also important.
Season		Season may be a causative factor due to extremes of hot or cold temperatures. In seasonally calving herds the risk also rises towards the end of the calving season.
Congenital defects		An increasing number of inherited conditions are being recognised e.g. complex vertebral malformation (CVM). These are breed specific. Risks will increase with a higher degree of inbreeding. Congenital defects can also be caused by infectious agents earlier in gestation, e.g. Schmallenberg disease.
Trace element imbalance		The most evidence is for iodine and selenium, although others (copper, zinc) may influence subsequent calf health.
Dam BCS		The risk may increase in dams calving with very low ≤1.5 or high ≥ 4 BCS at calving (on a five-point scale).
Intrauterine growth retardation		This is defined as a full term calf >280 gestational days but with a bodyweight less than the mean − 2xSD for the herd/breed.
Pre-calving movement of dam		If cows have not been moved before labour starts, moving them in stage 1 labour increases the risk compared with 'just-in-time' movement during stage 2.
Premature placental separation		This may be due to intrauterine infection or be caused by prolonged calving. The calf will become anoxic if the blood supply to the placenta is interrupted.
Post parturient trauma		This includes anything causing direct damage to the newborn calf, for example colostrum aspiration.

Source: Information in the table is derived from a number of sources (8,11,20–24,26,27).

isolate some potential risk factors, as stillbirth and calving difficulty are caused by an interaction of many factors in the calf and the dam. It can therefore be hard to determine whether the provision of assistance and the associated trauma and delay was a factor in the calf being stillborn, or whether a calf already dead or malformed *in utero* necessitated the assistance. Reported rates of providing calving assistance also vary greatly between 9–37% in different studies (21, 25). This discrepancy could reflect differences in management policy regarding the time point of intervention and/or under-recording by some farmers.

In summary, many factors can lead to high mortality rates. On farms with a consistently high incidence, there is a danger that this can become accepted as 'normal'. Risks can be divided into modifiable and non-modifiable, with many risks being at least partly under the control of the farm management, particularly those which are associated with increased risk of dystocia (28). These include age at first calving, choice of sire, calving management, feto-maternal health status and gestational nutrition. The increased use of sexed semen is also influential, while genomic testing of herds is providing an increasing amount of information on selection of sires with reduced risks of perinatal mortality and identifying genetic causes

of congenital defects (see Chapter 1). Primiparity, twinning and extremes of weather remain unavoidable risks, but can still be mitigated by the consistent provision of excellent management around calving.

IDENTIFICATION OF CALVES

If there is a group calving pen, and large number of animals are calving, there is a risk of recording the incorrect dam for a calf due to mis-mothering. This can affect future decision making about a calf, and should be avoided if possible.

> **Legal requirement for identification of dairy calves in the UK**
>
> - The primary ear tag must be applied within 36 hours of birth.
> - The secondary tag must be in the other ear by 20 days of age.

Each calf needs to be identified by one primary and one secondary ear tag, with most people fitting both tags at the same time. In the UK, these tags identify the farm of origin by displaying a county

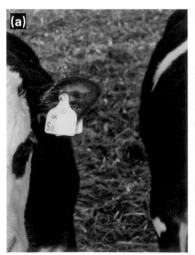 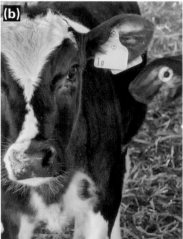 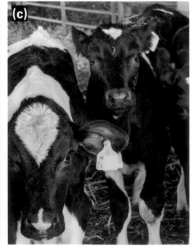

FIGURE 2.19 Correct and incorrect placement of ear tags in calves: (a) correct (between the ear cartilages); incorrect (b) too high (above the cartilage); (c) too low and wide in the ear.

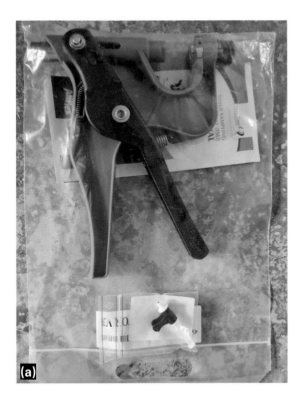

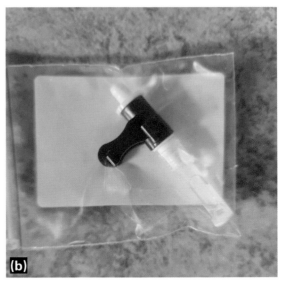

FIGURE 2.20 Specialist (a) ear tag and (b) receptacle for collecting tissue samples from ear notches.

parish holding (CPH) number as well as an individual identification number for the calf. The secondary tag can also contain management information. Flag tags or electronic identification (EID) button tags should be placed in the middle third of the ear between the ridges of auricular cartilage. If using metal tags, place them at the top of the ear, within the third closest to the head, making sure to leave ~0.8 cm space between the tag and ear edge to allow for ear growth.

In addition, in the UK the birth of the calf needs to be registered with the British Cattle Movement Service (BCMS) to attain a passport for it within 27 days of birth.

If an untagged calf dies before 36-hours old, the calf does not need to be ear tagged, but the farmer must record its date of birth and date of death against the dam number in the farm records.

Specialist ear tags can be purchased that allow collection of a notch of skin into a bar-coded vial on application of the tag (Figure 2.20). This can then be used for either genomic testing of calves

(see Chapter 1), or for infectious disease screening for BVDV. The samples can be stored at room temperature before posting to the testing laboratory where each sample is extracted before analysis of the DNA to reveal the genetic code.

REFERENCES

1. Kovács L, Kézér FL, Szenci O. Effect of calving process on the outcomes of delivery and postpartum health of dairy cows with unassisted and assisted calvings. J Dairy Sci 2016;99(9):7568–73.
2. Rørvang MV, Herskin MS, Jensen MB. Dairy cows with prolonged calving seek additional isolation. J Dairy Sci 2017 Apr 1;100(4):2967–75.
3. Saint-Dizier M, Chastant-Maillard S. Methods and on-farm devices to predict calving time in cattle. Vet J 2015 Sep;205(3):349–56.
4. Carrier J, Godden S, Fetrow J, Stewart S, Rapnicki P. Predictors of stillbirth for cows moved to calving pens when calving is imminent. In: Proceedings of the 39th ann Am assoc Bov pract 2006. p. 158–9.

5. Nagel C, Aurich C, Aurich J. Stress effects on the regulation of parturition in different domestic animal species. Anim Reprod Sci 2019;207:153–61.

6. Proudfoot KL, Jensen MB, Heegaard PMH, von Keyserlingk MAG. Effect of moving dairy cows at different stages of labor on behavior during parturition. J Dairy Sci 2013 Mar;96(3):1638–46.

7. Zerobin K, Spörri H. Motility of the bovine and porcine uterus and Fallopian tube. Adv Vet Sci Comp Med 1972 Jan 1;16:303–54.

8. Mee JF. Managing the dairy cow at calving time. Vet Clin North Am Food Anim Pract 2004;20(3): 521–46.

9. Beagley JC, Whitman KJ, Baptiste KE, Scherzer J. Physiology and treatment of retained fetal membranes in cattle. J Vet Intern Med 2010 Mar 1;24(2):261–8.

10. Gier HT, Marion GB. Uterus of the cow after parturition: Involutional changes. Am J Vet Res 1968;29(1):83–96.

11. Mee JF, Sánchez-Miguel C, Doherty M. Influence of modifiable risk factors on the incidence of stillbirth/perinatal mortality in dairy cattle. Vet J 2014;199(1):19–23.

12. Mee JF. Newborn dairy calf management. Vet Clin North Am Food Anim Pract 2008;24(1):1–17.

13. Hindson JC. Quantification of obstetric traction. Vet Rec 1978 Apr 15;102(15):327–32.

14. Tyler H. Calf development and birth. Midwest Plan Service; North Central Regional Extension Publication NCR-205. 2003.

15. Mee JF. Bovine perinatal mortality and parturient problems in Irish dairy herd. Dublin, Ireland: National University of Ireland; 1991.

16. Szenci O. Role of acid–base disturbances in perinatal mortality of calves: A review. Vet Bull 2003;73(7): 7–14.

17. Uystepruyst C, Coghe J, Dorts T, Harmegnies N, Delsemme MH, Art T, Lekeux P. Sternal recumbency or suspension by the hind legs immediately after delivery improves respiratory and metabolic adaptation to extra uterine life in newborn calves delivered by caesarean section. Vet Res 2002;33(6):709–24.

18. Mee JF. Resuscitation of newborn calves-materials and methods. Cattle Pract (United Kingdom) 1994;2:197–210.

19. Gladden N, Ellis K, Martin J, Viora L, McKeegan D. A single dose of ketoprofen in the immediate postpartum period has the potential to improve dairy calf welfare in the first 48 h of life. Appl Anim Behav Sci 2019 Mar 1;212:19–29.

20. Johanson JM, Berger PJ. Birth weight as a predictor of calving ease and perinatal mortality in Holstein cattle. J Dairy Sci 2003 Nov 1;86(11):3745–55.

21. Lombard JE, Garry FB, Tomlinson SM, Garber LP. Impacts of dystocia on health and survival of dairy calves. J Dairy Sci 2007 Apr 1;90(4):1751–60.

22. Brickell JS, McGowan MM, Pfeiffer DU, Wathes DC. Mortality in Holstein-Friesian calves and replacement heifers, in relation to body weight and I.G.F.-I concentration, on 19 farms in England. Animal 2009;3(8):1175–82.

23. Silva del Río NS, Stewart S, Rapnicki P, Chang YM, Fricke PM. An observational analysis of twin births, calf sex ratio, and calf mortality in Holstein dairy cattle. J Dairy Sci 2007 Mar 1;90(3):1255–64.

24. Mock T, Mee JF, Dettwiler M, Rodriguez-Campos S, Hüsler J, Michel B, et al. Evaluation of an investigative model in dairy herds with high calf perinatal mortality rates in Switzerland. Theriogenology 2020 May 1;148:48–59.

25. Whitaker DA, Kelly JM, Smith S. Disposal and disease rates in 340 British dairy herds. Vet Rec 2000 Mar 25;146(13):363–7.

26. Waldner CL. Cow attributes, herd management and environmental factors associated with the risk of calf death at or within 1h of birth and the risk of dystocia in cow-calf herds in Western Canada. Livest Sci 2014;163(1):126–39.

27. Cuttance EL, Mason WA, Laven RA, McDermott J, Phyn C. Prevalence and calf-level risk factors for failure of passive transfer in dairy calves in New Zealand. N Z Vet J 2017 Nov 2;65(6):297–304.

28. Mee JF, Sanchez-Miguel C, Doherty M. An international Delphi study of the causes of death and the criteria used to assign cause of death in bovine perinatal mortality. Reprod Domest Anim 2013 Aug;48(4):651–9.

29. Attupuram NM, Kumaresan A, Narayanan K, Kumar H. Cellular and molecular mechanisms involved in placental separation in the bovine: A review. Mol Reprod Dev 2016 Apr 1;83(4):287–97.

30. Ball PJH, Peters AR. Reproduction in cattle. 3rd ed. Wiley-Blackwell. p. 1–242; 2007.

31. MacDiarmid SC. Induction of parturition in cattle using corticosteroids: A review. Part 1. Reasons for

induction, mechanisms of induction, and preparations used. Anim Breed Abstr. 1983;51(6):403–19.

32. Peters AR, Laven RA. Treatment of bovine retained placenta and its effects. Vet Rec 1996 Nov 30;139(22):535–9.

33. Stephen CP, Johnson WH, Leblanc SJ, Foster RA, Chenier TS. The impact of ecbolic therapy in the early postpartum period on uterine involution and reproductive health in dairy cows. J Vet Med Sci 2019;81(3):491–8.

34. Newby NC, Leslie KE, Dingwell HDP, Kelton DF, Weary DM, Neuder L, et al. The effects of periparturient administration of flunixin meglumine on the health and production of dairy cattle. J Dairy Sci 2017 Jan 1;100(1):582–7.

35. Swartz TH, Schramm HH, Bewley JM, Wood CM, Leslie KE, Petersson-Wolfe CS. Meloxicam administration either prior to or after parturition: Effects on behavior, health, and production in dairy cows. J Dairy Sci 2018 Nov 1;101(11):10151–67.

36. Dai Y, Ivell R, Liu X, Janowski D, Anand-Ivell R. Relaxin-family peptide receptors 1 and 2 are fully functional in the bovine. Front Physiol 2017 Jun 6;8:359.

37. von Keyserlingk MAG, Weary DM. Maternal behavior in cattle. Horm Behav 2007;52(1):106–13.

38. Meagher RK, Beaver A, Weary DM, von Keyserlingk MAG. Invited review: A systematic review of the effects of prolonged cow–calf contact on behavior, welfare, and productivity. J Dairy Sci 2019 Jul 1;102(7):5765–83.

39. Jensen MB. The early behaviour of cow and calf in an individual calving pen. Appl Anim Behav Sci 2011 Nov 15;134(3–4):92–9.

40. Fröberg S, Lidfors L. Behaviour of dairy calves suckling the dam in a barn with automatic milking or being fed milk substitute from an automatic feeder in a group pen. Appl Anim Behav Sci 2009 Mar 1;117(3–4):150–8.

41. Fröberg S, Gratte E, Svennersten-Sjaunja K, Olsson I, Berg C, Orihuela A, et al. Effect of suckling ('restricted suckling') on dairy cows. Udder health and milk let-down and their calves' weight gain, feed intake and behaviour. Appl Anim Behav Sci 2008 Sep 1;113(1–3):1–14.

Chapter 3

Colostrum management

Claire Wathes

CHAPTER CONTENTS

The structure of the cow's placenta does not allow transfer of protective immunoglobulins (Ig) from the dam to the fetus before birth. This means that the calf is born without any circulating gamma globulins (IgG), a state referred to as being agammaglobulinaemic. Immediately after birth calves are confronted with many potentially pathogenic microorganisms. At this age, cellular components of the adaptive immune system are in a naïve state and are slow to respond (1). This makes young calves very susceptible to pathogens until their immune system develops sufficiently. The calf does not make significant amounts of its own IgGs until 2–4 weeks after birth and these do not approach adult levels until at least 4 months of age (2). Passive transfer of Ig must therefore be obtained via ingestion of colostrum in the first 24 hours after birth. Colostrum also contains many other bioactive ingredients that offer both nutritional and immune benefits. Providing calves with an adequate intake of high quality colostrum is widely recognised as being a key step to promote their health and survival. Getting the calf off to a good start also has long-term benefits including lower mortality and improved growth rates. This chapter includes information on the best ways to collect, store and administer colostrum, and then how to check that the system used on farm has been successful in ensuring that all calves achieve adequate levels of passive transfer.

WHAT IS COLOSTRUM?

Bovine colostrum contains mammary gland secretions together with serum proteins derived from the dam's blood, in particular Ig. These accumulate in the mammary gland during the dry period in the last 2 months before calving. Production of colostrum stops at birth so the concentration of most of the components is greatest in the first milking after calving, then declines steadily in the transition milk before reaching the lower concentrations normally found in whole milk after about six milkings. The mean concentration of fat in colostrum is around 6–7% and the total protein content is around 14%, so these essential nutrients are both present in significantly higher concentrations than is found in milk, in which the concentrations of both are usually in the range of 3–4% (3). The lactose concentration is, however, lower in colostrum at around 2.7% compared with 5% in whole milk (4). The main constituents of colostrum and their functions are summarised in Table 3.1. It can be seen from this list that although the IgG content is usually taken as the main assessment of quality, colostrum contains many more components which all have important functions in promoting the health and growth of the neonatal calf.

DAM FACTORS THAT INFLUENCE COLOSTRUM QUALITY

High quality colostrum has been defined as having an IgG concentration >50 mg/mL. Large scale studies of colostrum reported mean values of IgG of 68.8 mg/mL (3) and 74.4 mg/mL (8), but with extreme variability between the samples collected (3, 9). In these three studies 23%, 29% and 44% of the samples analysed contained <50 mg/mL IgG. This means that it is important to measure colostrum quality on farm and to understand some of the factors which might influence it.

Timing and volume of first milking

There is general agreement that the IgG concentration in colostrum is highest immediately after calving and then decreases, so that it is 17% lower at 6 hours and 27% lower by 10 hours post-calving (10). This is because a finite amount of IgG is transferred from the maternal blood into the mammary gland before calving, and this gradually becomes diluted as milk synthesis is upregulated. This also partly explains why few high producing cows (yield >8.5 kg at first milking) have high quality (>50 mg/mL) colostrum (11), although there is not a consistent relationship between colostrum yield and quality (12).

Dry period length

Because of the way in which IgG accumulates in the mammary gland before calving, the concentration in colostrum is reduced if the cow has a short dry period (<3 weeks (13)). Colostrum yield is also lower in cows with short (40 day) compared with conventional (60 day) dry periods (14). It is also important to reduce the risk of any intramammary infections during the dry period by applying correct drying off procedures, as infected quarters will produce less colostrum (Figure 3.1).

TABLE 3.1 Main constituents of colostrum.

Constituent	Comments/function
Fat	The calf is born with little body fat or glycogen reserves, so is highly dependent on the lipids in colostrum as a source of energy. This is particularly important for thermogenesis during cold weather.
Lactose	Lactose is the primary carbohydrate in colostrum and provides energy. It also regulates the water and osmotic content of the colostrum.
Protein	The main proteins present are IgG (see below), casein and albumin. Amino acids are mainly required for growth and can provide some energy.
Immunoglobulins	Over 80% of these are IgG together with some IgA and IgM. IgG is absorbed across the gut to provide circulating antibodies in the first 24 hours of life; IgA provides local immunity within the gut.
Maternal leukocytes	These migrate into the calf's circulation, providing immunological memory of specific pathogens to which the dam has been exposed.
Growth factors	These include IGF-1, insulin, EGF and TGFβ. These act locally to influence the differentiation of the epithelial cells of the gastrointestinal tract and increase villus size, resulting in enhanced absorptive capacity.
Antimicrobial factors	These include lactoferrin, lysozyme and lactoperoxidase, which suppress bacterial growth. There is also a range of other antimicrobial peptides present including β-defensins, complement, cathelicidin and calgranulins. These contribute to the local mucosal immune defence system and assist with pathogen recognition.
Oligosaccharides	These are thought to act as competitive inhibitors to prevent pathogen binding to epithelial surfaces of the intestine.
Vitamins	Colostrum supplies the calf with vitamins A, D and E, which do not cross the placenta in significant amounts. Carotene, riboflavin, vitamin B12 and folic acid are among others also present.
Minerals and trace elements	These include calcium, magnesium, zinc and selenium. Calcium is required for bone development. They all have a variety of other functions including acting as co-factors for enzymes.

Source: Collated from (3,5–7).

Breed

A comparison of five dairy breeds reported a range of 4.1% (Holstein) to 6.6% (Jersey) of IgG in colostrum (15), although this difference between Holsteins and Jerseys was not replicated in another more recent study (3). It is not, therefore, known if the reported difference was genetic or due to other potential variables between herds. However, a genome wide association study within the Jersey breed has produced preliminary evidence of loci which are associated with colostrum quality and quantity, suggesting that in future, genomic selection for these traits may become possible (16).

Age of dam

There is a trend for multiparous cows to have a somewhat higher IgG concentration compared to primiparous cows (11), with average values of 42.4, 68.6 and 95.9 mg/mL for cows in their first, second, or third and subsequent lactations, respectively (17). These differences are thought to reflect greater exposure to pathogens as animals' age. Nevertheless, some primiparous cows do produce good quality colostrum, so it is always worth testing it before deciding whether or not to use it.

Other US studies have similarly found better colostrum quality associated with more pre-partum days above 23°C (18) and higher colostrum yields in summer than in winter (19). In contrast, cows calving in the winter months in Northern Ireland produced colostrum with greater IgG concentration than cows calving in the autumn and spring months (9). Such potential seasonal differences therefore require determining for individual herds.

Dry cow nutrition

Views are mixed on whether it is possible to influence colostrum quality by changing the pre-partum diet (12). In general no relationship is found between dry cow nutrition and colostrum IgG concentration (9, 20). Rations which meet National Research Council (2001) guidelines and supply sufficient DM intake are, however, always recommended.

Pre-partum vaccination of the dam

Dam vaccination may be used as a strategy to increase concentrations of protective antibodies in colostrum against specific pathogens likely to cause problems for young calves (12). For example, cows immunised against salmonella have greater IgG concentrations than non-immunised cows (58.7 mg/mL vs 51.1 mg/mL) (9). It is unclear whether this does, however, benefit the offspring. A large scale study to evaluate the efficacy of a combination rotavirus-coronavirus/*Escherichia coli* vaccine on disease and death rates failed to detect any benefit, even though at least one of the three potential pathogens was found on every farm in the trial (21). Although the scientific evidence is lacking, in the authors experience, use of dam vaccination can have a positive impact on early calf health, especially when dealing with neonatal diarrhoea caused by infectious agents.

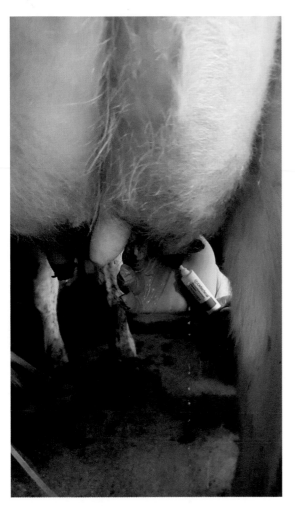

FIGURE 3.1 Sealing of the teats at drying off to reduce the risk of pathogens entering the udder and causing mastitis.

Season

Seasonal effects will clearly depend on the extremes of climate to which the cows are exposed in different geographical locations and may be hard to separate from differences in nutrition and day length. A high THI value in the month before calving significantly influences colostrum quality, with IgG concentrations highest (72.6 mg/mL) for THI $\geq$70 and lowest (64.2 mg/mL) for THI <40 (8). This was hypothesised to be due to more transfer of IgG to the udder during the dry period associated with greater vasodilation in warmer weather.

Milk somatic cell count

The somatic cell count (SCC) in the first milk sample tested after calving is significantly higher in cows producing colostrum of inferior quality. Cows having a SCC >50,000 cells/mL are 1.7 times more likely to have produced colostrum with an IgG content of <30 mg/mL than cows with a SCC <50,000. There is, however, no association between colostral IgG and the SCC measured in the previous lactation (22).

Summary

- Collecting colostrum as soon after calving as possible (<6 hours) will consistently maximise its' quality.
- The IgG content is likely to be higher in dams of ≥3 lactations.
- There is, however, significant variation in samples collected from different cows, much of which remains unexplained. It is therefore strongly advisable to test each sample on a routine basis before feeding to calves.
- Colostrum quality is also influenced by the way in which it is collected and stored.

COLLECTION AND STORAGE OF COLOSTRUM

Infectious agents such as *Mycoplasma* spp., *Salmonella* spp. or *Mycobacterium avium* subsp. *paratuberculosis* may be present in colostrum. The latter is the etiological agent causing Johne's disease (23). Such microorganisms multiply quickly, particularly in warm colostrum, with total coliform counts (TCC) rising rapidly during the first 24 hours, with the potential for the numbers present to double every 20 minutes (24). It is therefore essential to collect colostrum hygienically and then either to feed it promptly within 1 hour after collection or to store it appropriately within 1–2 hours by refrigeration or freezing. Pasteurisation or the addition of an appropriate preservative can also be used to reduce the bacterial load.

The recommended industry standard for colostrum at the time of feeding with respect to its microbial content is for the total plate count (TPC) to be <100,000 colony-forming units (cfu)/mL, with a TCC <10,000 cfu/mL (25). Two surveys found that only around one-half of samples tested met this standard (3, 26). Not only does this expose calves directly to potentially harmful infectious agents, but high levels of bacteria in colostrum also interfere with the ability of the calf to absorb the beneficial IgG through the gut (27).

Hygienic collection

The starting point is to ensure that the colostrum remains as clean as possible during the collection process to minimise the initial microbial load. This can be done cow-side using a portable milking machine, or in the parlour (Figure 3.2).

Tips for hygienic collection of colostrum

- Do not collect colostrum from diseased cows who are Johne's positive or are suffering from post-calving conditions.
- Ensure udder cleanliness. Remove any teat sealant and adopt an effective teat disinfectant routine to remove bacteria.
- Have clean hands and wear gloves to avoid contaminating the colostrum yourself.
- Sanitise cluster and pipework, both inside and out, after every use.
- Use a clean, sanitised dump bucket and transfer the colostrum to a clean sanitised bucket with a lid on.

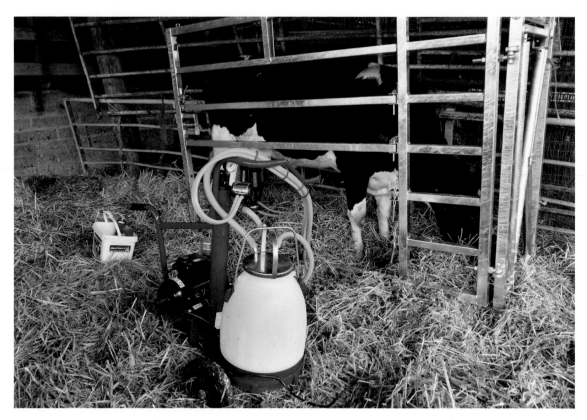

FIGURE 3.2 A portable milking machine allowing a freshly calved cow to have colostrum collected soon after calving.

Pooling colostrum

Pooling of colostrum samples between cows should be avoided as it dilutes IgG and other protein levels. This is not unexpected, as poorer quality colostrum is generally present in a larger volume so will dilute the good quality colostrum (28). Pooled samples also have more bacterial contamination reflected in higher TPCs (3). Use of pooled colostrum also increases the risk of transmission of Johne's disease to the calf (23).

Refrigeration of colostrum

Colostrum should be stored at 4°C, and the temperature of the refrigerator must be checked regularly. It is best to use sanitised 1–2 L containers for storage and to remember that when a large volume of warm liquid is placed into a refrigerator it will take some time for the temperature to drop. In refrigerated colostrum without preservative, the bacterial load still shows a steady increase over time and so should not be kept for more than 1 day (24).

Freezing of colostrum

Colostrum may be frozen and stored at –18 to –20°C for up to 1 year as long as repeated multiple freeze–thaw cycles do not occur and the freezer temperature is checked regularly (29). Commercially available single use bags should be used which are flat to allow easier storage and have a higher surface area for defrosting – a thin bag defrosts much more quickly than a block. It is important to ensure that all stored colostrum

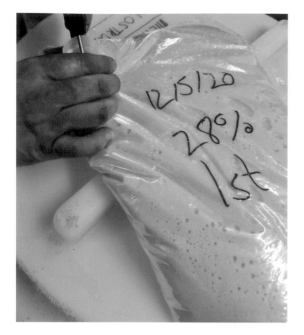

FIGURE 3.3 Labelling the bag of any stored colostrum is important – it should contain the date it was collected, the quality and the ID of the cow it was collected from (although the ID is not seen on this bag).

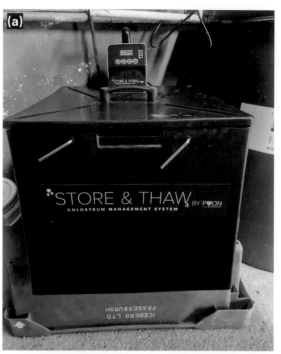

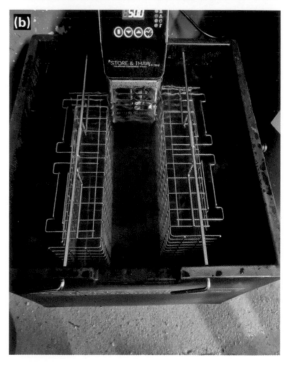

FIGURE 3.4 Use of a colostrum thawer can help ensure the preparation time is quick (~45 minutes to defrost and warm up) and efficient (the cages keep the bags of colostrum fully submerged and the water circulating).

is clearly labelled with both the collection date and cow identity, in case the donor cow later tests positive for Johne's disease (Figure 3.3). When thawing frozen colostrum ready for use, producers should avoid overheating or the crucial IgG may become denatured. The colostrum temperature should reach around 42°C to allow for a slight cooling before it reaches the calf but should not exceed 60°C. The best option for thawing is to use a water bath at a maximum temperature of 50°C. Microwaves should not be used as they destroy the IgG. Temperatures should be checked using a thermometer and once warmed the colostrum should be used immediately. One possible disadvantage of using either frozen or pasteurised colostrum is that both processes kill the maternal leukocytes present (12). These are known to be able to modulate the subsequent immune responses in the calves, but at present the clinical relevance of this remains uncertain.

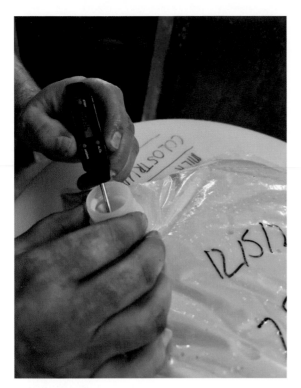

FIGURE 3.5 Use of a thermometer to check the temperature of the colostrum prior to feeding. By the time this colostrum has been decanted into a bottle and taken to the calf, the temperature will have cooled slightly.

Pasteurisation of colostrum

Pasteurising colostrum reduces the bacterial load and is able to decrease or eliminate certain pathogens (e.g. *Mycobacterium bovis*, *Escherichia coli*, *Salmonella enteritidis*) that can potentially cause diarrhoea in young calves (30). Both the TCC (1.15 vs 3.95 $\log_{10}$cfu/mL) and the TPC values (1.18 vs 3.62 $\log_{10}$cfu/mL) are significantly lower immediately after heat treatment in comparison with raw colostrum (31). If the treated colostrum is not going to be used straight away then it still needs to be chilled or frozen as the TCC values will quickly increase again. It is also important to note that pasteurisation does not make low quality or highly contaminated colostrum fit to be fed.

The main concern with the pasteurisation process is that it can cause a reduction in IgG content. This loss is minimised by ensuring that the temperature does not exceed 60–63°C for more than 30–60 minutes (20). This heat treatment generally reduces colostrum IgG levels by approximately 5%, but this is compensated for as blood IgG levels are improved when feeding colostrum treated in this way. It is important to refer to the manufacturer's instructions for the type of pasteuriser being used with regard to batch quantities. In general, however, smaller volumes are better as they reach the required temperature more quickly and this helps to preserve the maximum amount of IgG. Batches of 8–16 L provide the highest amount of IgG to the calf (27, 32). There is evidence that use of pasteurised colostrum improves the efficiency of passive transfer (33) as bacteria in colostrum can bind to antibodies before they can be absorbed in the gut, therefore reducing the number of bacteria leaves more IgG available for absorption (34).

Use of preservatives in colostrum

Some preservatives can be added to colostrum to increase its' shelf life. The most common is potassium sorbate (E202) at a final dilution of 0.5%. This preservative is widely used in human food and drink manufacture for its antibacterial and antifungal properties (35) and is approved for treating colostrum by the US Food and Drug Administration. In raw colostrum there is a steady increase in TPC even when it is refrigerated, with average bacterial counts reaching unacceptably high levels (TPC >100,000 cfu/mL) after 2 days. However, the combination of refrigeration at 4°C with potassium sorbate is able to maintain the average colostrum TPC below 100,000 cfu/mL for 6 days (24). A variety of other chemical additives (e.g. formic acid) have also been tested to reduce bacterial growth, particularly using acidification with or without refrigeration. These do, however, tend to reduce palatability (36).

Colostrum collection and storage – key points

- Minimise bacterial contamination of colostrum by cleanliness during collection.
- Ensure that colostrum is stored in an appropriate way to minimise microbial proliferation before feeding.
- Do not guess – check the temperatures of colostrum and fridges/freezers with a thermometer.

FEEDING COLOSTRUM: THE 3 QS

The goal when feeding colostrum is to achieve an adequate passive transfer of immunity (APT) from dam to calf. The traditional measure of success has been a blood level of >10 mg/mL IgG, although there is now increasing awareness that more IgG may be better (12, 37). Calves that do not reach this level are said to suffer a failure of passive transfer (FPT). There is universal agreement that newborn calves should all receive sufficient good quality colostrum as soon as possible after birth. The UK Welfare of Farmed Animals (England) Regulations (2007) state that this should be given to each calf as soon as possible after it is born and in any case within the first 6 hours of life. Opinions vary, however, as to how much should be fed and how often. Advice on this is frequently summarised as the 3 Qs: Quantity, Quality and Quickly. A fourth Q, Quietly, is also covered in the following section on how to feed colostrum.

Quantity

In order to achieve adequate passive transfer, calves must first consume a sufficient mass of IgG in colostrum. The actual amount required has been variously estimated at between 150 to 300 g IgG (12). The average IgG content of colostrum is around 70 mg/mL, so achieving APT requires consumption of at least 2 L. The calculations are complicated by the fact that colostrum quality can vary enormously and that the ability of the calf to absorb the IgG goes down rapidly over time. An amount which is adequate to achieve APT at 2 hours might therefore be insufficient if not fed until a later time point (38). A number of trials have measured circulating IgG in calves after feeding various volumes of colostrum and it is clear that the risk of FPT decreases progressively as the volume fed is increased from 2 L to 3 L to 4 L (6). It should also be noted that the amount required depends on the size of the calf, so another recommendation is that calves are fed 10% to 12% of their bodyweight as colostrum at first feeding. This works out at 3–4 L for a Holstein calf, but would be proportionately less for a smaller Jersey calf.

Quality

As the aim is for the calf to receive a sufficient amount of IgG, the quality of the colostrum is equally important as the quantity. There is a limitation to the volume of colostrum which a newborn calf can physically consume, so it is not possible to fully compensate for poor quality by continually increasing the volume. It is therefore recommended that colostrum fed to calves has a minimum of 50 mg/mL of IgG (11, 12, 38). In practice this concentration is very variable between individual cows (see above) and the only way of knowing the concentration is to measure it. This can be done using either a colostrometer or a Brix refractometer as outlined below.

The other really important aspect of colostrum quality is for the bacterial count at the time of feeding to be <100,000 cfu/mL (25). Collection and storage in a hygienic manner, using thoroughly cleaned equipment is therefore essential. Again, the only way to be confident that this standard is being achieved is to have the colostrum tested periodically. This can be arranged through a veterinary practice. In order for it to be representative, the sample should be taken just before it is fed to the calf. It is then sent to a laboratory for bacterial culture.

Quickly

The epithelial cells of the gut are initially able to absorb intact protein macromolecules including IgG, but this ability decreases rapidly after birth, ceasing completely by about 24 hours. This is referred to as gut closure (28, 39). The secretion of digestive enzymes also increases, so degrading IgG prior to absorption (40). Standard advice is therefore to ensure that colostrum is provided as soon as possible after birth. A number of studies have measured serum IgG in calves fed a standard batch of colostrum at different time intervals. These consistently show that the highest rates of absorption occur in the first 4 hours after birth but then the rate decreases with each 4 hour increment. Some limited absorption may still be possible between 12–24 hours, but no serum IgG was detected in some calves first fed at 12 hour (39, 41, 42). More recently, a large-scale survey of US dairies found that delaying first feeding until after 4 hours increased the risk of FPT by 2.7-fold (43).

Feeding immediately after birth is not always considered practical on farm, for example when cows calve at night and/or outside and staff availability may be limited (Figure 3.6). Some industry advice therefore recommends that a 6 hour window of time is acceptable, with the best results achieved if first feeding is within 2 hours of birth. It should be noted that the newborn calf has high levels of adrenaline and a strong impulse to suckle within 30–90 minutes of birth. In the authors' experience, this time frame provides the best opportunity to get the calf to suckle large volumes of colostrum from a teat bottle.

The condition of the calf in its first few hours of life also affects its' ability to absorb IgG (12). For example, respiratory or metabolic acidosis are more likely to occur following a difficult calving (28, 44) and such animals require additional supportive care. This could include the provision of

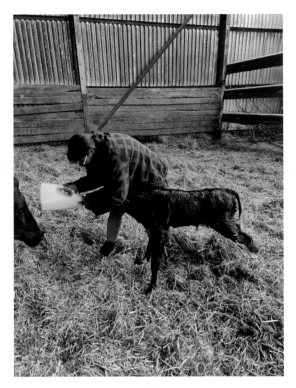

FIGURE 3.6 Bottle feeding colostrum into a calf soon after it was born. The calf is still wet and has only just started standing.

pain management in the form of a non-steroidal anti-inflammatory agent, which can improve calf vigour and IgG absorption (45).

Extended feeding of colostrum

In terms of passive transfer, the initial feed is the most important. Nevertheless, continuing to feed at least some colostrum or transition milk over the first couple of weeks of life is undoubtedly beneficial (12, 46). Colostrum contains many other bioactive components apart from IgG, and these can have an important role in epigenetics and developmental/metabolic programming (discussed in Chapter 1) (47). These substances include lactoferrin, lactoperoxidase and lysozyme, all of which suppress bacterial growth. There are also a number of other antimicrobial peptides including β-defensins, complement, cathelicidin and calgranulins. Together these assist with pathogen recognition and support local immunity within the gut (48). This can help to prevent or reduce the severity of bacterial and viral infections that cause enteritis in early life (49, 50), leading to a reduced need for antimicrobial therapy (51). These components also help the digestive tract of the newborn to mature (52) and to establish a beneficial gut microflora (53).

The newborn calf is reliant on the lipids and lactose in colostrum as a source of energy. The subsequent glucose absorption stimulates endogenous insulin secretion, which in turn helps to promote gut development (54). The lower critical temperature for a newborn calf is about 15°C. When external temperatures are below this then the calf requires extra energy to maintain its own body temperature (55) and its ability to absorb IgG is reduced (56). Feeding colostrum to calves at an environmental temperature of 10°C stimulated an 18% increase in heat production in the following hour (57). If this energy is not available then the calf is at risk of hypothermia. Rectal temperatures drop to a greater extent in the first hour after a difficult birth, so such calves are particularly vulnerable (43, 57). In addition to the colostrum feed, drying the calf, using supplemental heat and supplying deep straw bedding are also beneficial, particularly during cold weather.

HOW TO TEST COLOSTRUM

Testing colostrum is an important task that should be undertaken at every collection. The results are necessary in order to make an informed decision as to whether the colostrum is good enough to be fed or should be discarded. For consistency, the colostrum should be tested at a fixed temperature and a room temperature of 22°C is ideal. Body temperature straight from the dam is too warm and a sample just removed from the refrigerator is too cold.

Colostrometer

This measures the specific gravity of the colostrum and has the advantage of being cheap to buy and quick to use, but careful handling is needed as it is fragile. The colostrometer itself and any containers used must be clean and free from any obvious contaminants, such as faecal material. The colostrum is first collected into a bucket and a sample is then taken in a jug and poured into a sufficiently tall measuring cylinder to allow the colostrometer to float. There should not be any froth. Once the colostrometer has been floated in the colostrum it needs to be left for 1 minute before taking a reading. This is the value at the surface of the liquid (Figure 3.7). This reading correlates with the actual IgG concentration as measured by radial immunodiffusion assay (the gold standard), with r values in the range 0.5 to 0.7 reported (28, 58). The reliability of the classification is therefore reasonable but not perfect.

Refractometer

Refractometers measure the extent of light refraction of transparent substances in a liquid and this provides information on the concentration of

---

Colostrum feeding – top tips

- Test colostrum for quality and only feed if it contains >50 mg/mL IgG.
- Maintain cleanliness during collection and storage so that the bacterial count is <100,000 cfu/mL.
- Ensure that 3–4 L is consumed in the first feed (dependent on the size of the calf).
- Provide the first feed as soon as possible, but definitely within 6 hours of birth.
- Continuing to feed colostrum/transition milk over the next few days is beneficial, providing energy and local immunity within the gut.
- Vulnerable calves may need extra care such as warming or pain management to aid IgG absorption.

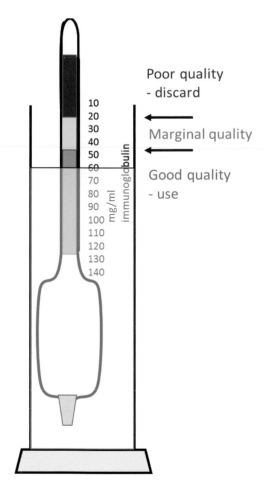

Poor quality
- discard

10
20
30
40
50
60
70
80
90
100
110
120
130
140

mg/ml immunoglobulin

Marginal quality

Good quality
- use

FIGURE 3.7 Use of colostrometer. Readings in the green zone indicate >50 mg/mL of immunoglobulin. This is good quality colostrum, which can be used or stored. Readings in the red zone indicate <20 mg/mL of immunoglobulin. This is poor quality and should be discarded. Readings in the amber zone indicate marginal quality, whose use should be avoided if possible.

both types of refractometer for use in colostrum measurement found that both were acceptable. The IgG concentration as measured by radial immuno-diffusion assay was positively correlated with both digital ($r = 0.79$) and optical ($r = 0.74$) Brix refractometer measurements (59). Refractometers do not, however, work well in assessing the quality of colostrum that has been pasteurised. The correlation of the readings with the actual IgG concentration was only 45% with each type of refractometer when colostrum had been heat-treated at 63°C for 60 minutes (59).

Using both types of refractometer, the glass prism where the sample is placed needs to be clean and not cracked and the equipment must be calibrated before each use. This involves putting 2–3 drops of distilled water onto the glass surface and lowering the sample cover so that the water spreads across the entire surface without any air bubbles or dry spots. The reading is taken after 15 seconds to allow the sample to adjust to room temperature. With optical refractometers a circular field is seen with graduations down the centre (Figure 3.8). For correct calibration the scale should read zero where the light and dark areas meet. If not this is adjusted using the calibration screw. The glass surface is then wiped clean and dried with a soft cloth. A couple of drops of colostrum (about 300 µL) are placed onto the glass prism and the reading process is repeated. High quality colostrum, which has a reading above 23% (equivalent to 50 mg/mL immunoglobulin), can be used or stored whereas colostrum with a reading below 18% should not be used as first feed colostrum (12, 58). The glass prism then needs to be cleaned using water and a cloth so that it is ready for the next time.

HOW TO FEED COLOSTRUM

Suckling from the dam

Suckling may appear as the most natural solution, but several studies have shown that there is a significantly increased risk of FPT if dairy calves are

dissolved substances within the sample. They can be used for many different purposes, so for colostrum it is important to select one with a scale in the range 0–32%. With traditional optical refractometers the reading is taken using natural (not fluorescent light) while looking through a magnifying eyepiece. With digital handheld refractometers light from an LED light source is used and the result is displayed on a digital readout scale. Evaluation of

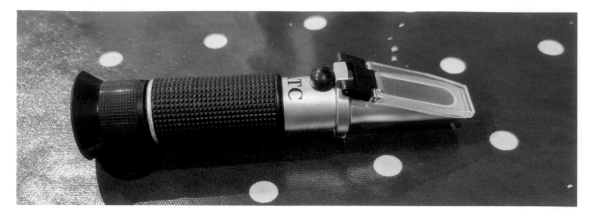

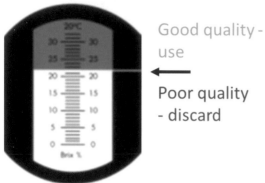

Good quality - use

← Poor quality - discard

FIGURE 3.8 Use of an optical Brix refractometer with a scale from 0% to 32%. A reading of 23% on the Brix scale is equivalent to a colostrum concentration of 50 mg/mL immunoglobulin.

just left with their dams (Figure 3.9). One study found that 61% of Holstein calves left with their dams had FPT at 48 hours (60). A more recent study similarly found that approximately one-third of Holstein calves fail to suck from the dam unaided and that calves left with their dams were at 2.4 times the risk of FPT in comparison with hand feeding (43). These issues are more likely to arise following a difficult calving, with weak calves less able to get up and suckle adequately in a timely fashion (61).

The structure of the mammary may cause problems if the udder is pendulous or the teats are too fat. Maternal behaviour can also be influential. Some dams may avoid or attack their calves, particularly those calving for the first time, while mis-mothering can be a problem in communal calving pens. Another issue with suckling is that the colostrum quality is not monitored and, as described above, this may not always be adequate.

A final consideration is the risk of the calf acquiring pathogens from the environment of the dam, in particular Johne's disease which may be in the colostrum but is mainly passed on through ingestion of faecal material which may be covering the dam's teats (62). When this is a concern, it is advised to snatch the calf from the pen as soon as possible after delivery to minimise the risk of transmission.

Concern over insufficient natural intake of colostrum from the dam together with an increased disease risk has prompted the recommendation that colostrum should be hand fed to the calf. This can be done using either a teat/nipple bottle or an oesophageal tube.

Teat/nipple bottle

Use of a teat/nipple bottle is generally considered the first choice method of hand feeding

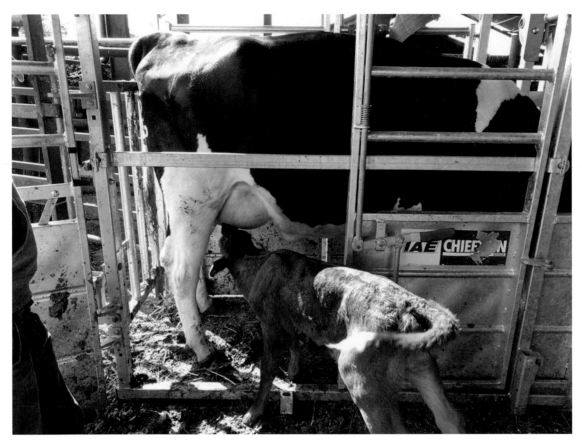

FIGURE 3.9 A cow restrained in a crush so that the calf may suckle from her.

(Figure 3.10). It is less stressful, and feeding a calf in this way promotes closure of the oesophageal groove, which allows the colostrum to enter the abomasum or 'true' stomach where digestion takes place (63). As mentioned above, calves are driven to suckle shortly after birth, so ensuring the colostrum is offered within 30–90 minutes of birth leads to the greatest success of getting the calf to ingest large volumes – the author finds that these calves will generally voluntarily consume 3–4 L of colostrum when offered within this time frame. However, calves that have been born for a few hours or have already tried to suckle their dam are often more resistant to teat feeding, as are calves that have had difficult calvings. This means it may be necessary to top up the extra volume required to achieve APT using an oesophageal tube. Another consideration is that in some cases getting the calf to suck from

the bottle may require a significant amount of staff time, but it does result in early training of the calf for feeding from an artificial teat which is a benefit when the calf is moved to the rearing pens.

Oesophageal tube

If done properly, feeding with an oesophageal tube is a reliable method to ensure that the calf receives an adequate volume of colostrum in a timely fashion. The technique does not stimulate reflex closure of the oesophageal groove, so colostrum enters the rumen rather than the abomasum and this increases the transit time to the small intestine by around 2–4 hours (64). This does not, however, appear to have a large impact on the success of passive transfer, so is not thought to be

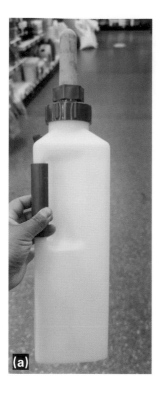

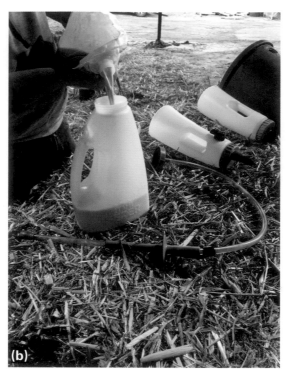

FIGURE 3.10 (a) An example of a nipple bottle that may be used to feed colostrum. (b) Pouring colostrum into a bottle that has both a teat and also an oesophageal tube attachment that can fit onto it.

a major concern (60, 65). Feeding colostrum in this way is a skilled technique that requires training and care to ensure the correct placement of the tube. This is essential to avoid any injury to the calf (Figure 3.11).

Preparation for oesophageal tube feeding

The method requires a feeding tube (plus a spare), a bag of at least 3 L of good quality colostrum warmed to 38–40°C, and either tape or a pen to mark the tube. The equipment to be used must have been thoroughly cleaned and disinfected and be in good working order. Any sharp edges or disintegrating rubber can harbour bacteria and may cause direct internal damage to the calf. Correct handling of the calf is important and comes back to the fourth 'Q' of colostrum management, which is to ensure that the whole procedure is performed quietly and calmly to minimise any possible distress. If the calf is still in the calving pen then it is also necessary to keep an eye on the dam who has a maternal instinct to protect her calf. The calf

should be backed into a corner of the pen, with one hand under its muzzle to keep its head and neck upright. Tube feeding should not be performed with the calf in lateral recumbency as milk can enter the lungs causing aspiration pneumonia or even death. If the calf cannot stand then it should be positioned on its sternum with the head held up and supported between the operator's legs. The head and neck must remain above stomach level throughout the feeding in order to prevent aspiration of fluids. Before inserting the tube, the length from the tip of the calf's nose to the point of the elbow behind the front leg should be measured and this point marked, to ensure that the correct length is inserted.

Inserting the tube

The end of the tube should first be moistened with either warm water or colostrum. The calf's head is raised gently and the sides of the mouth squeezed to open it. The tube can then be inserted slowly and gently over the tongue to the back of the mouth. It

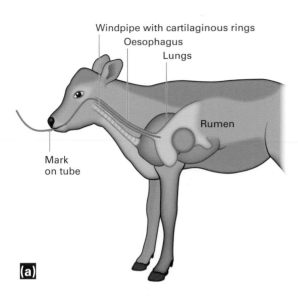

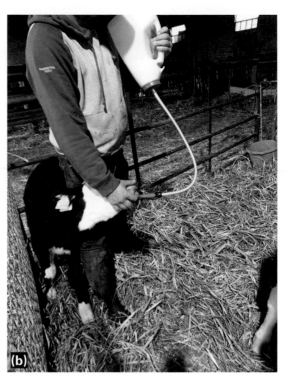

FIGURE 3.11 (a) Diagram showing the correct positioning of the tube inside the oesophagus. (b) Feeding of colostrum through an oesophageal feeder.

should then enter the oesophagus, which is directly above the trachea (windpipe). Extreme care is needed at this point to ensure that the tube is positioned correctly. It should never be forced, so if any resistance is felt it must be pulled out slightly and redirected. The windpipe is surrounded by cartilaginous rings which can be felt through the skin, whereas the oesophagus is soft and collapsible. When the tube is in the correct position inside the oesophagus then both structures can be felt (Figure 3.9a). The tube is then pushed in until the mark is reached.

Administering the colostrum

This should only begin once the operator is confident that the tube is positioned correctly and that the calf is comfortable and swallowing. The colostrum should be fed at a temperature of 38–40°C. The flow rate is controlled by gravity through raising or lowering the bag. Using a slow rate is better for the calf as it minimises the risk of regurgitation. Once the colostrum is finished then the

tube is kinked and withdrawn in one swift movement. Removing the tube prematurely while it still

Feeding colostrum – summary

- When a calf is left to suckle from the dam then it is not possible to be certain that sufficient colostrum has been consumed.
- Leaving the calf with the dam also increases the risk of disease transmission.
- A nipple bottle is the first choice method for hand feeding colostrum, with highest success levels when this is done within 30–90 minutes of life.
- Use of an oesophageal tube ensures delivery of the correct amount in a timely fashion.
- Any staff using tube feeding must be properly trained in this technique to avoid potentially serious injury to the calf.

contains liquid, may cause colostrum to enter the lungs. Once withdrawn, the feeding tube should be rinsed immediately, thoroughly cleaned and disinfected, and hung up to drain and dry in a clean, dry environment. It will then be ready for next time. If any residues are left on it then these provide breeding grounds for microorganisms, which will inadvertently be fed to the next calf.

USE OF COLOSTRUM SUPPLEMENTS AND REPLACERS

Good quality colostrum is the best feed for newborn calves, but alternatives may be needed if this is not available or the dam is likely to be a source of *Mycobacterium avium* subsp. *paratuberculosis*. It is, however, necessary to read the label carefully as the list of ingredients varies between brands and may be incomplete. The most important consideration is the IgG content. Some products just supply basic nutrients, such as energy and lactose, and contain little or no IgG. These are classified as supplements. Licenced colostrum replacers in the USA and Canada must contain a minimum of 100 g of IgG per pack derived from bovine colostrum and provide sufficient amounts of other nutrients to support the metabolic needs of the calf in the first day of life. They also have to be processed using accepted protocols to guarantee efficacy, safety and purity (12). Other unlicensed products available in the United States may contain immunoglobulins derived from various sources including milk, whey, bovine serum or plasma. In the UK market it is hard to source freeze dried colostrum, due to previous concerns that it may pose a disease risk, with commercially available products often being relatively expensive. Supplements which do not contain IgG may have some benefit but will not provide passive transfer. For those products which do contain IgG, the amount per packet is important. In order to supply the recommended 150–300 g IgG dose then two or three packets may be required and even then not all calves will achieve adequate passive transfer (12).

EVALUATING SUCCESS

Both dairy producers and their veterinary surgeons have become increasingly aware of the long-term benefits derived from every calf receiving an adequate supply of colostrum. Nevertheless, large scale on – farm surveys continue to report significant numbers of calves with FPT (e.g. USA 13% (66), UK 26% (67), 20.7% (31)). The effectiveness of the procedures used on farm can only be known by measuring the outcome. The success with which the calf has acquired passive immunity is typically evaluated by measuring IgG (or a proxy for it) in calf serum. It should be noted that this does not take full account of the other benefits in addition to passive transfer which the calf obtains from being fed colostrum and transitional milk over several days.

How to evaluate

The IgG concentration in the calf's blood can be measured directly using either radial immunodiffusion or an enzyme-linked immunosorbent assay (ELISA) (28). These methods are considered the gold standard but require that the samples are submitted to a laboratory and are also quite expensive to run. Other tests available provide estimates of the serum IgG concentration based on the concentration of total globulins or other proteins whose passive transfer is statistically associated with that of IgG. One of these is the zinc sulphate turbidity test, in which zinc sulphate forms a precipitate with IgG. The most frequently used alternative test is, however, to measure the serum total protein. This can be used as a proxy for IgG because IgG makes up a large fraction of the serum total protein in the calf's first week of life. Total solids are analysed with a refractometer using either the total protein or the Brix specific gravity percentage scales. This method is cheap, quick and can be performed on farm. A large number of studies have reported strong linear relationships between serum IgG and total solids, with r^2 values usually in the range 0.7–0.9 (12, 28).

When to evaluate

Measurements can be made from 24 hours after birth, after which time passive transfer ceases. The period from 1 to 5 days is ideal as beyond this the IgG levels may start to decay. In practice, sufficiently reliable measurements can be obtained within the first week of life (37, 68). This has the advantage that all calves born in a particular week can be assessed on the same day, for example during a routine veterinary visit. Ideally all calves would be evaluated, but failing this then sufficient animals should be sampled to be able to assess the adequacy of passive transfer at different times of year, for example with respect to climate, start or end of the breeding season or numbers of cows calving.

Sources of variation

The results of serum IgG measurements are known to be less reliable in sick calves, in which the readings may be either over- or underestimated (69). Calves with diarrhoea are likely to become dehydrated, resulting in raised total protein in serum. Others suffer from protein loss, which is reflected as a low total protein reading. The correlation between IgG and total protein readings reduces from $r^2 = 0.76$ in healthy calves to only $r^2 = 0.37$ in calves with watery diarrhoea (37). Another factor causing variation in the measurements is the use of colostrum replacers as opposed to natural colostrum. The manufacturing techniques used can also alter the level of absorption of both Ig and non-Ig proteins resulting in inaccurate assessment of passive transfer.

Interpreting the results

Very many studies have measured serum IgG levels to assess passive transfer and have then related these to the subsequent mortality and morbidity of the calves. Calves have historically been defined as having FPT if the serum IgG measured

between 24–48 hours of age was <10 mg/mL, based on an increased mortality risk below this threshold (28, 70). An alternative approach has been to use receiver operator curves (ROC) to decide on the best cut-off point to apply. For example, a cut-off of 57 mg/mL total protein has been found most effective at reducing false positives and false negatives, but values as low as 50 mg/mL have also been suggested (71).

More recently, it has become apparent that this failure or success approach to passive transfer using cut-points is not the most informative. First, choice of the cut-points to be adopted has a major impact on the proportion of calves classified as either adequate or failed and this is turn affects the perceptions of the producer as to how well they are performing. Second, and more importantly, there is evidence with respect to calf morbidity that there is a progressive reduction in disease incidence as the circulating IgG level increases. In a UK study, increasing IgG from 5.6 to 34.6 mg/mL (representing the 10th to 90th percentile of the measurements made) was associated with a fall in probability of bovine respiratory disease in pre-weaned calves from 0.54 to 0.30 (Figure 3.12) (37).

A group of calf experts in the USA met in 2018 to re-assess the data and determine if changes to the passive immunity standards were necessary to reduce calf morbidity (68). They evaluated four options based on the observed statistical differences between categories with respect to estimated morbidity and mortality. Consensus agreement proposed the use of four serum IgG categories at the individual calf level: excellent, good, fair and poor. The serum IgG levels together with the equivalent total protein and percentage Brix levels in each category are summarised in Table 3.2. The group also proposed that an achievable herd standard would be to have >40, 30, 20 and <10% of calves placed in the excellent, good, fair and poor categories, respectively.

As part of the evaluation, the suggested new categories were applied to a longitudinal study of 2360 calves from 104 dairy operations located in 13 US states which had been investigated in the

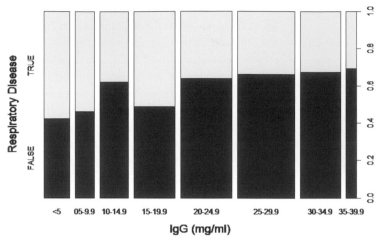

FIGURE 3.12 The probability of a pre-weaned dairy calf contracting bovine respiratory disease (BRD) in relation to the measurement of serum IgG in the first week of life. Each block is proportional in size to the number of individual calves within it. The light grey shading shows the proportion of calves within each block diagnosed with BRD (TRUE) and the dark grey indicates the proportion of calves without BRD (FALSE). The range of serum IgG concentrations in 5 mg/mL increments is shown along the X-axis. The study included 726 calves from 13 farms (37).

TABLE 3.2 Proposed categories of immunoglobulin G levels and equivalent total protein and Brix measurements to assess passive transfer rates in dairy calves (72).

Category	Proposed IgG levels (mg/mL)	Equivalent serum total protein (mg/mL)	Equivalent serum Brix levels (%)	Proposed proportion of calves in each category (%)
Excellent	≥25	≥62	≥9.4	>40
Good	18.0–24.9	58–61	8.9–9.3	30
Fair	10.0–17.9	51–57	8.1–8.8	20
Poor	<10.0	<51	<8.1	<10

TABLE 3.3 Percentage of dairy heifer calves experiencing pre-weaning morbidity and mortality when classified into four suggested categories of passive transfer (66,72,73).

Category	Total calves		Calf morbidity[a]		Calf mortality[b]	
Number of calves	2360		809		75	
	Serum IgG (%)	Serum total protein (%)	Serum IgG (%)	Serum total protein (%)	Serum IgG (%)	Serum total protein (%)
Excellent	35.5	38.7	28.5	29.3	2.5	2.5
Good	25.7	19.4	34.8	32.9	1.5	2.8
Fair	26.7	27.0	36.1	35.3	3.8	2.7
Poor	12.0	14.8	46.1	47.3	7.4	6.3

Notes: [a]Based on producer records; [b]based on number of live calves at 24 hours after birth.

National Animal Health Monitoring System Dairy 2014 study (66, 73). These results did indeed show progressive increases in morbidity (from 28% to 46%) and mortality (from 2.5% to 7.4%) between the excellent and poor passive transfer categories (Table 3.3).

WHAT COLOSTRUM CAN AND CAN'T ACHIEVE

The increasing amounts of data available that show the benefits of achieving adequate passive transfer are indeed encouraging producers to implement colostrum management plans on farm. There is, however, a danger in thinking that once this is achieved it is 'job done' regarding steps to be taken to ensure optimum health in pre-weaned calves. It is therefore also useful to appreciate the limitations.

What colostrum can do

Receiving an adequate amount of colostrum undoubtedly helps to get calves off to a good start. The short-term benefits have already been discussed. A number of prospective studies have also reported longer term benefits to achieving a high level of passive transfer.

Benefits of colostrum feeding

- Provides passive transfer of antibodies to the blood. This helps reduce the risk of diseases that occur in the whole calf (e.g. septicaemias, pneumonia or joint ill).
- Provides an extremely high energy food.
- If given over several days helps reduce the chance of diarrhoea. This relies on antibodies (IgA) and antimicrobial proteins to be present in the gut, not the blood.
- Reduces the risk of pre-weaning and post-weaning mortality.
- Improves weight gain in the first 6 months of life.
- Associated with higher first lactation milk production.

What colostrum can't do

It must be remembered that the transfer of immunity from mother to calf via the colostrum is only possible before gut closure, so the amount of IgG provided is finite. As mentioned above, the calf does not make significant amounts of its own IgGs until 2–4 weeks after birth and these do not approach adult levels until at least 4 months of age (2). Furthermore, the organisms causing diarrhoea act locally within the gut rather than systemically and so circulating IgG is not protective.

Limitations of colostrum feeding

- Passive transfer cannot supply an unlimited number of antibodies. The protection can be quickly used up in dirty, unhygienic environments in which the calf is exposed to a high pathogen challenge.
- Passive transfer of IgG does not provide complete protection against diarrhoea.
- Calves with good passive transfer can still catch respiratory disease, despite having a reduced risk.

MANAGEMENT PLAN

Colostrum management has consistently been shown to have a profound and lasting impact on calf health and survival. Mortality rates in pre-weaned calves are generally of the order of 3–5%, while disease incidence is much higher, with 48.2% of 492 calves born on UK farms diagnosed with diarrhoea and 45.9% with respiratory disease (31). These are unacceptably high levels, which not only reduce production efficiency but also impact on calf welfare. On many farms the individual(s) responsible for overseeing the birth and colostrum management of the calf are not the same as the one(s) who then take on the rearing process. If any health issues do arise in the pre-weaned calves it is not uncommon for a 'blame game' to develop between them. It is therefore in everyone's best interests (including the calf) to have robust procedures in place regarding colostrum feeding and for the early events in a calf's life to be documented for future reference. This requires: (i) the farm staff and veterinary practice to develop a realistic management plan tailored for each farm; (ii) to ensure that the reasons behind the plan are explained to all those who are required to implement it; (iii) that these staff receive adequate resources, time and training to put the plan into practice; and (iv) that the outcomes are recorded and monitored. The components of a colostrum management plan include the following.

- Establish an easy-to-use system for recording birth information on every calf born.
- Ensure that appropriate facilities and equipment are in place for collecting and feeding colostrum.
- Ensure that good washing and disinfection facilities are in place so that all the equipment used is kept scrupulously clean.
- Have written standard operating procedures (SOPs) for key aspects including colostrum collection, monitoring, storage and feeding.
- Provide staff training in procedures.
- Ensure that someone takes responsibility for collecting and analysing the data, for example, on colostrum quality, passive transfer, calf morbidity and mortality rates by age.
- Set up regular meetings between farm staff and the veterinary practice to review the data and agree realistic goals for improvement.

One suggestion is that every calf should have its own birth certificate produced using check boxes to record the key information (68) – the reference paper provides a useful example which can be copied or adapted.

Colostrum management plan – summary

1 Record details of the calf's birth:
   a ID of calf, dam and sire, sex, breed
   b calving details: time, area, dystocia, birth weight, number of calves born
   c navel treatment
   d time of removal from dam to calf pen.

2 Record details of the colostrum fed: time and number of feeds, source, quality test, method used to administer, volume given at each feed.

3 Keep health records for the calf: passive transfer, vaccinations, other test results, for example, for BVDV, mortality.

4 Write SOPs for colostrum collection and processing, colostrum administration and equipment cleaning procedures.

5 Provide staff training, for example, on the safe use of oesophageal tubes.

6 Review the data regularly and adapt the plan accordingly, setting realistic performance targets.

REFERENCES

1. Firth MA, Shewen PE, Hodgins DC. Passive and active components of neonatal innate immune defenses. Anim Health Res Rev 2005 Dec;6(2):143–58.

2. Chase CCL, Hurley DJ, Reber AJ. Neonatal immune development in the calf and its impact on vaccine response. Vet Clin North Am Food Anim Pract 2008;24(1):87–104.

3. Morrill KM, Conrad E, Lago A, Campbell J, Quigley J, Tyler H. Nationwide evaluation of quality and composition of colostrum on dairy farms in the United States. J Dairy Sci 2012 Jul;95(7):3997–4005.

4. Godden S. Colostrum management for dairy calves. Vet Clin North Am Food Anim Pract 2008;24(1):19–39.

5. Godden SM, Lombard JE, Woolums AR. Colostrum management for dairy calves. Vet Clin North Am Food Anim Pract. W. B. Saunders 2019;35(3):535–56.

6. Patel S, Gibbons J. Ensuring optimal colostrum transfer to newborn dairy calves [Internet]; 2014. Available from: http://www.volac.com/news/agriculture-news/news176/.

7. Ganz S, Bülte M, Gajewski Z, Wehrend A. Inhaltsstoffe des bovinen Kolostrums – Eine Übersicht. Tierarztl Prax Ausgabe G Grosstiere – Nutztiere. 2018 Jun 1;178–88.

8. Shivley CB, Lombard JE, Urie NJ, Haines DM, Sargent R, Kopral CA, et al. Preweaned heifer management on US dairy operations: Part II. Factors associated with colostrum quality and passive transfer status of dairy heifer calves. J Dairy Sci 2018 Oct 1;101(10):9185–98.

9. Dunn A, Ashfield A, Earley B, Welsh M, Gordon A, Morrison SJ. Evaluation of factors associated with immunoglobulin G, fat, protein, and lactose concentrations in bovine colostrum and colostrum management practices in grassland-based dairy systems in Northern Ireland. J Dairy Sci 2017 Mar 1;100(3):2068–79.

10. Moore M, Tyler JW, Chigerwe M, Dawes ME, Middleton JR. Effect of delayed colostrum collection on colostral IgG concentration in dairy cows. J Am Vet Med Assoc 2005 Apr 15;226(8):1375–7.

11. Pritchett LC, Gay CC, Besser TE, Hancock DD. Management and production factors influencing immunoglobulin G1 concentration in colostrum from Holstein cows. J Dairy Sci 1991;74(7):2336–41.

12. Godden SM, Lombard JE, Woolums AR. Colostrum management for dairy calves. Vet Clin North Am Food Anim Pract. W. B. Saunders 2019;35(3):535–56.

13. Dixon FJ, Weigle WO, Vazquez JJ. Metabolism and mammary secretion of serum proteins in the cow. Lab Invest 1961;10:216–37.

14. Grusenmeyer D, Ryan C, Galton D. Shortening the dry period from 60 to 40 days does not affect colostrum quality but decreases colostrum yield by Holstein cows. J Dairy Sci 2006;89:336.

15. Muller LD, Ellinger DK. Colostral immunoglobulin concentrations among breeds of dairy cattle. J Dairy Sci 1981 Aug 1;64(8):1727–30.

16. Kiser JN, Cornmesser MA, Gavin K, Hoffman A, Moore DA, Neibergs HL. Rapid communication: Genome-wide association analyses identify loci associated with colostrum production in Jersey cattle1. J Anim Sci 2019 Mar 1;97(3):1117–23.

17. Morrill KM, Conrad E, Lago A, Campbell J, Quigley J, Tyler H. Nationwide evaluation of quality and composition of colostrum on dairy farms in the United States. J Dairy Sci 2012 Jul 1;95(7):3997–4005.

18. Cabral RG, Chapman CE, Aragona KM, Clark E, Lunak M, Erickson PS. Predicting colostrum quality from performance in the previous lactation and environmental changes. J Dairy Sci 2016 May 1;99(5):4048–55.

19. Gavin K, Neibergs H, Hoffman A, Kiser JN, Cornmesser MA, Haredasht SA, et al. Low colostrum yield in Jersey cattle and potential risk factors. J Dairy Sci 2018 Jul 1;101(7):6388–98.

20. Heinrichs AJ, Jones CM, Erickson PS, Chester-Jones H, Anderson JL. Symposium review: Colostrum management and calf nutrition for profitable and sustainable dairy farms. J Dairy Sci. Symposium review: Colostrum management and calf nutrition for profitable and sustainable dairy farms. Elsevier Inc. 2020;103(6):5694–9.

21. Waltner-Toews D, Martin SW, Meek AH, McMillan I, Crouch CF. A field trial to evaluate the efficacy of a combined rotavirus-coronavirus/Escherichia coli vaccine in dairy cattle. Can J Comp Med 1985;49(1):1–9.

22. Gulliksen SM, Lie KI, Sølverød L, Østerås O. Risk factors associated with colostrum quality in Norwegian dairy cows. J Dairy Sci 2008;91(2):704–12.

23. Doré E, Paré J, Côté G, Buczinski S, Labrecque O, Roy JP, Fecteau G. Risk factors associated with transmission of Mycobacterium avium subsp. paratuberculosis to calves within dairy herd: A systematic review [Internet]. J Vet Intern Med 2012;26(1):32–45.

24. Stewart S, Godden S, Bey R, Rapnicki P, Fetrow J, Farnsworth R, et al. Preventing bacterial contamination and proliferation during the harvest, storage, and feeding of fresh bovine colostrum. J Dairy Sci 2005;88(7):2571–8.

25. McGuirk SM, Collins M. Managing the production, storage, and delivery of colostrum. Vet Clin North Am Food Anim Pract 2004;20(3):593–603.

26. Houser BA, Donaldson SC, Kehoe SI, Heinrichs AJ, Jayarao BM. A survey of bacteriological quality and the occurrence of Salmonella in raw bovine colostrum. Foodborne Pathog Dis 2008 Dec 1;5(6):853–8.

27. Johnson JL, Godden SM, Molitor T, Ames T, Hagman D. Effects of feeding heat-treated colostrum on passive transfer of immune and nutritional parameters in neonatal dairy calves. J Dairy Sci 2007;90(11):5189–98.

28. Weaver DM, Tyler JW, VanMetre DC, Hostetle DE, Barrington GM. Passive transfer of

colostral immunoglobulins in calves. J Vet Intern Med 2000;14(6):569–77.

29. Foley JA, Hunter AG, Otterby DE. Absorption of colostral proteins by newborn calves Fed Unfermented, Fermented, or buffered colostrum. J Dairy Sci 1978 Oct 1;61(10):1450–6.

30. Godden S, McMartin S, Feirtag J, Stabel J, Bey R, Goyal S, et al. Heat-treatment of bovine colostrum. II: Effects of heating duration on pathogen viability and immunoglobulin G. J Dairy Sci 2006 Sep 1;89(9):3476–83.

31. Johnson KF, Chancellor N, Burn CC, Wathes DC. Prospective cohort study to assess rates of contagious disease in pre-weaned UK dairy heifers: Management practices, passive transfer of immunity and associated calf health. Vet Rec Open 2017 Apr 1;4(1).

32. Godden SM, Smith S, Feirtag JM, Green LR, Wells SJ, Fetrow JP. Effect of on-farm commercial batch pasteurization of colostrum on colostrum and serum immunoglobulin concentrations in dairy calves. J Dairy Sci 2003;86(4): 1503–12.

33. Elizondo-Salazar JA, Heinrichs AJ. Feeding heat-treated colostrum to neonatal dairy heifers: Effects on growth characteristics and blood parameters. J Dairy Sci 2009 Jul 1;92(7):3265–73.

34. Gelsinger SL, Jones CM, Heinrichs AJ. Effect of colostrum heat treatment and bacterial population on immunoglobulin G absorption and health of neonatal calves. J Dairy Sci 2015 Jul 1;98(7): 4640–5.

35. Stopforth JD, Yoon Y, Barmpalia IM, Samelis J, Skandamis PN, Sofos JN. Reduction of Listeria monocytogenes populations during exposure to a simulated gastric fluid following storage of inoculated frankfurters formulated and treated with preservatives. Int J Food Microbiol 2005 Apr 1;99(3):309–19.

36. Uzmay C, Kaya I, Kaya A. Utilisation possibilities of surplus colostrum by acidification with formic acid in rearing calves II. Performance of calves fed acidified colostrum stored at summer ambient temperatures or in a refrigerator. Pak J Biol Sci 2002;6(14):1214–22.

37. Johnson K. Managing UK dairy heifers for optimum health and survival. PhD Thesis University of London; 2016.

38. Chigerwe M, Tyler JW, Schultz LG, Middleton JR, Steevens BJ, Spain JN. Effect of colostrum administration by use of oroesophageal intubation on serum IgG concentrations in Holstein bull calves. Am J Vet Res 2008;69(9):1158–63.

39. Bush LJ, Staley TE. Absorption of colostral immunoglobulins in newborn calves. J Dairy Sci 1980 Apr 1;63(4):672–80.

40. Quigley JD, Drewry JJ. Nutrient and immunity transfer from cow to calf pre- and postcalving. In: J Dairy Sci. American Dairy Science Association 1998;81(10):2779–90.

41. Stott GH, Marx DB, Menefee BE, Nightengale GT. Colostral immunoglobulin transfer in calves. III. Amount of absorption. J Dairy Sci 1979 Dec 1;62(12):1902–7.

42. Matte JJ, Girard CL, Seoane JR, Brisson GJ. Absorption of colostral immunoglobulin G in the newborn dairy calf. J Dairy Sci 1982 Sep 1;65(9):1765–70.

43. Beam AL, Lombard JE, Kopral CA, Garber LP, Winter AL, Hicks JA, Schlater JL. Prevalence of failure of passive transfer of immunity in newborn heifer calves and associated management practices on US dairy operations. J Dairy Sci 2009 Aug 1;92(8):3973–80.

44. Besser TE, Szenci O, Gay CC. Decreased colostral immunoglobulin absorption in calves with postnatal respiratory acidosis. J Am Vet Med Assoc 1990;196(8):1239–43.

45. Evans NJ, Murray RD, Carter SD. Bovine digital dermatitis: Current concepts from laboratory to farm. Vet J 2016;211:3–13.

46. Kargar S, Roshan M, Ghoreishi SM, Akhlaghi A, Kanani M, Abedi Shams-Abadi AR, Ghaffari MH. Extended colostrum feeding for 2 weeks improves growth performance and reduces the susceptibility to diarrhea and pneumonia in neonatal Holstein dairy calves. J Dairy Sci 2020 Sep 1;103(9): 8130–42.

47. Bagnell CA, Steinetz BG, Bartol FF. Milk-borne relaxin and the Lactocrine hypothesis for maternal programming of neonatal tissues. Ann N Y Acad Sci 2009 Apr 1;1160(1):152–7.

48. Wheeler TT, Smolenski GA, Harris DP, Gupta SK, Haigh BJ, Broadhurst MK, et al. hosts. Host-Defence-related proteins in cows' milk. Animal 2012;6(3):415–22.

49. van der Tol PPJ, Metz JHM, Noordhuizen-Stassen EN, Back W, Braam CR, Weijs WA. The vertical ground reaction force and the pressure distribution on the claws of dairy cows while walking on a flat substrate. J Dairy Sci 2003;86(9): 2875–83.

50. Berge ACB, Besser TE, Moore DA, Sischo WM. Evaluation of the effects of oral colostrum supplementation during the first fourteen days on the health and performance of preweaned calves. J Dairy Sci 2009 Jan 1;92(1):286–95.

51. Chamorro MF, Cernicchiaro N, Haines DM. Evaluation of the effects of colostrum replacer supplementation of the milk replacer ration on the occurrence of disease, antibiotic therapy, and performance of pre-weaned dairy calves. J Dairy Sci 2017 Feb 1;100(2):1378–87.

52. Blum JW, Hammon HM. Bovines Kolostrum: Mehr als nur ein Immunglobulin-lieferant. Schweiz Arch Tierheilkd 2000 May 1;142(5):221–8.

53. Malmuthuge N, Guan LL. Understanding the gut microbiome of dairy calves: Opportunities to improve early-life gut health. J Dairy Sci 2017 Jul 1;100(7):5996–6005.

54. Hammon HM, Steinhoff-Wagner J, Schönhusen U, Metges CC, Blum JW. Energy metabolism in the newborn farm animal with emphasis on the calf: Endocrine changes and responses to milk-born and systemic hormones. Domest Anim Endocrinol 2012;43(2):171–85.

55. National Research Council. Nutrient requirements of dairy cattle. 7th ed. Washington, DC: National Academies Press; 2001.

56. Olson DP, Papasian CJ, Ritter RC. The effects of cold stress on neonatal calves II. Absorption of colostral immunoglobulins. Can J Comp Med 1980;44(1): 19–23.

57. Vermorel M, Dardillat C, Vernet J, Saido N, Demigne C. Energy metabolism and thermoregulation in the newborn calf [Internet]. Ann Rech Vet 1983;14(4):382–9.

58. Bartier AL, Windeyer MC, Doepel L. Evaluation of on-farm tools for colostrum quality measurement. J Dairy Sci 2015 Mar 1;98(3):1878–84.

59. Elsohaby I, Mcclure JT, Keefe GP. Evaluation of digital and optical refractometers for assessing failure of transfer of passive immunity in dairy calves. J Vet Intern Med 2015 Mar 1;29(2):721–6.

60. Besser TE, Gay CC, Pritchett L. Comparison of three methods of feeding colostrum to dairy calves. J Am Vet Med Assoc 1991;198(3):419–22.

61. Broom DM. Cow-calf and sow-piglet behaviour in relation to colostrum ingestion. Ann Rech Vet 1983;14(4):342–8.

62. Radia D, Bond K, Limon G, Van Winden S, Guitian J. Relationship between periparturient management, prevalence of MAP and preventable economic losses in UK dairy herds. Vet Rec 2013 Oct 12;173(14):343.

63. Hegland RB, Lambert MR, Jacobson NL, Payne LC. Effect of dietary and managemental factors on reflex closure of the esophageal groove in the dairy calf. J Dairy Sci 1957 Sep 1;40(9):1107–13.

64. Lateur-Rowet HJM, Breukink HJ. The failure of the oesophageal groove reflex, when fluids are given with an oesophageal feeder to newborn and young calves. Vet Q 1983 Apr 1;5(2):68–74.

65. Adams GD, Bush LJ, Horner JL, Staley TE. Two methods for administering colostrum to newborn calves. J Dairy Sci 1985 Mar 1;68(3):773–5.

66. Urie NJ, Lombard JE, Shivley CB, Kopral CA, Adams AE, Earleywine TJ, et al. Preweaned heifer management on US dairy operations: Part V. Factors associated with morbidity and mortality in preweaned dairy heifer calves. J Dairy Sci 2018 Oct 1;101(10):9229–44.

67. MacFarlane JA, Grove-White DH, Royal MD, Smith RF. Identification and quantification of factors affecting neonatal immunological transfer in dairy calves in the UK. Vet Rec 2015 Jun 13;176(24): 625.

68. Lombard JE, Garry FB, Urie NJ, McGuirk SM, Godden SM, Sterner K, et al. Proposed dairy calf birth certificate data and death loss categorization scheme. J Dairy Sci 2019 May 1;102(5):4704–12.

69. Godden S. Colostrum management for dairy calves. Vet Clin North Am Food Anim Pract 2008;24(1): 19–39.

70. Windeyer MC, Gamsjäger L. Vaccinating calves in the face of maternal antibodies: Challenges and opportunities. Vet Clin North Am Food Anim Pract. W. B. Saunders 2019;35(3):557–73.

71. Windeyer MC, Leslie KE, Godden SM, Hodgins DC, Lissemore KD, LeBlanc SJ. Factors associated with morbidity, mortality, and growth of dairy heifer calves up to 3 months of age. Prev Vet Med 2014 Feb 1;113(2):231–40.

72. Lombard J, Urie N, Garry F, Godden S, Quigley J, Earleywine T, et al. Consensus recommendations on calf- and herd-level passive immunity in dairy calves in the United States. J Dairy Sci 2020 Aug 1;103(8):7611–24.

73. Urie NJ, Lombard JE, Shivley CB, Kopral CA, Adams AE, Earleywine TJ, et al. Preweaned heifer management on US dairy operations: Part I. Descriptive characteristics of preweaned heifer raising practices. J Dairy Sci 2018 Oct 1;101(10):9168–84.

Chapter 4

Calf housing and the environment

Tom Shardlow and Sophie Mahendran

CHAPTER CONTENTS

The environment in which calves are housed can have significant effects (both positive and negative) on health and performance. Suboptimal housing is at least a partial factor in most outbreaks of disease (obvious or otherwise), especially in young calves. This inevitably will affect growth rates (and therefore future performance), mortality rates and welfare of the animals involved.

The main components of the environment that must be considered are ventilation, moisture control, temperature, hygiene, group sizes and stability. These factors are closely interlinked, and above all will be affected by the local climate and weather in which the building is situated within. It is also important to ensure that calf buildings comply with relevant animal welfare regulations.

While it may be ideal to aim for the use of specially designed and purpose built facilities for calf housing, consideration must be given to the monetary investment required. Carrying out a cost–benefit assessment of the investment into calf housing (new buildings or adaptations of pre-existing ones) is a valuable exercise that will inform decision making (see Table 4.1). Although some factors are difficult to predict accurately this is still a useful exercise before investment is made. The likely impacts on and costs of disease, mortality rates and poor performance are best assessed with the help of a vet or consultant.

TYPES OF CALF HOUSING

The type of housing that is selected will be influenced by the available space, calving pattern and management choices on an individual farm.

TABLE 4.1 Outline of considerations when assessing cost–benefit for adapting calf housing or building a new facility.

Assessing costs	Assessing benefits
Capital expenditure required (and ongoing additional running costs)	Likely impact on disease level
Estimated longevity of building/adaptation	Financial benefit of disease reduction
Number of calves to use the facility in this period	Likely impact on mortality rate
Cost per calf	Financial impact of mortality rate
	Likely impact calf performance metrics (e.g. growth rate)
	Likely impact on future performance (e.g. milk yield/days to slaughter)
	Benefits if reduced time spent on daily tasks (e.g. different feeding/hygiene regimes)
	Welfare benefits

There are many different options available, with summaries of each main type given below.

Calf hutches and igloos

Calf hutches are available for housing both individuals, pairs or small groups of calves, and are a housing solution that was initially developed in the USA. They provide a small covered housing zone with a penned outdoor area, allowing the calf to choose its preferred environment. The main benefits to this housing type is the improved biosecurity and reduced spread of disease between hutches, and some flexibility in the layout and positioning of the hutches. The hutches are also very long lasting

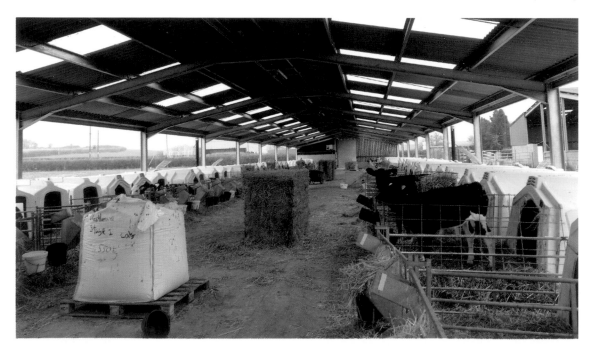

FIGURE 4.1 Individual calf hutches underneath a roof.

due to the plastic fabrication, and although they can be a costly initial investment, they will last for a long time.

One of the main misconceptions surrounding hutches is the idea that they are designed to be outside in the climates that experience high rainfall. In the UK, although it varies by region, it rains for approximately 150 days a year, meaning that the outside area of hutches become sodden, unhygienic and dirty. Driven rain may reach inside of the hutch depending on the direction of the wind and the size of the entrance into the hutch, which can allow calves themselves to become wet, and in the winter months, cold. Hutches should be situated so that the outside area is under a roof, so providing protection from the rain, and also providing shelter in the summer months from the sun. The hutches can be placed entirely under the roof (Figure 4.1), or have the hutch itself situated outside and just the penned area underneath the roof. Some commercially available systems come with a veranda built in, providing a solution that does not require erecting a whole roofed area.

Another consideration with hutches is the ground upon which they are placed. Concrete provides the ideal base, allowing thorough cleaning and disinfection once the hutch is removed. Use of hardcore will allow some drainage underneath the hutch, but again the area is difficult to clean, and without an adequate angle/ run for drainage, pooling of moisture can occur in wet weather conditions.

A disadvantage of hutches is the increased labour required to feed, bed and check each pen on a daily basis, especially in bad weather conditions. Where there is no roof, workers will be exposed to the wind and wet, which usually results in a poorer job being done and a resultant negative impact on calf rearing.

Individual housing

As well as the more traditional calf hutches (Figures 4.1 and 4.5), there are other types of individual calf

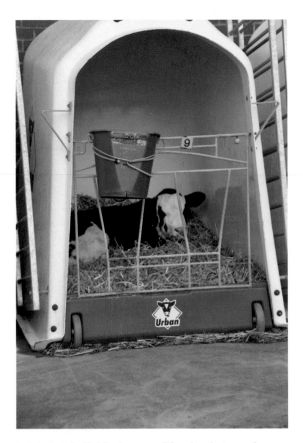

FIGURE 4.2 Individual pens with wheels to make movement of pens easy.

housing available (Figures 4.2–4.5). These often consist only of an indoor covered area where the calf is kept for the first couple of weeks of life.

The individual housing of calves was traditionally thought to reduce the spread of disease (diarrhoea and respiratory disease) through a reduction in contact in comparison to group housing (1), while the use of housing modules offers easier cleaning and disinfection (2). However, more recent studies into the behaviour and welfare needs of calves have shown isolation as a calf has negative impacts on social learning and cognitive performance. Calves learn by social learning and facilitation, with the ability to watch and copy others being important, especially for behaviours such as ingestion of concentrate feeds (3). The presence of at least one other calf also helps them deal with stressful situations (4), allowing them to develop

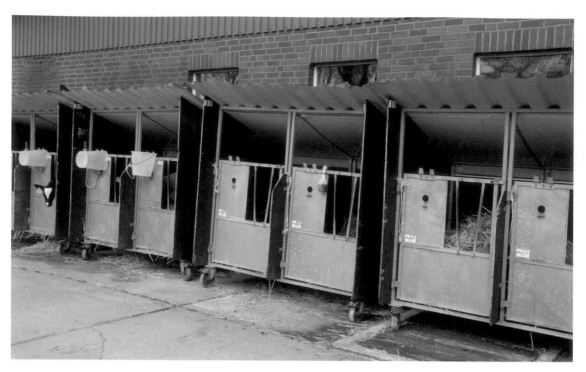

FIGURE 4.3 Individual pens raised off the ground and well bedded with straw for insulation.

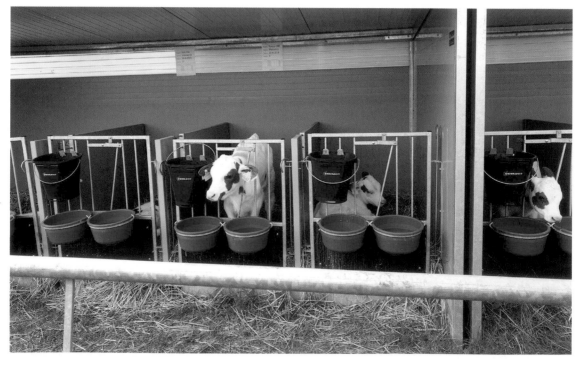

FIGURE 4.4 Individual calf pens with solid partitions between pens, and holders on the front gate for water, concentrates and a milk feeding bucket.

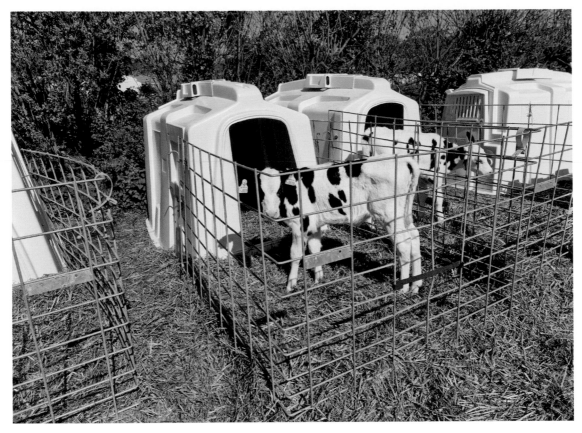

FIGURE 4.5 The more traditional individual calf pen with a plastic hutch and a metal perimeter for an outside area.

behavioural flexibility which is important for them as adults entering the milking herd (3).

The Welfare of Farmed Animals (England) Regulations 2000

- No calf shall be confined in an individual stall or pen after the age of 8 weeks unless a veterinary surgeon certifies that its health or behaviour requires it to be isolated in order to receive treatment.
- The width of any individual pen for a calf shall be at least equal to the height of the calf at the withers, and the length shall be at least equal to the body length of the calf (measured from the nose to the caudal edge of the pin bone, multiplied by 1.1).
- Individual stalls or pens for calves (except for those isolating sick animals) shall have perforated walls which allow calves to have direct visual and tactile contact.

Housing of calves in pairs rather than individual pens is one compromise to achieve the benefits of housing calves socially without the risks associated with increased group sizes (Figures 4.6 and 4.7). Pair housed calves have demonstrated better growth rates compared to individually housed calves (5, 6), especially around the weaning period when growth rates have been reported at 0.41 kg/day for individuals compared to 0.67 kg/day for pair housed calves (7, 8). This supports the idea that social housing helps with a smooth transition at weaning (9), probably due to increased solid feed intakes.

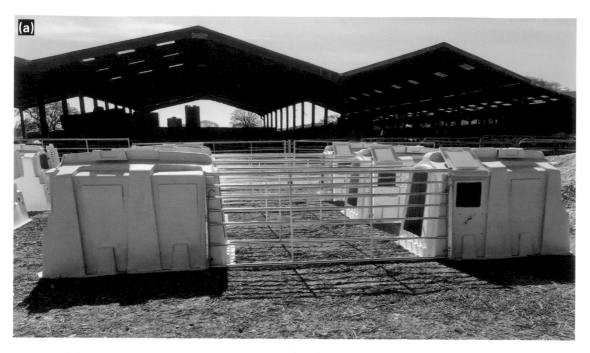

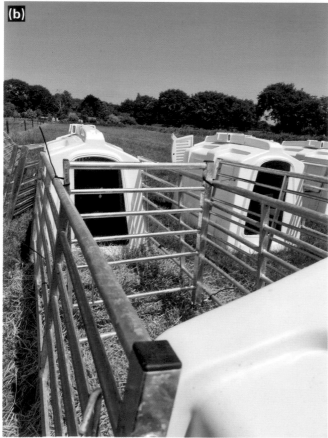

FIGURE 4.6 (a) Conversion of individual calf hutches into pairs by utilising 10 ft (3.05 m) gates between them. (b) A smaller gate can be placed between if you wish to start the calves off individually, and then removed at a couple of weeks old to allow them to become a pair.

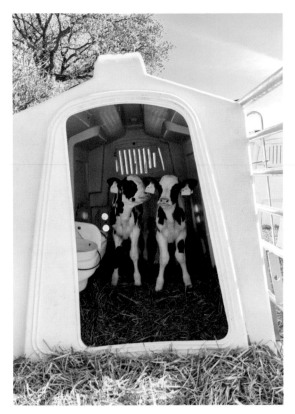

FIGURE 4.7 A pair of calves housed within a single calf hutch.

Cross sucking is often seen as one of the disadvantages of housing calves together. This activity is a non-nutritive sucking behaviour that is driven by a calf's innate need to suckle, and can result in hair loss and inflammation of the sucked area, usually around the navel (10). If an inappropriate feeding method is used that allows the calf to drink its milk too quickly, the calf will be motivated to look for other objects to suckle on, so provision of a teat on the wall of the pen will allow the calf to direct its motivation to suckle onto the teat rather than another calf (11). There is varying evidence about the effect of housing type on cross sucking, with two studies indicating no link with the type of housing (pair compared to individual) during weaning or post-weaning (12, 13), and one study indicating an increase in cross sucking in pair housed calves (14).

Calf sheds

The final option for housing calves is the use of a shed, within which calves can be housed as individuals, pairs or groups. These sheds can be purpose built, usually being lower and narrower compared to adult livestock sheds (Figure 4.8), or they can be existing buildings that have been re-purposed for housing calves (Figure 4.9). It is this latter type of building that often causes the greatest problems in terms of optimising the environmental conditions to promote good health.

Calf sheds should be designed so as to allow an all-in, all-out system for cleaning. Practically speaking, this means that calves can be removed from a specific area of the shed for thorough cleaning prior to repopulation. Other considerations for these sheds include easy access for both people and machinery to bring in equipment such as the Milk Taxis (they roll better over concreted areas), and

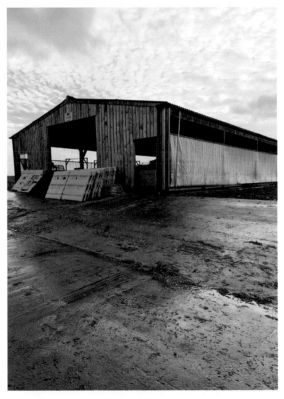

FIGURE 4.8 A specifically designed calf shed, with adjustable curtain sides for air flow control.

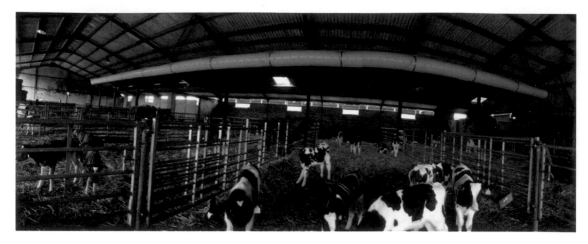

FIGURE 4.9 A large shed that has been retro-fitted to house groups of calves. Improvements in this shed design would include solid partitions between the pens to reduce disease transmission and offer draft protection at the calf level.

tractors for bringing straw to bed down and also to muck out. Ensuring this access is easy and convenient will make the job of calf rearers much more pleasurable! Something else to ensure is that calf housing is not in the same air space as adult cattle, as they can act as sources of respiratory viruses (15).

Group housing of calves

Housing of calves in groups is mostly influenced by the feeding method chosen, for example, automatic calf feeders (ACFs) or multi-teat milk feeders. Grouping also reduces the amount of labour required per calf, but can be more challenging to manage due to it being harder to identify sick animals, and a careful eye is needed to ensure that all animals in the group are getting the expected feed level – smaller calves or calves with a weak suck reflex may struggle to compete with stronger calves when milk feeding at group feeders.

The size of groups is an important consideration, with many recommending a maximum of 12 calves per group. It is generally considered that the risk of disease increases in line with the group size, so aim to keep group sizes as low as possible (17). Other research has also shown that calves in

larger groups grow more slowly and suffer from more respiratory disease (18). Larger groups may be needed on ACFs in order to utilise them efficiently, but while many are sold with the recommendation of one teat being able to cope with groups of 30 calves, in the authors' experience groups of no more than 20 calves should be fed via a single teat.

Other aspects to consider are the stocking density of the group pen, minimum recommendations for space are given in Table 4.2, but again the more area you can provide per calf, the better the environment will cope and the less any infection pressures will be. A recommendation of 4–5m² per calf will give optimum hygiene and comfort levels. Higher stocking rates have also been shown to reduce the air quality within a shed (19), as well as increasing levels of air moisture and airborne bacterial counts (20).

The age range of calves within a group pen should be kept as small as possible, ideally with no more than 2 weeks between the oldest and youngest calves. Older calves will act as sources of infection for younger animals, and may also bully younger animals which will affect their feed intakes and growth rates (21). In addition, avoiding nose-to-nose contact between groups will help reduce disease spread (20).

TABLE 4.2 The minimum required and recommended space allowances for a calf.

Approximate age and size of calves	Minimum legal area (m²/calf)	Minimum recommended area (m²/calf)
0 months or ~45 kg	1.5	2.0
0–2 months or ~45–100 kg	1.5	3.0
3–5 months or ~100–150 kg	1.5	4.0
5–7 months or ~150–200 kg	2.0	5.0
>7 months or >200 kg	3.0	6.0

Source: Adapted from AHDB (16).

Another factor that can cause problems in group housing is not maintaining group stability. Once you have formed a group of calves, they should remain together without any changes until at least post-weaning. This reduces the level of aggressive behaviour within the group (22), with stable groups shown to have higher daily weight gains and fewer disease incidents than dynamic changing groups (23). The only caveat to this recommendation is that sometimes calves with a timid or quiet character (or who are physically quite small compared to their cohort), may struggle to compete effectively for food resources. These individuals often benefit from being moved into a group with younger calves, and will gain in confidence at accessing food resources, leading to improved growth rates and overall health for that individual. Before doing this, it is essential to be certain that the calf is not smaller due to infection, which will then be passed on to the younger group.

A final point to consider with group housing is the requirement to have an isolation area for sick calves. Leaving a calf with clinical signs of either diarrhoea or respiratory disease will just spread infectious agents to other calves, increasing the likelihood of a bigger disease outbreak.

Keeping calves at grass

In spring block calving systems, it is not uncommon to find calves kept in fields while still on milk. In these situations, there tends to be a large group size of similarly aged calves, and being in a field can reduce the need for additional housing. Given the unreliable climate in the UK, it is important that calves at grass still have access to shelter (with dry bedding) that provides enough room for all calves to lie down. This shelter not only provides protection from the elements, but can be important in helping calves keep warm as there will be little nestling ability on grass. Due consideration must also be given to monitoring worm burdens via faecal egg counts in the calves, as grazing will begin at a few weeks of age, thereby reducing the age at which exposure and therefore anthelmintic treatments might be needed.

VENTILATION OF CALF HOUSING

Ventilation is the provision of fresh, clean air to an enclosed space. This fresh air displaces stale, dirty air, which can harbour bacteria, dust and noxious gases (24, 25) (Box 4.1). This is why inadequate ventilation in a calf environment leads to poor respiratory health (19) with knock-on detrimental effects on growth rates and performance.

The Welfare of Farmed Animals (England) Regulations 2000

Within housing, air circulation, dust levels, temperature, relative air humidity and gas concentrations must be kept within limits which are not harmful to the animals.

Box 4.1 Substances effectively removed from calf buildings by adequate ventilation

1 Disease-causing pathogens – pathogens can be transmitted through the air to allow spread of infections from one individual to another.

2 Particulate matter (dust) – dust settles in the lower respiratory tract causing irritation, can harbour pathogens (bacteria) and create an environment conducive to pathogen proliferation.

3 Moisture – a humid atmosphere promotes the survival of environmental pathogens. Moisture is also a good thermal conductor (drawing heat away from the calf) so can create cold environments.

4 Noxious gases – ammonia (the most commonly referred to noxious gas), hydrogen sulphide, carbon monoxide and methane. They irritate the mucosa (especially of the eyes and respiratory tract), making calves more susceptible to infections. Exposure to ammonia at levels of 25 ppm for prolonged periods can result in irritation and inflammation of the respiratory tract (humans can smell ammonia at 20 ppm). Carbon dioxide becomes irritant at levels >3000 ppm, hydrogen sulphide is toxic at levels >50 ppm.

5 Heat – the upper critical environmental temperature of a calf is 25°C, but this is also affected by humidity levels. Provision of shade or even cooling systems may be required during hot periods, with heat stress increasing mortality levels in calves. Calves are most at risk of developing heat stress during short periods of high temperatures as it does not allow them to adapt to environmental conditions.

Calf buildings are optimally ventilated when the total air volume is replaced with fresh air ~8 times per hour in cooler months, increasing up to 60 air changes per hour in the summer months (26, 27). Fresh air into a shed should then be evenly distributed across the housing to avoid stagnant areas. This should be achieved without exposing calves to air speeds of over 0.5 m/s (and ideally less than 0.3 m/s) (21). Air speed can be measured using a handheld anemometer, which is relatively inexpensive to purchase. Exposing calves to air speeds higher than this can result in a chilling effect.

Types of ventilation

The energy required to drive ventilation within a calf's environment can be provided naturally by either the wind, the stack effect or mechanical ventilation.

Natural ventilation

Utilising wind for natural ventilation is the cheapest option, but a farmer's ability to do this can vary depending on the geography within which the building is situated, and the position of surrounding buildings. The prevailing wind predominantly comes from the west or south-west in the UK, with housing best orientated at right angles to drive air through the shed (i.e. with the long axis of the housing perpendicular to the wind).

Inlet apertures (to allow air into the shed) need to be evenly spaced around the building and be designed to allow air to enter in a controlled way (thus preventing excesses of air speed at the animal level). Generally, this is provided by walls that have a solid barrier that is at least as high as the animals' housed, topped by porous material. There are several options for the porous material.

• Space boarding – wooden boards with gaps between them (Figure 4.10). Gaps wider than 25 mm between boards may let too much rain or high speed wind pass through.

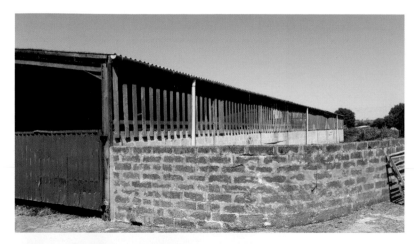

FIGURE 4.10 Removal of additional boarding from the building sides may improve air entry, but this must be done in conjunction with provision of air outlets.

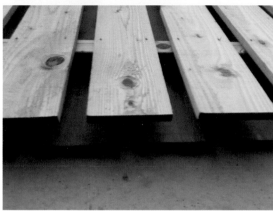

FIGURE 4.11 Yorkshire boarding is a double row of offset boards (as opposed to a single row in space boarding). This provides superior protection from the weather, and allows boards to be spaced wider apart, improving inlet.

- Yorkshire boarding – two rows of wooden boards which can have wider gaps between them (Figure 4.11). This type of cladding is useful on very exposed sides that receive a lot of wind or driving rain.
- A proprietary porous fabric – often with a roller design to allow lifting for large machinery to enter a shed, or to increase air inlet areas on still days that have little natural air movement (Figure 4.12).
- Perforated metal cladding – is good at providing rain protection, although the air inlet area provided is usually small.

Whatever the material type used, it is important to keep the air inlets clear of dirt and debris that could hamper air flow, such as ivy growing up the side of older sheds.

In order to prevent a draft at calf level within a building, use of solid sided pen walls (Figure 4.13) or provision of shelter, such as that offered by straw bales (Figure 4.14), can be helpful. Care should be exercised to ensure such calf level shelter does not lead to microenvironments being created within the pen due to lack of localised air movement. Microenvironments are at a higher risk of becoming contaminated with poor quality air (26). This problem can be overcome through use of mechanical ventilation systems (see below).

Attention should also be paid to gaps under doorways or pen dividers that allow air to move around at calf level. These can be managed by ensuring there are minimal gaps, or filling them with plastic sheeting such as that used to line parlour walls.

The stack effect

Housing that is ventilated without the aid of mechanical devices relies on the physical property of warm air rising to drive the ventilation. This is known as the stack effect. The fundamental principle of the stack effect is that warm air generated by the animals leaves the building via apertures in the roof which creates a negative pressure drawing

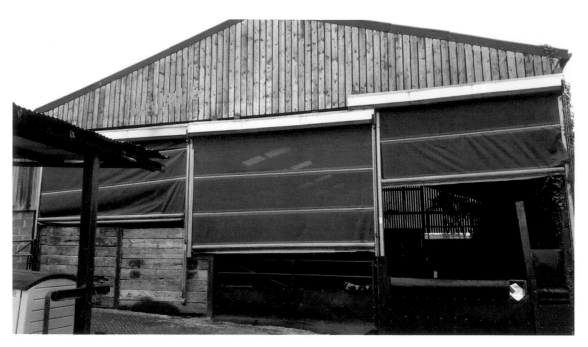

FIGURE 4.12 Porous fabric allows air and light into a building and can be mounted on rollers to allow machinery access. Above the rollers, space boarding has been placed.

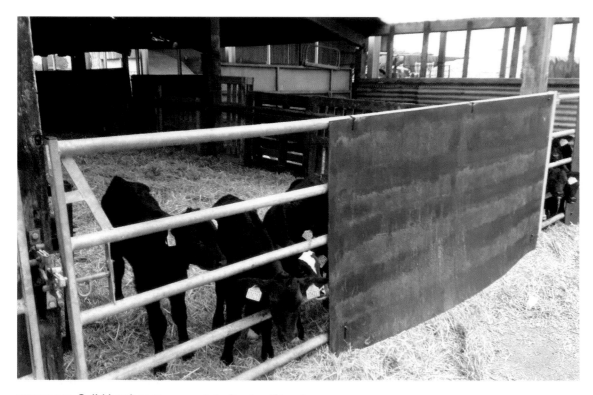

FIGURE 4.13 Solid barriers to prevent drafts at calf level.

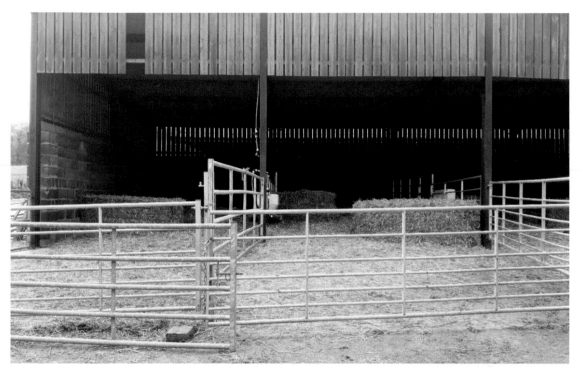

FIGURE 4.14 Use of bales in exposed areas to prevent drafts at calf level.

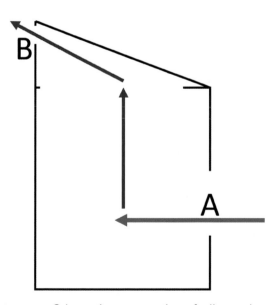

FIGURE 4.15 Schematic cross-section of a livestock building ventilated by the stack effect. Stale air is heated by the stock and rises (red arrow), escaping through apertures above eaves height (B). This draws fresh air (blue arrow) into the building through apertures in the side walls (A).

fresh air in through apertures in the sides of the building (Figure 4.15).

Optimising stack effect ventilation requires several factors to be present. The main factor being that the animals must generate adequate heat in the shed to warm the air around them sufficiently. This can be problematic when young calves are housed as they do not start to produce enough heat until they weigh ~100 kg. There is also often a low ratio of heat generated to overall volume of air in the building, meaning that it is nearly impossible to achieve a stack effect unless the air volume is reduced, such as with the case with calf hutches.

Additional requirements for a stack effect are that there are sufficient apertures (openings) in the sides/below the eaves of the building to provide an inlet for fresh air into the building, as well as sufficient apertures in the roof/above the eaves of the building to provide outlets for air to escape from the building (Figure 4.16). These apertures should be distributed across the whole of the building in

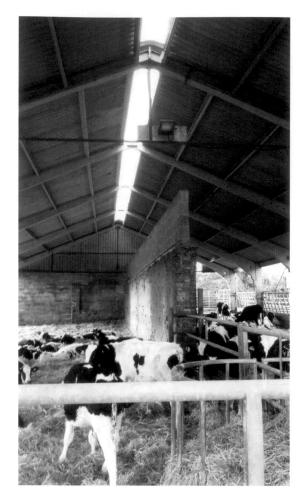

FIGURE 4.16 Removal of the building ridge as has occurred in this picture will significantly improve outlet and ventilation. A cover may be required in areas of high rainfall or where young calves are being housed.

both the roof and the sides to avoid creating dead zones. Lastly, the pitch of the roof should ideally be 22°, with anything less than this resulting in air being deflected downwards and back into the building. Low pitched roofs are more common in buildings that are >10 m wide, resulting in difficulties getting consistent air flow across the whole width of the shed.

It is important to note that if any of these factors are suboptimal in a given building, attempts to compensate by further improving other factors will not necessarily have the desired effect. An example of this

is where the ridge outlet is inadequate, but improvements are attempted by increasing the apertures in the sides of the building to increase air inlet (Figures 4.17 and 4.18). This will not improve ventilation on a still day and may expose calves to excess air speed and moisture in windy and rainy conditions.

Mechanical ventilation

Mechanical ventilation is warranted when either there is no temperature differential between inside and outside a building (i.e. when there is insufficient weight of animal to heat the airspace), or when it is not possible to provide adequate, evenly spaced inlet apertures.

In almost all cases, positive pressure ventilation (PPV) systems (that blow air into a shed) have advantages over negative pressure (NPV) systems that forcibly remove air from a shed (21).

In calf housing, mechanical PPV systems generally involve one or more fans pumping air into the building via a cylindrical duct (usually a polythene tube) with intermittent holes that runs the entire length of the shed. The purpose of the duct is to disperse fresh air to all areas (and dispel stale air from all areas). The tube must be designed with bespoke air outlet holes specific for each building (Figures 4.19 and 4.20), if not they have the potential to be ineffective or even detrimental to calf health (26). Important considerations for fitting a PPV system to a calf shed include the following.

1. Ensuring the fan is of sufficient capacity to replace the air volume in the building between 4 and 8 times per hour.
2. Ensuring that the duct diameter and hole diameters are such that there is even output of air down the length of the tube.
3. Ensuring that the holes in the tube are of a location and size that prevent excessive air speed at calf level.

When purchasing a PPV system, specialist advice should be sought to get these design features correct. This includes the use of computer

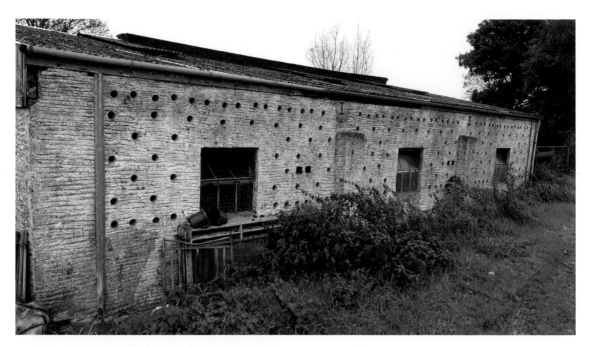

FIGURE 4.17 Ingenious solution to an absence of inlets involved drilling holes into the breeze block side walls to allow air into the building.

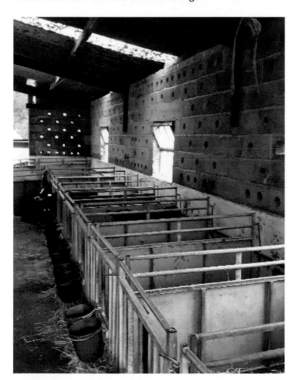

FIGURE 4.18 The inside of the shed shown in Figure 4.17, with air inlets created along the entire length of the side wall.

programs that take into account fluid dynamics of air movement to allow calculation of the correct measurements for a PPV tube. This ensures the system has a positive effect on calf health (28). These systems will cost £1000–1500 to purchase, and will cost ~£1 per day to run.

NPV systems use extractor fans to remove air from a shed. However, they will not remove stale air evenly over the entire airspace unless it is a sealed, controlled climate building with strategically placed, limited inlet holes (e.g. as employed with most chicken sheds). Air will take the path of least resistance to an extractor fan, meaning that if sited in a space boarded wall it will simply draw air from the immediate vicinity, thus leaving the majority of air in the shed unaffected.

Assessing ventilation in cattle housing

The best time to assess ventilation in a building is on a still, cold day. Assessments made during windy

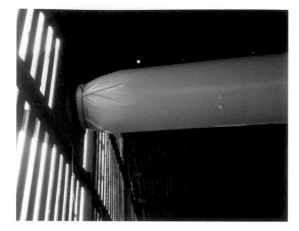

FIGURE 4.19 A fan mounted on the outside of this building blows fresh air into a duct with holes down the length which disperse the air evenly over the calves.

and/or warm conditions are more likely to mask deficiencies in building design, and not provide a true representation of the air movements within a shed. Animals should also be present in the building to simulate normal stocking conditions and

ensure any effects of body heat produced by the animals can be assessed (Box 4.2).

Box 4.2 Practical assessment of the ventilation using the human senses

- **Smell** – A strong smell of ammonia (causing stinging of the eyes and nose), and excessive particulate build-up in the air which can cause coughing or sneezing due to irritation of the nose and throat suggest poor ventilation.
- **Sight** – Spiders will not build cobwebs in areas of high air movement, so presence of them is suggestive of a poorly ventilated building (Figure 4.21).
- **Feel** – Suboptimal ventilation can be indicated by excessive humidity, which can manifest as condensation on surfaces or a damp feeling.
- **Animal observation** – Calves avoiding poorly ventilated areas of the building,

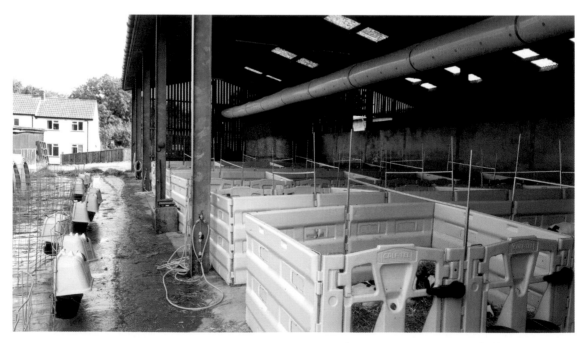

FIGURE 4.20 This fan and duct system has been designed to replace the air inside the calf shed four times per hour in a way that disperses it evenly and does not chill the calves.

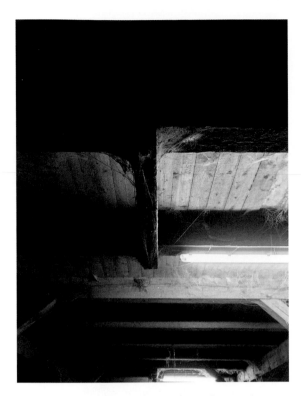

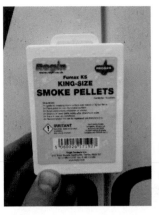

FIGURE 4.22 Smoke pellets generate several minutes of smoke to assess building ventilation.

FIGURE 4.21 Cobwebs in the ceiling of a poorly ventilated calf shed.

or congregating at the building periphery near air inlets indicates a non-uniform circulation of air in the building.

Further assessment of ventilation can be conducted using smoke from either a disposable cartridge (Figure 4.22) or a commercially available smoke machine (Figure 4.23). A propane gas powered insect fogger can also be converted to a smoke machine by using mineral oil or liquid paraffin in place of insecticide. It is important to use cool smoke generated in this way, as opposed to smoke generated from combustion of something like straw, which will rise of its own accord. The smoke allows visualisation of how quickly stale air is eliminated from a building – the smoke should be completely eliminated from the building in 2–3 minutes and there should be no stale areas where it remains.

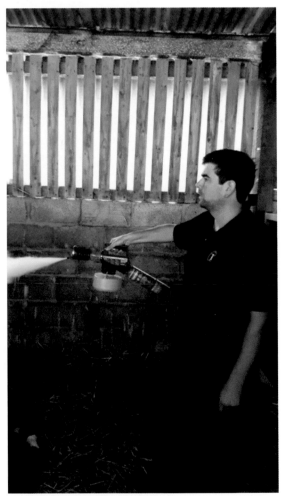

FIGURE 4.23 Generating 'smoke' (aerosolised liquid paraffin or mineral oil) from a propane insect fogger to assess building ventilation.

Calculating ventilation requirements

Calculating a building's ventilation requirements based on the number and size of animals it contains can be done relatively easily by taking a few measurements (Box 4.3). These figures are then processed using sources such as those provided by AHDB (16) to give you the total area for inlets and outlets that a building requires. In general, though, at least 0.04 m^2 ridge outlet per calf up to 100 kg bodyweight is required, rising to 0.1 m^2 per adult animal (but this will vary according to the roof pitch and stocking density). Inlet apertures in the building sides need to be at least twice the ridge outlet area, and optimally four times the outlet area.

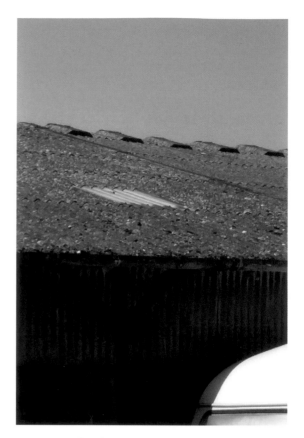

FIGURE 4.24 Cranked ridge tiles do not provide adequate outlet for optimal ventilation of livestock buildings.

> **Box 4.3** Calculating required inlet and outlet areas
>
> Calculations to determine optimal inlet and outlet area requirements are relatively simple and require computation of the following variables:
>
> - the **maximum** number of cattle to be housed in the building
> - the **maximum** average weight of these animals
> - the difference in height between the eaves and the ridge (if not known or difficult to measure this can be calculated with the pitch angle and roof span via trigonometry)
> - the total covered floor area of the building (calculated from the length and width).

Outlet apertures are generally provided at the ridge as this promotes the stack effect. However, buildings housing animals above 150 kg bodyweight can also benefit from a 'slotted roof' where a gap of 10–20 mm is left between roof tiles. The heat generated by animals of this size acts to overcome the likelihood of rain ingress.

Traditional cranked ridge tiles (Figure 4.24) provide insufficient outlet (generally around 20% of what is required) and so outlet is invariably optimised by use of a continuous open ridge along the entire building length. If the open ridge is directly over bedded areas or is particularly wide (especially over 35 cm width) then a cover may be needed over the ridge (this will depend on the average rainfall for the locality of the calf building). Ridge coverings should be designed so that they do not limit air flow.

In mono-pitched buildings (where the roof slants in a single direction (Figure 4.25)), the principles of ventilation are the same as in a gabled roof. The effective outlet is at the top of the roof and is unlikely to be a limiting factor. However, inlets may be limiting if there are not enough evenly distributed holes in the back wall and the stack effect

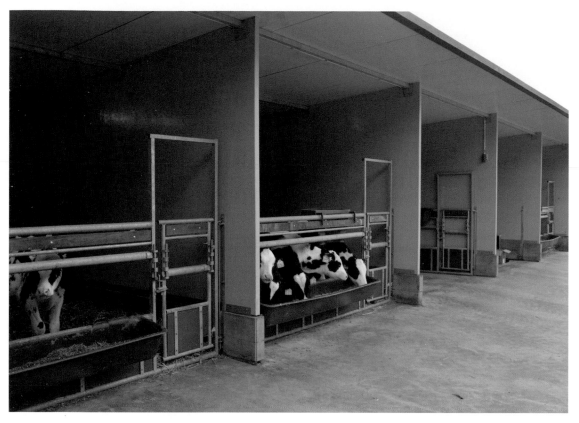

FIGURE 4.25 A modern mono-pitched design calf housing unit, more commonly seen in Europe.

may not occur if the roof pitch is below 15° and/or the building is greater than 9 m in depth.

HUMIDITY AND MOISTURE CONTROL

High humidity levels (>70%) in a calf environment (both in the atmosphere and on surfaces) are linked to both disease and poor performance due to the promotion of pathogen survival and transmission, as well as conduction of heat away from calves. Sources of moisture are numerous and include rain, urine, faeces, sweat, spilt milk and water from drinkers – these can total ~7 L per calf per day! Identifying the unnecessary ingress of water into buildings is a useful first step in preventing moisture build-up. This can include rain from leaking roofs or blocked/inadequate guttering, leaking

water troughs/drinkers or excessive use of water when cleaning the environment (Figure 4.26).

Moisture is effectively removed from the calf's environment by ensuring good drainage and ventilation. Floor design to facilitate adequate drainage is essential to ensure that deposited moisture can escape the building as quickly as possible (21). Sloped, concrete flooring will facilitate drainage and is also easy to clean. Beneath bedding, and in areas where moisture is expected to pool, a minimum 1:20 slope is required (see Figure 4.29). A 1:60 slope is sufficient in scraped areas or passageways.

Drainage channels of 75–100 mm diameter can help remove excessive moisture away from areas where dirty water collects, and a perforated metal covering helps prevent them becoming blocked with bedding. Drainage channels are particularly effective at the edge of passageways, which can be constructed with camber to direct water to them.

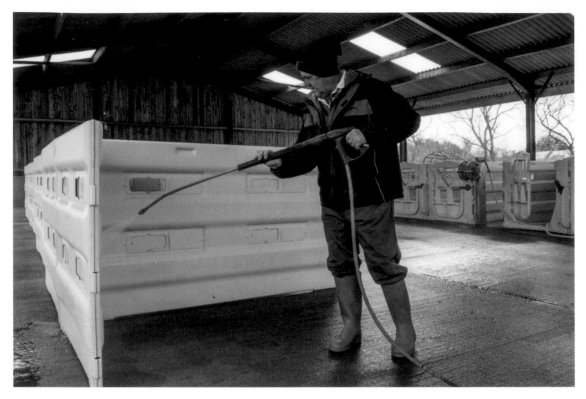

FIGURE 4.26 Water used for cleaning and disinfection has the potential to build up in calf sheds. Surfaces should only be cleaned using a pressure washer if there are no calves in the airspace. These lightweight, mobile calf pens are being cleaned while the shed has been de-stocked.

Strategic use of slatted areas can also be used effectively in areas of particular moisture accumulation, for example, around automatic milk feeders (Figure 4.27). These feeding systems provide challenges with moisture control as calves will consume large volumes of milk and congregate in the same area to urinate and defecate (Figure 4.28).

It is important to remember that it is a legal requirement to provide fresh drinking water to all calves at all times (UK Legislation for calf feeding – Welfare of Farmed Animals (England) Regulations 2000). Non-compliance is, however, quite common with one UK survey reporting an incidence of around 20% of UK farms (29). This is a welfare issue and also reduces the ability of the calf to cope with diarrhoea, so potentially worsening dehydration and increasing the risk of mortality.

Careful consideration of pen design with respect to drinkers and milk feeders will reduce the amount of moisture on bedding. It is sensible to locate liquid feeding equipment at the front of (and ideally outside of) sloped pens to avoid water or milk from running back under bedding (Figures 4.29–4.31).

In addition to ensuring good drainage of the pen, bedding should be added frequently enough so that calves are always kept dry. In pens with low stocking density, this may only be required every couple of days, but in a wet environment, this can escalate to bedding twice daily. A quick way of checking pen moisture levels is to kneel on the bedding – you should have completely dry knees when you stand up, otherwise the pen bedding is too damp.

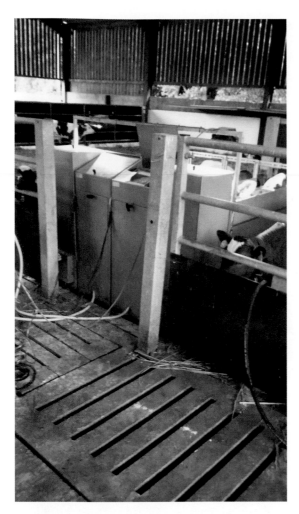

FIGURE 4.27 These automatic calf milk feeders have been placed on a slatted area to ensure adequate drainage beneath an area of significant moisture production.

HOUSING TEMPERATURE

Extremes of ambient temperature (high or low) impact on calf health and performance by causing stress, immunosuppression and higher disease incidence (30, 31). To facilitate optimum calf health and performance, ambient temperature should be maintained in the calf's thermoneutral zone (TNZ) (30). The TNZ is the range of temperatures at which the calf does not have to direct energy away from important but non-critical functions (e.g. growth, immune function) to achieve thermoregulation.

The TNZ is bounded by the lower critical temperature (15°C in calves <3-weeks old) and the upper critical temperature (>25°C) (32). As calves get older and their rumen develops, the lower critical temperature drops, reaching around −15°C as an adult (in dry conditions).

Placement of a min/max thermometer in the calf shed will enable monitoring of the temperature at a glance, enabling suitable management changes to be made when temperature thresholds are met (Figure 4.32).

Avoiding cold stress

Physical signs of cold stress include increased lying times, calves huddling together (when group housed), avoidance of areas where there are draughts and reduced growth rates. The ability of calves to 'nest' in deep beds of straw provides thermal insulation from their surroundings and gives protection from drafts. This is associated with lower levels of respiratory disease (33), and it follows that the provision of ample bedding (so the calf's legs are not visible on the straw) is an effective way to keep a calf's environment above the lower critical temperature. Avoiding calf contact with thermal conductors (e.g. concrete, metal) will help, and this can be done by use of thermal insulators (e.g. plastic) to line walls. Environmental moisture will also act as a thermal conductor drawing heat away from the calf. Ensuring that the environment is as dry as possible therefore has the effect of reducing cold stress.

An increase in air speed has the effect of increasing the lower critical temperature (making calves more prone to cold stress at temperatures as high as 17°C). As described in the previous section on ventilation, air speeds of less than 0.5 m/s and ideally 0.3 m/s are desirable at calf level (32). This can be achieved by providing solid barriers at calf level, with porous material above calf level to allow in fresh air. When high velocity air hits porous material, turbulence reduces its speed.

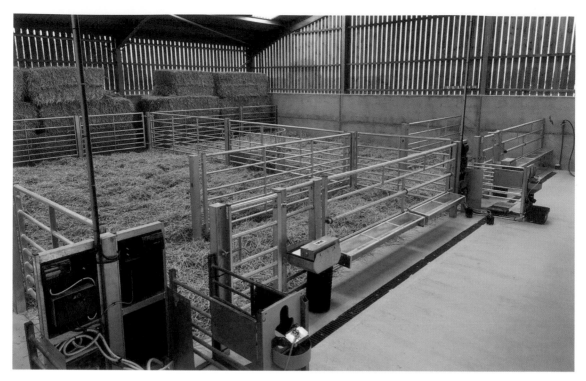

FIGURE 4.28 A well designed calf shed with a drainage system at the front of the pen.

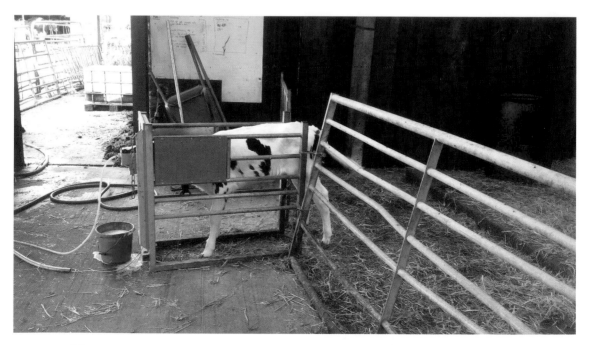

FIGURE 4.29 This automatic milk feeding station has been placed away from the bedded area, next to a scrapable surface demarcated with a railway sleeper. This prevents moisture from the feeder contaminating the bedding.

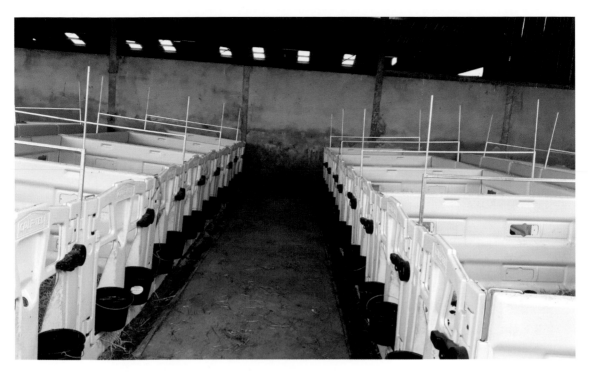

FIGURE 4.30 Drainage has been considered in this design of these calf pens. They have been sited on a 1 : 20 slope from back to front, with drainage channels cut in the passageway in front of the pens. Camber on the passageway directs water to the drainage channels.

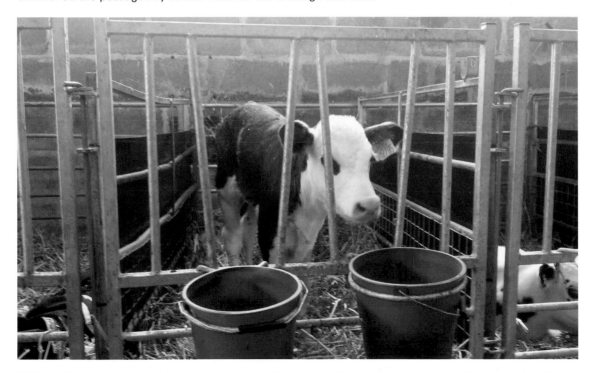

FIGURE 4.31 Buckets and drinkers placed outside the front of these pens to reduce spillage onto bedding.

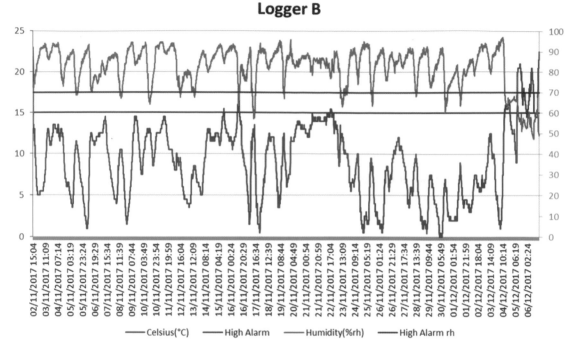

FIGURE 4.32 Graph showing the range of temperature and humidity on a UK farm in November. The humidity is constantly above the recommended 70% level, and the temperature below the lower TNZ of 15°C.

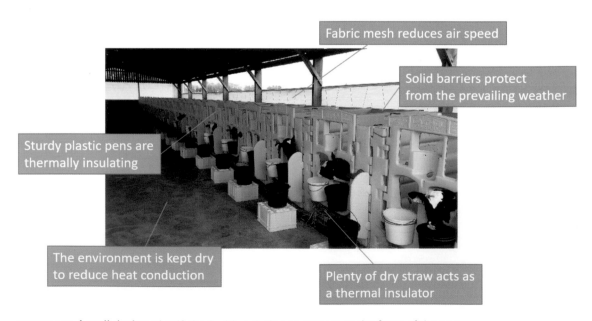

FIGURE 4.33 A well designed calf shed with a drainage system at the front of the pen.

Calf jackets

Another way to tackle cold stress is to reduce heat loss from calves using insulating jackets (Figure 4.34). The best calf jackets are made from breathable material that allows moisture to wick away from the surface of the calf, and should have adjustable fasteners that allow the size of the jacket to be increased as the calf grows (34). These jackets must be used with care as they can become fomites for disease transmission if they become dirty and covered in faecal material – ensuring they are thoroughly washed prior to use on another animal is critical. There is inconclusive scientific evidence as to whether there is any improvement in growth rates in calves wearing jackets (35), but when used correctly they can keep calves warm and dry. Jackets should be used in calves <3-weeks old when the night time temperature reaches as low as 8–10°C for three consecutive nights. It is important to make sure that the straps on calf jackets are adjusted as the calf grows otherwise it can lead to pressure on the chest and abdomen which will make the calf uncomfortable (Figure 4.35).

Use of heaters

Heat may also be provided to calves using heaters. Placement of 1500 W quartz linear heaters along walls will provide warmth to anything the radiating waves come into contact with (rather than just heating the air). However, these heaters only have a limited range, and utilise relatively large amounts of electricity. In more enclosed sheds, warming of the air on entry to the shed via heat exchangers can be very effective, but this set-up is more common in fully enclosed, environmentally controlled sheds found in the USA (21).

Avoiding heat stress in calves

Owing to climate change, heat stress in calves is becoming a more significant problem as environmental temperatures increase during the summer

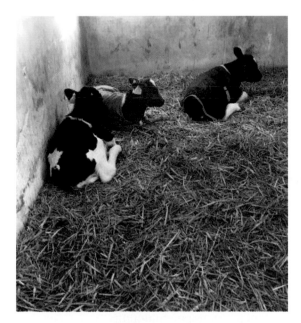

FIGURE 4.34 Calves wearing jackets, but still exposed to cold concrete walls with inadequate straw bedding that doesn't allow nestling.

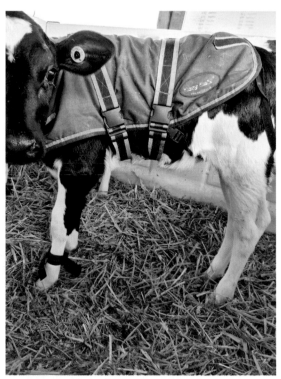

FIGURE 4.35 A calf that has outgrown its calf jacket – the belly straps are extended as long as possible, but they are still tight across the bottom of the abdomen.

months. Physical signs of heat stress can be more obvious to spot than for cold stress, with calves having increased respiratory rates or panting, sweating, spending more time standing, drinking less milk and less water. Ensuring calves are provided with shade, away from direct sunlight is vital, along with adequate supplies of clean drinking water. Additional cooling can be provided by fans to increase the airflow within a building, aiming for an air speed of 1 m/s to help reduce heat stress. One study from America has demonstrated that summer cooling with fans improved growth rates and lowered respiration rates of calves (31), with positive pressure ventilation tubes being able to assist with this. Another way to reduce the risk of heat stress is to reduce stocking densities within a pen.

The other thing to consider in hot weather is irritation caused by flies and the risk of fly strike occurring around the perineal area of calves with dirty bottoms. Again, air movement over calves will deter flies, but use of chemical fly repellents may be necessary (e.g. synthetic pyrethroids).

LIGHTING

> ### The UK Welfare of Farmed Animals (England) Regulations 2000
>
> Where animals are kept in a building, adequate lighting (whether fixed or portable) shall be available to enable them to be thoroughly inspected at any time.

As with adult dairy cows, provision of sufficient light (especially during the winter months) is important for both the people working in the shed, and also for the animals living within it. Calves should ideally have 14 hours of light at a level of 200 lux, with just 6 hours of low light (~20 lux) overnight. Provision of good lighting encourages calves to get up and feed, increasing intakes and having a positive effect on growth rates. It also

allows staff better observation of the calves to check for signs of ill health such as faecal staining around the perineal area, or nasal discharge.

HYGIENE OF CALF HOUSING

Maintaining a clean environment includes both the housing (walls and bedding), and the feeding equipment (milk feeding, concentrate feeding, water buckets and forage source). Allowing any of these areas to become contaminated with faecal material and dirt increases the risk of disease transmission, especially of diarrhoea causing pathogens. Many surfaces within calf housing are not easy to clean, and this includes any porous material, organic flooring (dirt floors) or broken surfaces. Walls can be rendered or epoxy resin paints applied to improve cleanability (36).

The most hygienic systems are those that work on an all-in, all-out basis enabling complete removal of organic matter, cleaning, disinfecting and drying prior to reuse. The majority of bedding can be removed using machinery, with corners and edges often needing finishing off by hand (Figure 4.36). Pens should then be pressure washed or steam cleaned (although not if the shed still has calves housed within it as this can lead to spread of contamination and excess moisture into the air), ideally with a detergent included to help remove biofilms. A suitable disinfectant should be applied prior to allowing the pen to dry.

One of the most common diarrhoea pathogens associated with poor hygiene is *Cryptosporidium* spp., which is a genus of protozoal parasite whose eggs are shed in calf faeces. These eggs (oocysts) can remain viable in the environment for prolonged periods of time, and can be unwittingly consumed by the calf when investigating contaminated bedding, or ingesting contaminated feed or water. Killing of oocysts can only be achieved by certain disinfectants with a specific licence for action against *Cryptosporidium* spp., and these include hydrogen peroxide, KenoTMCox, Kilcox, Keracox and Neopredisan. Note must

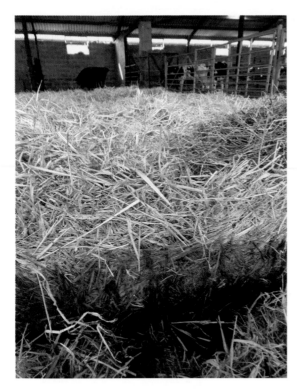

FIGURE 4.36 Deep straw bedding showing accumulation of liquids and faeces at the bottom of the straw pack.

be taken of the required concentrations and contact time that each product needs to ensure optimum effectiveness.

If dirt or hardcore flooring is used for calf housing, placing a layer of hydrated lime directly onto the surface, or a thick layer of sand can help reduce calf exposure to any pathogens that remain on the ground due to an inability to clean it properly.

REFERENCES

1. Sischo WM, Atwill ER, Lanyon LE, George J. Cryptosporidia on dairy farms and the role these farms may have in contaminating surface water supplies in the northeastern United States. Prev Vet Med 2000 Feb 29;43(4):253–67.
2. Wells SJ, Dee S, Godden S. Biosecurity for gastrointestinal diseases of adult dairy cattle. Vet Clin North Am Food Anim Pract 2002;18(1):35–55, v.
3. De Paula Vieira A, von Keyserlingk MAG, Weary DM. Effects of pair versus single housing on performance and behavior of dairy calves before and after weaning from milk. J Dairy Sci 2010 Jul 1;93(7):3079–85.
4. Grignard L, Boissy A, Boivin X, Garel JP, Le Neindre P P. The social environment influences the behavioural responses of beef cattle to handling. Appl Anim Behav Sci 2000 May 5;68(1):1–11.
5. Lundborg GK, Oltenacu PA, Maizon DO, Svensson EC, Liberg PGA. Dam-related effects on heart girth at birth, morbidity and growth rate from birth to 90 days of age in Swedish dairy calves. Prev Vet Med 2003 Aug 8;60(2):175–90.
6. Warnick VD, Arave CW, Mickelsen CH. Effects of group, individual, and isolated rearing of calves on weight gain and behavior. J Dairy Sci 1977;60(6):947–53.
7. Miller-Cushon EK, DeVries TJ. Effect of social housing on the development of feeding behavior and social feeding preferences of dairy calves. J Dairy Sci 2016 Feb 1;99(2):1406–17.
8. Liu S, Ma J, Li J, Alugongo GM, Wu Z, Wang Y, et al. Effects of pair versus individual housing on Performance, Health, and behavior of dairy calves. Animals (Basel) 2019 Dec 25;10(1):50.
9. Jensen MB, Duve LR, Weary DM. Pair housing and enhanced milk allowance increase play behavior and improve performance in dairy calves. J Dairy Sci 2015 Apr 1;98(4):2568–75.
10. Rushen J, de Passillé AM. The motivation of non-nutritive sucking in calves, Bos taurus. Anim Behav 1995;49(6):1503–10.
11. Veissier I, de Passillé AM, Després G, Rushen J, Charpentier I, Ramirez de la Fe AR, Pradel P. Does nutritive and non-nutritive sucking reduce other oral behaviors and stimulate rest in calves? J Anim Sci 2002;80(10):2574–87.
12. Costa JHCC, von Keyserlingk MAGG, Weary DM. Invited review: Effects of group housing of dairy calves on behavior, cognition, performance, and health. J Dairy Sci 2016 Apr 1;99(4):2453–67.
13. Wormsbecher L, Bergeron R, Haley D, de Passillé AM, Rushen J, Vasseur E. A method of outdoor housing dairy calves in pairs using individual calf hutches. J Dairy Sci 2017 Sep 1;100(9):7493–506.
14. Chua B, Coenen E, van DJ, Weary DM. Effects of pair versus individual housing on the

behavior and performance of dairy calves [Internet]. J Dairy Sci. American Dairy Science Association 2002;85(2):360–4.

15. Mars MH, Bruschke CJM, Van Oirschot JT. Airborne transmission of BHV1, BRSV, and BVDV among cattle is possible under experimental conditions. Vet Microbiol 1999 Apr 13;66(3):197–207.

16. AHDB. Youngstock and heifers [Internet]. Dairy housing: A best practice guide. 2015.

17. Hänninen L, Hepola H, Rushen J, De Passillé AM, Pursiainen P, Tuure VM, et al. Resting behaviour, growth and diarrhoea incidence rate of young dairy calves housed individually or in groups in warm or cold buildings. Acta Agric Scand A 2003;53(1):21–8.

18. Svensson C, Liberg P. The effect of group size on health and growth rate of Swedish dairy calves housed in pens with automatic milk-feeders. Prev Vet Med 2006 Jan 16;73(1):43–53.

19. Wathes CM, Howard K, Jones CDR, Webster AJF. The balance of airborne bacteria in calf houses. J Agric Eng Res 1984 Jan 1;30:81–90.

20. Lago A, McGuirk SM, Bennett TB, Cook NB, Nordlund KV. Calf respiratory disease and pen microenvironments in naturally ventilated calf barns in winter. J Dairy Sci 2006 Oct 1;89(10):4014–25.

21. Nordlund KV, Halbach CE. Calf barn design to optimize health and ease of management. Vet Clin North Am Food Anim Pract Mar 1, 2019 p;35(1):29–45. https://doi.org/10.1016/j.cvfa.2018.10.002.

22. Mounier L, Dubroeucq H, Andanson S, Veissier I. Variations in meat pH of beef bulls in relation to conditions of transfer to slaughter and previous history of the animals1. J Anim Sci 2006 Jun 1;84(6):1567–76.

23. Pedersen RE, Sørensen JT, Skjøth F, Hindhede J. How milk-fed dairy calves perform in stable verses dynamic groups. Proc Br Soc Anim Sci 2006;2006:42–.

24. Kaufman J, Linington M, Osborne VR, Wagner-Riddle C, Wright TC. SHORT communication: Field study of air ammonia concentrations in Ontario dairy calf housing microenvironments. Can J Anim Sci 2015;95(4):539–42. Available from: http://www.nrcresearchpress.com.

25. Nordstrom GA, McQuitty JB. University of Alberta [Research Bulletin:1976. p. 76].

26. Nordlund KV. Practical considerations for ventilating calf barns in winter. Vet Clin North Am Food Anim Pract. Elsevier 2008;24(1):41–54.

27. Bates DW, Anderson JF. Calcualtion of ventilation needs for confined cattle. J Am Vet Med Assoc 1979 Mar 15;174(6):581–9.

28. De Paula Vieira A, von Keyserlingk MAG, Weary DM. Effects of pair versus single housing on performance and behavior of dairy calves before and after weaning from milk. J Dairy Sci 2010 Jul;93(7):3079–85.

29. Boulton AC, Rushton J, Wathes DC. A Study of Dairy Heifer Rearing Practices from Birth to Weaning and Their Associated Costs on U.K. Dairy Farms. Open J Anim Sci 2015;05(2):185–97.

30. Nonnecke BJ, Foote MR, Miller BL, Fowler M, Johnson TE, Horst RL. Effects of chronic environmental cold on growth, health, and select metabolic and immunologic responses of preruminant calves. J Dairy Sci 2009 Dec 1;92(12):6134–43.

31. Hill TM, Bateman HG, Aldrich JM, Schlotterbeck RL. Comparisons of housing, bedding, and cooling options for dairy calves. J Dairy Sci 2011 Apr;94(4):2138–46.

32. Wathes CM, Jones CDR, Webster AJF. Ventilation, air hygiene and animal health. Vet Rec 1983;113(24):554–9.

33. Lago A, McGuirk SMM, Bennett TBB, Cook NBB, Nordlund KVV. Calf respiratory disease and pen microenvironments in naturally ventilated calf barns in winter. J Dairy Sci 2006;89(10):4014–25.

34. AHDB. Calf management; 2018.

35. Scoley G, Rutherford N. Calf jackets and the importance of keeping calves warm [Internet]; 2019. Available from: https://www.foodandfarmingfutures.co.uk/Library/content/Detail.

Chapter 5

Feeding the pre-weaned calf

Esme Moffett and Sophie Mahendran

CHAPTER CONTENTS

Early life nutrition is one of the cornerstones of developing a strong foundation for the future of a calf. It has a direct impact on the growth of the calf, along with effects on the metabolic activity and immune system which affect both short- and long-term health and productivity. When feeding artificially reared calves, a balance must be struck between replicating the natural situation of the calf remaining with its dam, and the on farm practicalities and economics involved in achieving this. The milk fed should be close in composition to the mother's own milk, but unlike the suckler calf who feeds little and often throughout the day, the artificially reared calf is often expected to drink high volumes at low frequency, so there is inevitably a trade-off between mimicking nature and achieving targets.

The welfare of the calves must always be considered. The first of the Five Freedoms established by the UK Farm Animal Welfare Council in 1979 is 'freedom from hunger and thirst'. If feeding quality or quantity is not suitable, the calf will be nutritionally 'stressed', which is not acceptable. The nutrition provided by milk is not only required for maintenance and growth, but also warmth and immune function. Good feeding practices enhance good management and will prevent or reduce many other issues.

The main aims of the pre-weaning period are:

- to maximise growth rates at this important stage of development
- to ensure excellent development of the rumen so calves can thrive on a non-milk diet post-weaning
- to avoid disease.

The digestive tract maturation stage of the calf should also be considered when deciding on feeding regimes. Calves less than 3 weeks old have poorly developed digestive tracts, so the ingredient content of the milk fed to the calves is vital to ensure adequate digestion and to maximise growth (1). This means that younger calves will thrive in the first few weeks of life on a milk feed that is of similar nutritional content to that from the dam, but as they get older and the digestive tract matures and enzyme production increases, they are able to utilise a wider range of feed stuffs (2).

Legislation for calf feeding – Welfare of Farmed Animals (England) Regulations 2000

- All calves should be fed at least twice per day.
- A daily ration of fibrous food must be provided from 2 weeks of age.
- Calves should be provided with fresh drinking water at all times.

WHAT MILK TO FEED?

Essentially there are two choices of milk to rear calves on: whole milk or calf milk replacer (milk powder). Whole milk should ideally be from the bulk tank and therefore of saleable quality, however, it is not uncommon to still see waste milk being fed. Calf milk replacer (CMR) is used on many farms, but the choices on the market are vast so the product quality can be very variable.

Table 5.1 summarises the advantages and disadvantages of each option which are discussed in more detail below.

Calves thrive on consistency, which is essential for all aspects of management, but particularly so for milk feeding. Therefore, the best choice for an individual farm may be the one with which they can achieve the highest consistency and could be influenced by farm size, resources or labour. This should always be part of the conversation about milk choice; what is best on paper may not be best for the farm.

Whole milk

When talking about feeding whole milk, this is saleable milk that would otherwise be in the bulk tank – this is not the same as feeding waste milk or high somatic cell count milk (neither of which are advisable). Milk containing antibiotics should never be fed to calves as it promotes the development of antimicrobial resistant bacteria in the calf's gut that could pose a human health risk (3).

Whole milk is the original and most 'natural' food source for calves, but the pressures of modern farming can limit its benefits due to the dilution effect in high yielding cows. Although saleable tank milk should be fairly consistent, there will still be some variation in its day-to-day quality depending on stage of lactation of the cows in the herd, the season and the cows' diet. Whole milk is also deficient in many vitamins and minerals, especially vitamins B, D and E.

Whole milk generally has much higher fat

TABLE 5.1 Summary of the main advantages and disadvantages of whole milk and milk replacer feeding.

	Whole milk	**Calf milk replacer**
Advantages	Always available	Consistent
	Antibody protection	Less risk of disease transfer
	Less labour	Usually cheaper to feed (depending on milk price)
Disadvantages	Variable quality, especially of solid contents	More labour
	Disease risks to the calf, e.g. Johne's Disease	Quality varies between products

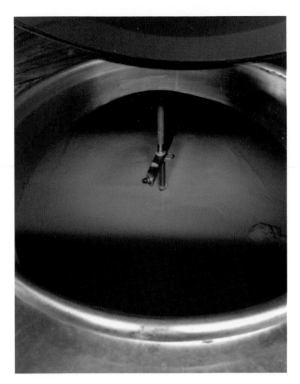

FIGURE 5.1 Feeding whole milk means milk that is suitable to be in the bulk tank.

(30–40%) and protein (20–30%) percentages than CMR, making it higher in energy. It is also presented to the calf at the most desirable concentration of approximately 13% solids, and along with it only containing natural milk protein, this enhances the overall digestibility for the calf. Whole milk also has the added advantage of being collected from cows exposed to the same pathogens as the calves. This means that their milk will contain farm-specific antibodies, which could help provide local intestinal immune protection for an extended period. Such localised protection has been shown to reduce the occurrence of calf disease, such as diarrhoea and respiratory disease (4). However, there is a disease risk associated with feeding whole milk due to shedding in the milk, specifically for transmission of Johne's disease, Mycoplasma or *Mycobacterium bovis* from adults to calves (5). This means that whole milk feeding should be avoided on farms where the risk of infection is high.

The cost of feeding whole milk compared to CMR is another factor to consider. Comparative calculations have shown that, with a milk price of 30 p/L for milk and a CMR cost of £1800 per tonne, CMR was estimated to be ~£17 cheaper for feeding a calf up to 10-weeks old (6). Although there is not necessarily a bill associated with feeding whole milk, it is certainly worth doing the maths to establish the true cost of feeding the calves – you will probably be surprised. Another issue to consider is that producers feeding bulk tank milk may want to limit the volume fed so as not to impact on milk sales too heavily. However, they will fail to see the cost–benefits of high-level milk feeding to young calves – better feed conversion rates, and better growth setting the calves up for a longer and more productive life.

There are alternative ways to feed whole milk other than just in its raw form.

Pasteurisation

Relatively small and affordable milk pasteuriser machines are now available to buy for use on farms (Figure 5.2). They tend to use the process of heating milk to 60–65.5°C, and holding it there for 30 minutes (7), allowing batches of milk to be pasteurised ready to be fed to the calves. It is also possible to get high-temperature, short-time (HTST) pasteurising units, which heat treat the milk at 71.7°C for just 15 seconds (8). The process of heating the milk has been shown to reduce the levels of bacterial contaminants, so is a good option for farms that are concerned about a disease risk from whole milk. However, pasteurisation does not make milk sterile, so starting with a high bacterial count batch of milk (waste milk) is still going to produce a product with a higher than acceptable pathogen level (9).

Milk should be stored appropriately (covered and cooled) if it is not going to be pasteurised immediately and likewise the same should apply post-pasteurisation if it is not to be fed straight away, as the bacterial count will rapidly rise again.

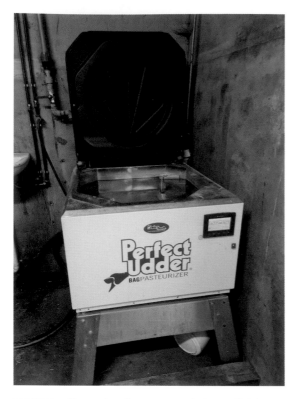

FIGURE 5.2 Example of a commercially available pasteurisation machine.

Cold acidified milk

Provision of large quantities of milk that are fed ad libitum to calves requires a method of preserving the milk while a batch is consumed (without the use of refrigeration) – this can be achieved by acidifying the milk so it can be kept for 1–3 days, and is more commonly seen in North America than in Europe. Provision of milk in this way encourages increased intakes, which is associated with increased weight gains and structural growth (10). It may be best suited to block calving herds where there are large batches of calves that need feeding, while limiting the capital cost of expensive equipment that will only be used for a short period of the year. This system can be set up with a plastic barrel to hold the milk, with teats and piping attached for the calves to suck from.

Adding organic acids (such as citric acid, propionic acid or formic acid) to whole milk lowers the pH level to around 4.5–5.5, and provides a way of preserving the milk without affecting the nutritional content (11). Many commercial preparations are available with the correct concentration of acid to be added to the milk. As with pasteurisation, if the bacterial count of the raw milk that is to be acidified is already high, then the acidified milk will be less well preserved.

Quick method for acidifying milk

- Take a commercially available preparation of 85% formic acid (highly irritant).
- Dilute 1 L of acid with 9 L of water.
- Add 30 mL of diluted solution per litre of cold milk to achieve a pH of 4.5.

Feeding cold acidified milk is best started once the calf is at least 1-week old and is already sucking strongly on warm milk, as the switch to cold milk can put them off feeding if they are too young. Other things to consider when preparing large volumes of acidified milk are to ensure the milk is stirred a few times a day to prevent separation, and the holding tank is covered to prevent fly access. The tank should be thoroughly cleaned between batches of milk, and any milk lines and teats cleaned daily.

It is now possible to heat up milk in ad lib feeding systems using commercially available products such as the Heatwave (Pyon). These products use a simple method that passes the cold milk close to a heating element to warm it up prior to ingestion. This makes the milk more appetising, especially for younger calves.

Yoghurt

Similar to acidification, this is a way of preserving milk to avoid excessive bacterial growth. It is not commonly done as it involves the production and maintenance of a starter culture, and can only start to be fed to calves from 7–14-days old. However, it may have its place on some units so should be

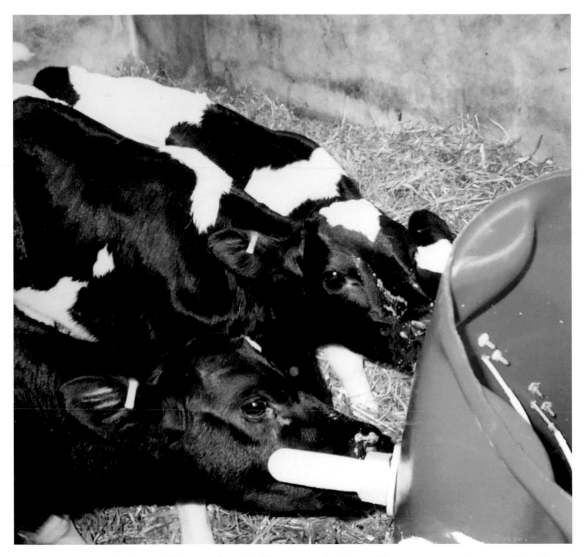

FIGURE 5.3 Calves drinking milk from a barrel with teats and tubing with non-return valves reaching down into the milk.

borne in mind if farms are wanting a way to preserve large volumes of milk for batch feeding. A basic guide to producing yoghurt from whole milk is to add three bottles of Actimel natural yoghurt to 1.1 L of warm milk, and leave it for 12 hours in a warm place to form your starter culture (12). This is then added to 13.5 L of warm milk and left for 24 hours until thick and sour. This in turn is added to 180 L of warm milk, and left for 12 hours before being ready to be fed to calves. This yoghurt can be fed through teats, buckets or troughs, but it can

take calves some time to get used to it due to the cold and thick consistency.

Calf milk replacer

There are many CMRs available commercially, with individual feed companies each producing several different options (Figure 5.4). This means choosing a powder that best suits the needs of an individual farm can be daunting. All CMR comes

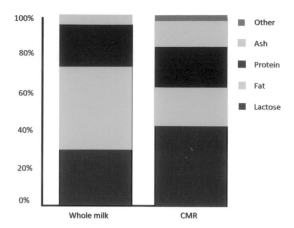

FIGURE 5.4 Comparison of the constituents of whole milk compared to CMR. Adapted from Trouw Nutrition.

in powdered form and has to be reconstituted with warm water at the correct concentration.

The following important considerations must be taken into account when choosing a milk powder.

- What age of calves is the CMR for?
- How is the CMR being mixed? Milk Taxi/automatic feeding machine/by hand.
- What is the desired growth rate?
- What is the budget?
- Testimonies: can the vet/farm advisor/other farmers recommend or provide feedback (both positive and negative) on certain products?

There is unlikely to be one product which fits all these criteria, so producers will need to compromise, but at least the selection will have been based on objective decision making rather than a lucky dip.

Protein in CMR

Protein supplies important amino acids to calves and is mainly required for growth of lean tissues, with only a small amount needed for maintenance (30–33 g/day (13)). There are two sources of protein used in CMR: dairy and non-dairy protein.

Dairy proteins are collected as by-products of processing and fall into either the skim milk powder or whey milk powder categories. Dairy proteins are highly digestible for all ages of calf and are the best choice for younger calves with a less developed digestive tract.

Skim milk powder is a by-product of butter and cream production, and contains both the milk proteins casein and whey (6). When these milk powders are digested by the calf, they form a milk clot in the abomasum, which allows thorough digestion of the casein protein (by rennet, pepsin and hydrochloric acid) prior to entry into the intestines. As skim milk is more expensive to produce, the proportion of the total protein content in CMR is usually 20–50%. Care must be taken if the CMR contains <6% skim powder as the low level of casein will not form a stable milk clot, and there is a high risk of nutritional diarrhoea being induced (14).

Whey milk powder is a by-product of cheese manufacture and is made up of lactose (a carbohydrate) and whey proteins (6). These milk powders do not form a clot in the abomasum (as they do not contain casein), but as whey protein is well digested by the intestines, this is not a problem for the calf. There are several methods of whey extraction which vary between manufacturing processes and include acid precipitation, high temperature drying techniques, crystallisation and ultrafiltration at lower temperatures (6). These different techniques lead to different qualities of whey protein being produced.

Non-dairy proteins are usually plant-based, and commonly include soya protein, hydrolysed wheat gluten and pea protein (6), which are quite cheap for manufacturers to source. Ideally, non-dairy proteins should not make up >50% of the total protein content of the milk powder. The most common type is wheat gluten, which is highly digestible, does not sediment out of solution, but lacks certain amino acids (lysine and threonine) so should not be used for calves <14-days old. Soy-based proteins can have reduced digestibility due to anti-nutrient factors such as trypsin, which will lead to diarrhoea, so again should not be fed to young calves <3-weeks old. Pea protein is a good quality, highly digestible protein that is high in lysine. However, it sediments out of solution easily so its use should be carefully considered depending on the mixing method used. If the overall content of plant proteins is quite high, this will be indicated by a CMR crude fibre content >0.15%.

Some powders also contain egg protein, and while it looks like this should be a good protein source due to the good amino acid content and high digestibility, these powders do not tend to perform well in real-life (15).

Protein can only be fully utilised by the calf if there is enough energy in the diet to support its digestion, with a high protein but low energy CMR resulting in energy limiting growth. It is important to check the label to ensure that good quality dairy proteins are the predominant protein source, with a target minimum level being at least >22% protein. Higher protein diets will result in greater growth rates (16), with the maximum available in the UK currently being 26%.

Energy in CMR

The energy in CMR comes from both fats/oils (in the UK these are vegetable oils) and carbohydrate (mostly in the form of lactose). Extra energy needs to be added to CMR due to the removal of butterfat during processing, with the aim being to replace this with short and moderate fatty acid chains that are found naturally in milk fat (6).

The carbohydrate, lactose, is a natural component of whey, but only has around half the energy value of fat. Calves can produce the enzyme lactase (needed for the digestion of lactose to glucose and galactose) from birth, whereas the enzymes needed to break down other types of carbohydrate only start to be produced as the calf ages. The level of lactose in CMR tends to be higher than that found in whole milk (42–50% vs 33–38% of dry matter (DM)) due to the historical availability of milk by-products (17). This gives a lower energy density and lower energy : protein ratio in CMR compared with whole milk, meaning calves provided with whole milk generally retain more fat. Care must

be taken if the level of lactose is too great as it has a high osmolality, resulting in a draw of water into the intestinal lumen content and resulting in diarrhoea (18).

Fat is the most concentrated energy source found in milk, but CMR tends to have lower levels of fat compared to whole milk (16–22% vs 30–40% of DM) (19). Young calves <2-weeks old are unable to digest non-milk fats very well, resulting in diarrhoea if levels are high in CMR. In the UK all fat sources are vegetable oils, with the most common sources being palm, coconut and soya. Coconut oil has good digestibility and a similar fatty acid profile to whole milk, but should only make up a maximum of 30% of the total fats/oils. The ideal target for fat levels in CMR is 20%, with higher fat levels known to suppress initial concentrate intakes (20). Some companies are now producing CMR with homogenised milk fats in them. This process decreases the size of the fat globules, which is thought to improve the solubility and increase the digestibility of the fat.

Calculating CMR energy content

When assessing a CMR, the actual energy content of the CMR is not listed on the packaging. However, it can be calculated using the nutrient listing and some mathematical equations.

First, you need to estimate the lactose content of the CMR:

Lactose estimation = 100 – crude protein% – fat% – ash%

You can then calculate the energy content (metabolisable energy (ME)) of the CMR:

ME (MJ/kg of DM) = {[0.057 × % crude protein] + [0.092 × % fat] + [0.0395 × % lactose]} x 3.77

Whole milk has an energy level around 21 MJ/kg of DM.

The last component of this exercise is to know the energy requirement of the calf you are feeling! This is the most complex part of the problem due to the energy requirements being affected by many different factors including the size of the calf (which affects the maintenance energy requirements), the target daily growth rate and the environmental temperature (as cold weather increases energy consumption and therefore maintenance energy requirement of the calf), and whether the calf is consuming any concentrate feed as well.

The basic equation for the energy a calf needs (at an environmental temperature of 15–20°C) is given by (21):

$$ME (MJ/day) = 0.1 \times BW^{0.75} + (0.84 \times BW^{0.344}) (ADG^{1.2})$$

where BW = bodyweight in kg and ADG = average daily growth in kg.

Further information can be found in the section 'How much CMR to feed'.

For a more straightforward approach to these calculations, there are online programmes available that can perform these calculations very quickly and easily, for example, that from AHDB (https://ahdb.org.uk/calf-milk-replacer-energy-calculator) (Figure 5.5).

Vitamins and minerals

A calf needs vitamins and minerals for all its metabolic processes, but they only have a very limited store of them in the body and so are dependent on dietary sources. The vitamin and mineral content is described as the ash content on CMR ingredient lists, which should ideally be <7.5% otherwise there is an increased risk of osmotic diarrhoea due to increased rates of abomasal emptying (6).

Usually vitamins A, D and E are supplemented in CMR as they are required for normal health and growth of the calf. Vitamin A is involved in maintaining epithelial tissue and mucous membranes, as well as being involved in sight and the immune function. Vitamin D is vital for proper calcium metabolism and therefore skeletal growth. Vitamin E is an antioxidant and is required for a healthy immune system. The main minerals that are usually included in CMR are iron (for red blood cell production), selenium (needed to support a healthy immune system), zinc (needed for enzymes involved in metabolism), iodine (important for a functioning immune system), manganese (needed for enzymes involved in normal bone formation) and copper (important for haemoglobin synthesis and enzymes involved in metabolism).

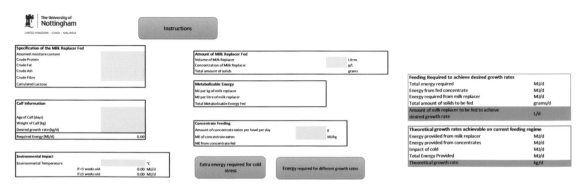

FIGURE 5.5 A screenshot of the AHDB CMR energy calculator that was designed in conjunction with the University of Nottingham. See the Appendix for a larger image.

Understanding the label

- Ingredients are listed in descending order of inclusion, but the label does not tell you actual proportions.
- No information is given on the energy content of the CMR, but you can calculate it.
- No information is given about physical properties of the CMR, for example, mixability or sedimentation.
- Seek out a powder with protein >22%, fat ~20%, ash <7.5% and fibre <0.3%
- Proteins from dairy sources tend to be better quality and more digestible.

Ask the company for more detailed specification of ingredients – they might not always give it to you!

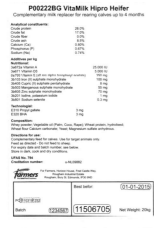

FIGURE 5.6 A list of constituents on a CMR bag. See the Appendix for a larger image.

Lactose estimation = 100 – crude protein%
– fat% – ash%

= 100 – 26 – 17 – 8.5

= 48.5%

The energy content of the CMR:

ME (MJ/kg of DM) = {[0.057 × %crude protein] + [0.092 × %fat] + [0.0395 × %lactose]} × 3.77

= [(0.057 × 26) + (0.092 × 17) + (0.0395 × 48.5)] × 3.77

= [1.482 + 1.564 + 1.916] × 3.77

= 18.7 MJ

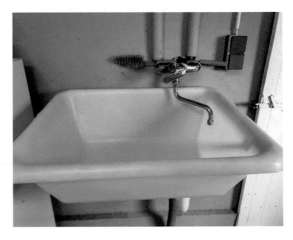

FIGURE 5.7 A hygienic sink with hot and cold water to allow cleaning of equipment.

Mixing CMR

Once the correct CMR has been selected for a particular farm, it is imperative that the optimum preparation guidelines are followed for mixing it up ready to be fed – if you get the reconstitution wrong, you can create a lot of nutritional problems in the calves (even if you have the most expensive CMR!), and consistency is key. Having a clean and organised area for preparing the milk can help with this, with a hot and cold water source and clean sink being vital to maintain hygiene of the equipment (Figure 5.7).

The first step is to measure out the correct amount of CMR for the concentration that you want to feed, ideally using scales (Figure 5.8). This can range between 125–150 g/L, with a value of 135 g/L mimicking the DM content of whole milk (13.5%). It is important to remember that the correct weight of CMR should have water added to make up 1 L of fluid. Powder should not be added to 1 L of water as this will give an incorrect (more dilute) concentration (Table 5.2). If using a scoop of a known size to measure out the CMR, make sure that it is clean and not covered in crusty powder as this will alter the amount of CMR measured out – the scoop weight should be re-calibrated with every new bag of CMR opened (Figure 5.9). If using a milk mixer

TABLE 5.2 An example of the amount of milk powder and water that need to be mixed together to give a 15% solution of CMR.

Litres of milk required	Milk powder required, grams	Approximate litres of water required
3	450	2.5
6	900	5.1
9	1350	7.6
12	1800	10.2
15	2250	12.7
18	2700	15.5
21	3150	17.8
24	3600	20.4
27	4050	22.9
30	4500	25.5

Source: Adapted from Volac Feed For Growth (www.feedforgrowth.com).

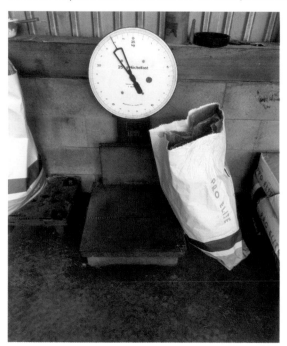

FIGURE 5.8 Weigh scales (either analogue or digital) can make measuring out CMR quick and easy.

CMR as this will also increase the osmolality to give an undesirable concentration.

Once the CMR is weighed out, it should be mixed with water at ~42°C (any hotter than 45°C may denature the proteins). Having a digital thermometer can help with this. Mixing the CMR at this temperature helps it to dissolve, and allows

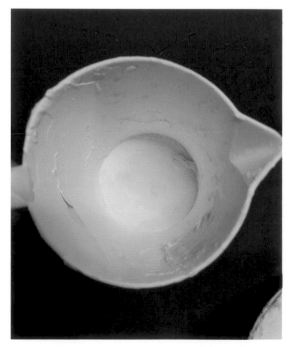

FIGURE 5.9 Scoop used to measure out CMR that has a layer of powder stuck to the inside which will be reducing the accuracy of measurements.

with volume markings on the side, do not assume that these volumes are correct for measuring out your water amounts (Figure 5.10).

If you want to feed more CMR, it is better to increase the volume fed rather than increasing the concentration per litre as the latter will increase the osmolality of the milk and can cause digestive problems. Similarly, do not add rehydration solution to

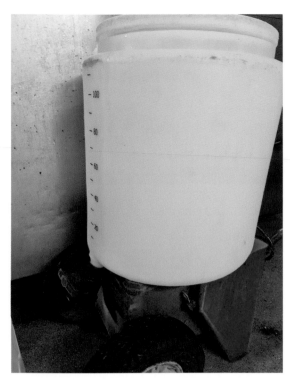

FIGURE 5.10 A Wydale milk mixer with marking on the side to indicate volume of fluid – these pre-printed markings are inaccurate and will lead to unknown concentrations of CMR being made.

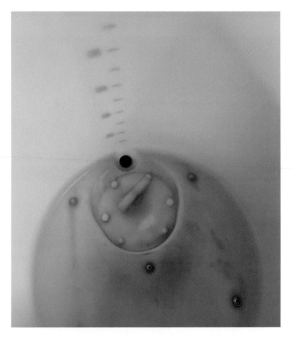

FIGURE 5.11 The inside of a Wydale milk mixer, showing the mechanism for mixing the powder and water.

for some cooling between mixing and delivery to ensure it is still fed to the calves at ~40°C. From the authors' experience, feeding the milk at this warmer temperature really improves palatability and encourages the calves to drink compared to trying to feed cooler milk.

Ensure that the CMR is mixed well with the water, either using a hand whisk or a mechanical mixer. Be aware of sedimentation, especially if mixing by hand (Figures 5.11 and 5.12). This can be reduced by mixing small volumes at a time and feeding it straight away before mixing more.

When investigating issues with calf rearing, always try and watch the staff make up the CMR feeds. This will often reveal where problems occur, and allows you to monitor their attention to detail.

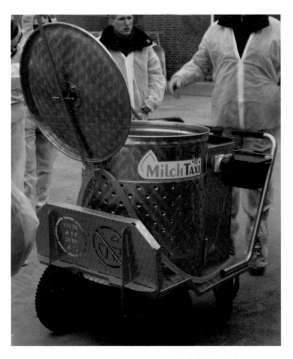

FIGURE 5.12 Some of the new Milk Taxi machines have inbuilt scales, which can help with speeding up accurate mixing of CMR.

Osmolality of CMR

Osmolality is a measure of the concentration of solute particles in solution. Whole milk has an osmolality of 300 mOsm/kg, but CMR tends to be higher, in the range of 400–600 mOsm/kg. One of the main determinants of osmolality in CMR is the sodium level. A high osmolality should be avoided as it will compromise gastrointestinal barrier function, it acts to draw fluid into the intestinal lumen resulting in diarrhoea, and it delays abomasal emptying which can increase the chance of bloat or abomasitis in calves.

Things that can increase the osmolality of the mixed milk include having a poor quality CMR, increasing the concentration of CMR per litre (levels of 180 g/L of CMR can be harmful), and adding rehydration solutions into CMR mixes.

AMOUNTS OF MILK TO FEED

As mentioned in the section on energy levels in CMR, there are specific equations that can be used to calculate the actual requirements for the amount of CMR that needs to be fed in order for a calf to receive enough energy for both maintenance and growth. It is possible to get an idea on calf satiety by observing the calves. Calves that are full of milk and content are more likely to be quietly lying down, whereas hungry calves are more likely to be on their feet and blaring when they see people.

Suckler calves that are left with their dam are known to consume up to 12 small milk meals a day of ~1 L at each feed, and this is what the normal physiology of a calf is designed to cope with. However, artificial rearing systems often impose human constraints on feeding, with many calves required to consume their milk intakes in just two feeds per day. Historically the recommendation for milk feeding was to provide calves with 10% of their bodyweight as milk (22), for example a newborn 40 kg calf would get 4 L of milk per day. However, this rough guide does not take into account the energy requirements for growth, or for keeping warm if the environmental temperatures were low.

It is now more generally recommended to feed 15–20% of bodyweight as milk, but again it is better to come up with a more specific feeding plan based on the milk being fed and the size of the calves – a guide is given in Table 5.3. Research studies have shown that offering higher volumes of milk (8 L) from birth (23) or even ad lib milk to calves results in better growth performance (24). When offered ad lib milk, the total amount consumed each day will vary, but over an 8-week period it will average out to ~10 L per day. Some people may refer to this as accelerated feeding programmes, but this is actually just restoration of biologically normal intakes of milk for a calf.

Although this may seem like a lot of milk, which will come at a cost to the farm, the feed conversion ratio of a calf is the best it will be within the lifetime of the animal (2 : 1 up to 10-weeks old compared to 10 : 1 at 8-months old) – for every 2 kg of food a calf consumes, they will grow by 1 kg. This means that in terms of growth efficiency, calves are the most productive animals on the farm, which should be capitalised on (Table 5.3). In conjunction with the fact that the pre-weaning period only makes up 10 weeks of a calf's life, nutrition should not be restricted here – this is false economy and can be detrimental to the future of the animal. These feeding strategies offer the best opportunity to reach the target 750–800 g/day growth rates that are recommended. There was some concern raised about high pre-weaning growth rates having a negative impact on fatty tissue development in the mammary gland which could impair future milk production (25). However, this has since been disproved, with higher growth rates in calves allowing heifers to reach puberty sooner, with greater development of mammary tissue and therefore higher yields in the first lactation (26).

It has to be remembered that higher levels of milk feeding must be used in conjunction with a strategic weaning programme to ensure a smooth transition onto solid feeds – this is ideally 8 weeks of high-level milk feeding followed by a 2-week

TABLE 5.3 A guide to the energy requirements for maintenance and growth at 0.8 kg/day for calves of different bodyweights.

Bodyweight of calf (kg)	40	50	60	70	80	90	100
Energy needed (MJ/day) for maintenance + growth at 0.8 kg/day	16.7	18.7	20.6	22.4	24.0	25.6	27.1
Extra energy (MJ/day) needed when temperature ≤5°C	1.8	2.1	1.2	1.4	1.5	1.6	1.8
Amount of milk to be fed per day (L) at an environmental temperature of 15°C	6.1	6.8	7.5	8.1	8.7	9.3	9.9
Amount of milk to be fed per day (L) at an environmental temperature of 5°C	6.7	7.6	8.4	9.1	9.8	10.5	11.2

Notes: An example of the amount of milk that would have to be fed is then calculated – this uses a 24% protein CMR with 18.3 MJ of energy per 1 kg, and fed at a concentration of 15%. It does not take into account concentrate intakes as the calf gets older. It is assumed that CMR has a 5% moisture level. Adapted from the AHDB CMR calculator.

weaning period where milk volumes are slowly reduced (see Chapter 6 on weaning).

A calf's abomasum can easily hold 3 L of milk in one go from birth, with this volume increasing to a capacity in excess of 5 L by 3 weeks of age (27). Farmers can be deterred from feeding higher volumes of milk to calves due to concerns over nutritional diarrhoea. Although it is true that a calf ingesting higher volumes of milk will have slightly looser faecal consistency, if a calf is drinking in the correct manner, this should not lead to clinical diarrhoea. The main causes of nutritional diarrhoea are milk being of a high osmolality or concentration, or milk ending up in the calf's rumen. Physiologically, the calf has an oesophageal groove which directs milk past the rumen, so that it enters into the omasum and then abomasum where it can be digested (28). Closure of this groove is vital to prevent milk entering the rumen and fermenting, and is encouraged by allowing calves to suckle their milk from a teat at ~0.6 m from the ground and making sure milk is warm.

The nutrient requirement for a calf increases with age, meaning they require more milk as they get older – this is a step-up system. Managing this in a manual feeding system requires organisation by the calf rearer, with systems such as coloured pegs/ tapes, or white boards with information on them being used to identify the amount of milk a pen needs. These systems can mean milk volumes are updated on a weekly basis, with excellent communication between staff needed to avoid confusion and ensure consistency for the calves.

In terms of how often milk should be fed to calves, European law stipulates that calves up to 4-weeks old must be fed at least two liquid feeds a day, with a recommendation to maintain this until weaning. Once-a-day feeding was promoted as a labour saving strategy, and while having a role to play in the weaning process, it is NEVER recommended as a feeding strategy for younger calves – it will leave them undernourished and vulnerable to disease (energy is a vital component of a fully functioning immune system). Most farms will provide milk feeds twice daily to calves, and although three times daily would help to increase milk intakes and enhance calf nutrition in manual feeding systems, it may not be logistically feasible on many units. Automatic calf feeders offer a mechanised way of milk delivery, and are discussed in more detail below.

The last matter to consider when deciding on quantities of milk to feed is the environmental temperature. The lower thermoneutral zone of a calf up to 3-weeks old is 15°C, below which a calf has to use energy to keep warm (see Table 5.3). This means that less energy is available for growth and to fuel the immune system. If feeding restricted quantities of milk, farms should consider increasing the amount of CMR fed during colder weather to ensure growth rates and health are not limited. This can be done by either increasing the volume or frequency of milk feeding or by slightly increasing the concentration of CMR used to make up the milk.

If calves become ill, it is important to maintain milk feeding – never withhold milk if a calf is willing to suckle it. Nutrition is vital to fuel the immune system and provide nutrients for the body to repair itself. Studies have shown that in calves with diarrhoea, maintaining milk feeding helps the small intestine villi to heal and promotes weight gain (29). If calves refuse to drink their milk, electrolyte solutions should be provided via an oesophageal tube feeder – milk should never be fed by this method as it leads to milk entering the rumen where it can ferment and cause bloat and death.

Teat or bucket delivery of milk

There are two ways in which the milk can be delivered to a calf – via a teat or via a bucket/trough. The method used is usually influenced by how calves are housed, and whether the farm feel that their current method of feeding is working or not. This should be confirmed by objective data collection such as counting the cases of bloat, assessing the amount of cross sucking, and the growth rates being achieved.

Feeding through a teat is the most 'natural' method for calves to suckle milk. It encourages production of plenty of saliva which is important for digestion and also helps stimulate rumen development (Figure 5.13).

Sucking results in closure of the oesophageal groove, which is important to ensure that milk is diverted away from the rumen, and into the abomasum where it can begin to be digested. This can be enhanced by ensuring the teat is ~0.6 m from the ground, and the calf's head is in an overstretched position to mimic sucking from an udder (Figure 5.14).

Calves have an innate desire to suck, so using teat feeders can help satisfy this need. It also allows larger milk volume feeds to be given in a controlled manner without the risk of milk entering the rumen, which is at an increased risk when calves consume milk too quickly (27). Teats must be good quality to ensure calves have to work to suck the milk – teats with valves in can work well and act more like a natural teat (e.g. Peach Teats).

If using feeders that allow multiple calves to feed from the same teats (e.g. Wydale/Milk Bar or auto-feeders), then hygiene must be paramount (Figure 5.15). Teats will need cleaning after every feeding session, and will need monitoring closely for signs of wear (such as the hole becoming too big and allowing milk to run freely) (Figure 5.16). This can create an aspiration risk for the calf, and also allows them to drink the milk too quickly.

Using buckets or troughs to feed calves is considered an easier way for people to manage feeding as it allows calves to drink milk very quickly, and minimises the amount of washing that needs to be done as buckets are quicker to wash than teats. Calves will need to learn to drink out of a bucket as it is not a natural feeding method, but they often pick this up quickly with some training. Drinking out of a bucket may not allow the oesophageal groove to close properly (30), which increases the risk of milk ending up in the calf's

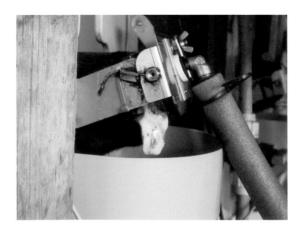

FIGURE 5.13 Saliva production from a calf sucking a teat.

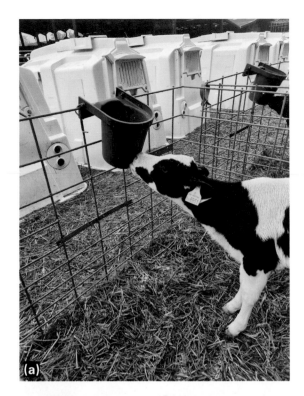

FIGURE 5.14 Individual teat feeders hung at ~0.6 m from the ground in two different systems.

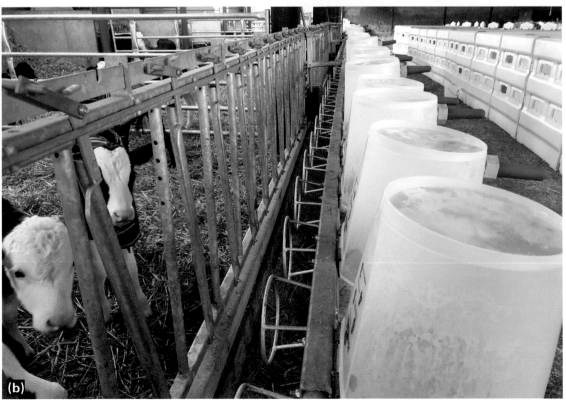

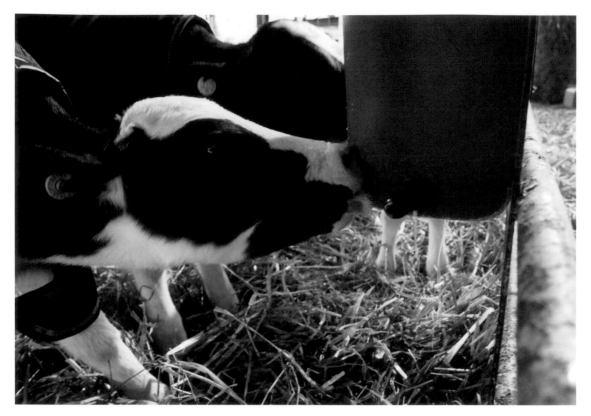

FIGURE 5.15 Example of a multi-teat calf feeder.

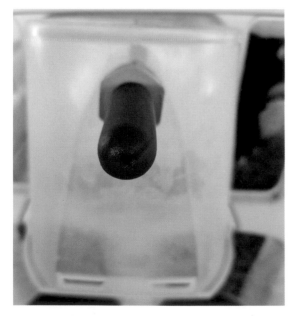

FIGURE 5.16 A worn out teat with a large hole that will allow milk to run into the calf's mouth and increases the risk of aspiration pneumonia.

rumen where it can ferment and cause bloat or diarrhoea. To help reduce the risk of this, the bucket base should be 30 cm off the ground. Some large rearing units feed milk in group buckets or troughs to reduce labour, but this makes it impossible to monitor how much milk each calf is consuming. This can be problematic as a reduction in voluntary feed intakes is a good early detection system for sick calves.

Drinking from a bucket allows calves to consume their milk allowance very quickly, often in 30–60 seconds depending on the volume fed. However, sucking times on ad lib teat systems have been reported to be as long as 13 minutes, showing a calf's natural preference for longer drinking times (31). In addition, in order for calves to feel satiated or full after a meal, they not only need to consume enough milk to provide them with the nutrients required, they also need to satisfy their desire to suckle. If this is not met, as in the case with bucket

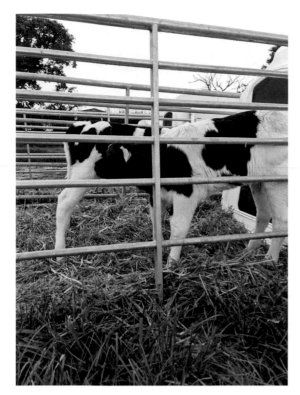

FIGURE 5.17 Two calves exhibiting cross sucking behaviours.

feeding, abnormal non-nutritive sucking behaviours (better known as cross sucking) will develop (see Figure 5.17).

Cross sucking

This usually manifests as a calf sucking on the navel of another calf, although they can use other parts of the body such as the stifle or ear (Figure 5.17). This can lead to hair loss, and in some cases can induce navel ill or skin infections. It is also very common to see non-nutritive sucking in calves fed on low rations of milk (32), and this, along with vocalisation, are indicators that calves are hungry (33). To address this problem in bucket rearing systems, provision of dry teats for the calf to suck on, attached to the wall of the pen can help, although they should be regularly cleaned to reduce the risk of them acting as a fomite for spread of disease.

AUTOMATIC CALF FEEDERS

Automatic calf feeders (ACFs) are becoming increasingly popular as mechanisation of the dairy industry accelerates. These machines have a powder hopper and water boiler that is able to reconstitute CMR in real-time when a calf enters a feeding station, with one machine able to service up to four teats at a time. They identify individual calves by either EID ear tags, or by neck collars that can be reused between calves. They provide continuous, automated and real-time monitoring of the calves, but their success still depends on excellent management, and there is a substantial initial investment required. The major benefits of an ACF is that they allow natural feeding to be mimicked, whereby calves can be fed small volumes throughout the day, but overall allowing much higher

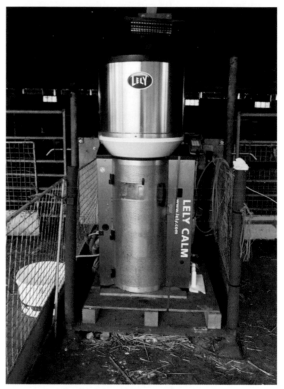

FIGURE 5.18 An example of an ACF that is readily available in the UK. Above the calf feeder is an infrared heat lamp which can be switched on in cold conditions to help reduce the chance of the water freezing in the machine and pipes.

volumes to be fed. If using CMR in an ACF it must be designed for this purpose, so check the label or directly with the manufacturer – some CMRs may become clogged when using in an ACF.

Often when tasks become automated there is a temptation to give the animals themselves less attention – this should not be the case. Rather than spending time preparing and manually feeding the calves, the stockperson will have to spend the time pen walking to make sure each calf is checked for signs of ill health. Changes in behaviour are often seen prior to seeing clinical signs, and this will be reflected in ill calves having fewer feeding visits and spending less time feeding per day – this will be indicated by the ACF (34).

ACF maintenance is important to ensure the machine is working as it should. The machines are programmed to run inbuilt daily cleaning cycles to flush pipes, but just like a milking parlour, an additional daily manual clean is also needed. This will include use of a strong alkali to wash through the pipe work, and manual cleaning of the teats to remove saliva and prevent biofilm development. It is also advisable to wash the walls of the stall daily to minimise disease spread from calves licking these surfaces. In addition, the pipework and rubber seals should be checked weekly for any build-up of dirt that will act as a reservoir for bacterial accumulation within the ACF system, increasing the risk of diarrhoea in the calves being fed. Calibrations of the powder dispensing and fluid volumes should also be done on a monthly basis.

Many ACFs are sold with a claim that they are able to feed approximately 30 calves per feeding station/teat, but in reality this is too many calves. Large group sizes are a risk factor for increased calf disease (35), especially as multiple calves are sharing a teat. The optimum group size is 10–15 calves, but more importantly it is vital that there is not more than a 2-week spread of age ranges within the group (36). Dynamic groups where the oldest calves are removed from a group and then younger ones added are much more likely to get disease problems, and the associated social changes are also very stressful for the calves.

It is best to have a period of adjustment after birth prior to introduction onto an ACF. Getting calves trained and feeding well off a manual teat feeding system will help them to learn how to use the ACF more quickly. It is generally recommended to introduce calves at 5–10-days old, but only as long as they are healthy (37). If calves fail to adapt to the ACF, take them off and manage them by manual feeding to improve their feeding vigour, then re-introduce to the ACF. Generally, you should not move calves between groups unless they are struggling – some calves have a timid personality and may struggle in a group of larger or more boisterous animals, so moving them into a group of younger calves can help to improve their health and well-being. This should never be done if the calf is exhibiting any disease symptoms. If a calf becomes ill, it is best to remove it from the group to reduce the spread of disease to the rest of the group – having a hospital pen set up and ready makes this isolation easier (38).

An important factor for setting up an ACF is the position and situation of the machine (Figure 5.19). A lot of fluid is created by these feeders due to the auto-wash cleaning cycles, spillage of milk when the calves are drinking, and also the urination and defaecation that tends to occur around the feeder. These all lead to increased environmental moisture levels, with good drainage required to ensure liquids do not pool (as this is a risk factor for cryptosporidiosis and coccidiosis) or drain into the lying area (which can increase humidity which is a risk factor for respiratory disease). Consideration should also be given to the distance between the mixer and the feeding stations, as the further the milk has to travel, the more likely it is to cool and the calves have to work harder to get the milk. Having the ACF boiler temperature set so milk is mixed at 42°C can help with this, as will insulating the pipes. There is also a risk of the machine freezing in cold weather, so provision of insulation to place around the machine, or an infrared heat lamp can help reduce this risk. However, there should always be a back-up plan for feeding the calves if the machine does freeze.

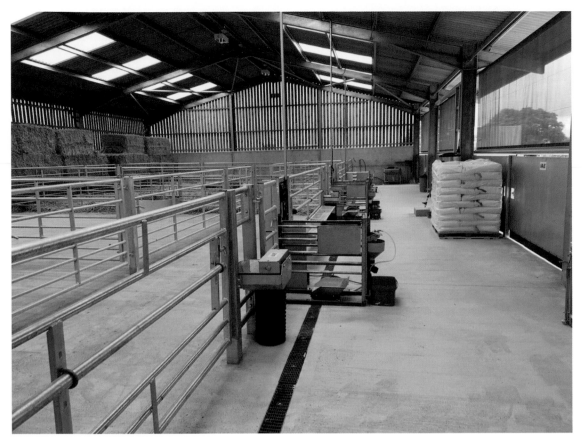

FIGURE 5.19 A calf barn designed for ACFs, which are positioned outside of the pen over good drainage.

A further benefit to using an ACF is the ability to have a well-controlled and gradual wean-down program. The machine is able to incrementally reduce the amount of milk a calf is given over a pre-set period of time (ideally 2 weeks), and this is the best way to encourage solid feed intakes while keeping nutritional stress to a minimum.

Training calves to drink in artificial rearing systems

When calves are artificially reared, they often have to be trained to feed using the chosen farm method. The speed and ease with which calves pick this skill up can vary greatly. Provision of the colostrum feeds through a teat bottle within 1 hour of birth can really help with training, as calves are usually very eager to suckle and then develop a strong positive association with people and the artificial teat. Calves that have been left to suckle their dam are often much harder to train, and may strongly resist sucking from artificial feeding methods.

Training calves to drink from a teat will be easier than an open bucket, but both can take time and require patience. Always handle calves in a gentle and calm manner to aid their learning, as if a calf is stressed by the handler's behaviour they will be scared and slower to learn. The best method is to let the calf suck your fingers (which also allows you to check the strength of the suck reflex) and then guide its mouth to the teat or the open bucket. Other tricks that may encourage a calf to suck is to gently scratch the calf's back or tail head, which mimics the nuzzling of the dam and can help to

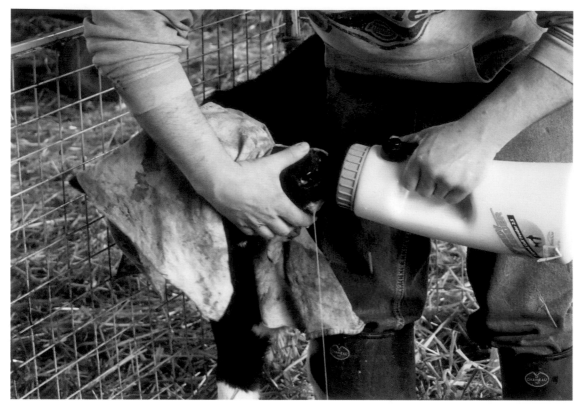

FIGURE 5.20 Placing a cloth over the eyes of a calf can help to calm them down and focus on drinking their milk

relax the calf and encourage them to suck. If a calf is quite stressed in its environment, covering its eyes with a cloth can help them to focus on the taste of the milk (Figure 5.20). Placing the teat into the calf's mouth and squirting a small amount of milk into the mouth can help them get the taste of the milk, but this must be done with care to ensure that milk in not inhaled. If the situation is becoming stressful, walk away and calm down, and this will also allow the calf to relax – then try again a short while later (e.g. 30 minutes).

Although you want the calf to be hungry for its meal, calves should not be purposefully starved to make the job easier. Also, never be tempted to feed a calf its milk through an oesophageal feeding tube if it will not suck from the teat or bucket – this will put milk directly into the rumen and be detrimental to the calf's health.

Hygiene

Hygiene and cleanliness of the feeding equipment is vital to keep bacterial counts in the milk as low as possible.

An example protocol for cleaning calf feeding equipment follows.

- Rinse with cold milk and strip out teats to remove milk residues.
- Soak with warm water and detergent to remove any residual fats.
- Scrub all surfaces to remove remaining milk residues.
- Rinse in water to remove remaining detergent.
- Leave upside down to drain and dry.
- Teats should be removed and washed separately once a day.

More tips for successful calf feeding

- It can be helpful to alert the calves to the fact it is feeding time, such as by encouraging calves to their feet so they are ready and eager to feed.
- Feed the calves at the same time each day – calves can become stressed when waiting for their food.
- Feed the calves in the same order each time – again this helps reduce stress.
  - If using shared feeding buckets between calves, move from the youngest to oldest calves to reduce the risk of spreading disease pathogens to the most susceptible animals.
- Ensure the milk is at the correct temperature 39–40°C to encourage drinking.
- Having the same staff manage the calves can help with ensuring the same routine is used, and allows the staff to get to know the calves – all animals are different, and getting used to how they are normally can help making spotting sick calves easier.

CONSISTENCY is KEY!!!!

- It can work well to have 2 sets of teats, allowing one set to soak in 3% hypochlorite solution to thoroughly disinfect them.
- Teats MUST be replaced once worn or broken.

THE NON-MILK DIET

Concentrates

Concentrate feed (often referred to as a starter pellet) is an important addition to the pre-weaned calf's diet to provide the nutrients (volatile fatty acids: butyrate and propionate) required for development of rumen papillae and microflora, thereby allowing the transition of a calf to become a ruminant (Figure 5.21). Calves should begin to be offered concentrate within the first week of life, but their solid feed intake is minimal until ~4 weeks of age. Historically it was thought that feeding lower amounts of milk would encourage younger calves to start eating concentrates sooner, but their ability to digest and extract energy at this age is very low, and recent studies have found that intensified/enhanced milk feeding regimens actually result in improved solid feed intakes overall (40).

Early introduction to concentrates will encourage the calf to investigate and 'play' with it before high intakes are required. Initially only a handful or two of concentrates should be offered and should be replaced daily to keep it fresh and maintain interest. Any uneaten feed can be given to older animals unless heavily contaminated. Once the calf begins to clear the concentrate they are fed each day, the amount offered can be increased. Calves should be eating at least 1.5 kg, ideally 2 kg, of concentrate per day for at least 3 consecutive days by weaning. It is not uncommon to find that in systems that feed high volumes of milk, these intakes are not achieved until the weaning process is started when the quantity of milk offered is slowly decreased.

The form of the concentrates can be coarse mix, pellets or pencils, and should have a crude protein level of around 18%. Evidence can be found to support all forms, so essentially it may well come down to farmer preference, availability or previous experience of the farmer or advisor. Whatever the form, the feed should be highly palatable, dust-free and clean, ideally with a diameter of at least 1.2 mm to reduce the risk of ruminal parakeratosis and bloat (Figure 5.22).

Forage

Provision of a forage fibre source has been shown to improve rumen pH level and feeding behaviour, with positive impacts on feed intakes and weight gain (39), as well as helping to develop the muscularity of the rumen wall and aid rumen health

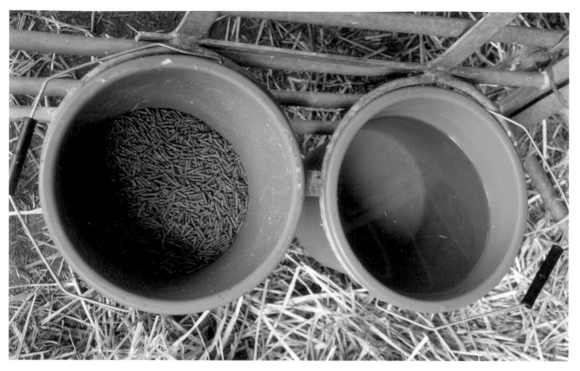

FIGURE 5.21 A typical system for holding buckets to supply both water and concentrates in a calf pen.

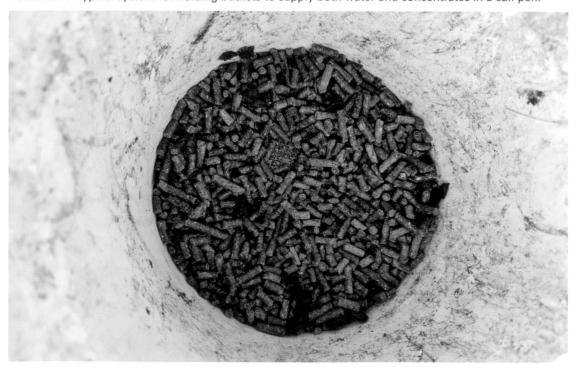

FIGURE 5.22 A bucket of calf pellets contaminated with rat faeces. This is unhygienic and will put the calves off consuming this solid feed.

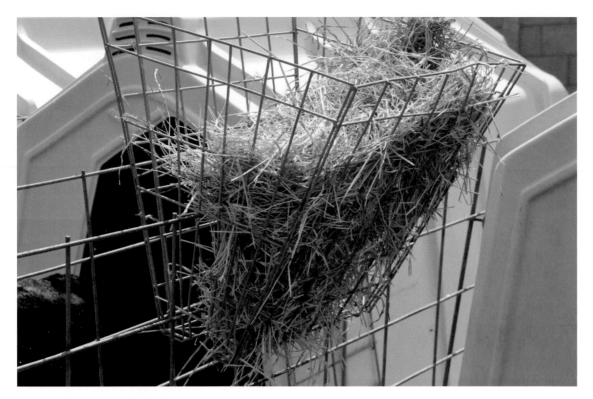

FIGURE 5.23 A small rack with good quality straw in it.

by preventing papillae clumping together (Figure 5.23). Development of the rumen and fibre intake can accelerate the expression of normal rumination behaviours, with calves observed to chew the cud from 3–4 weeks of age with the correct diet (41). It will also form a 'fibre mat' in the rumen which is essential for the function of some microbes (42). The commonly used forage sources in the UK are straw and hay, but it must be of good quality.

Problems with excessive fibre intake can be seen in calves that are fed very restricted milk diets, with their hunger driving them to eat large quantities of forage, resulting in calves with very pot-bellied appearances. This is therefore a milk feeding issue, and rarely caused by the type of forage being offered.

There are various ways forage can be incorporated into the diet. Some farms rely on the calf getting their forage requirements from the straw bedding. This is only acceptable if calves are individually housed and have fresh bedding provided daily, otherwise the disease risk from ingestion of

faeces is too high. Most farms provide forage in a rack that keeps it off the floor and is easy to access. Grass silage may be offered to older calves, but only in small amounts and it must be changed regularly to avoid spoilage.

It is common to see a calf chewing on a long piece of straw and think they are getting the forage they need, when in fact they are probably eating very little. The best method of forage provision is to provide the calves with chopped straw, either in its own bucket or trough, or mixed with the starter pellets. This has been shown to increase intakes of starter ration and will ensure rumen health is maximised (43, 44).

Water

A calf's body is made up of around 70% water, and therefore forms a vital part of the diet which is often overlooked in calf rearing. Unfortunately, many producers think that water is unnecessary for calves on milk, but this is wrong for two reasons. First, milk is a food, not a drink and, second, artificially reared calves are not fed enough milk volume to cover their hydration needs. Calves will drink around 150 mL/day from birth, and up to a few litres by weaning time. Water availability is also key to increasing concentrate intake, with calves deprived of water shown to have a 38% reduction in weight gain (45).

Water should be clean, fresh (replaced at least daily) and available ad libitum. This is especially important in hot weather or if a calf has diarrhoea, which will cause dehydration (Figure 5.24). If calves are group housed and expected to drink from a water trough, make sure they can reach it! It may be that a temporary step is needed when the calves are very small. Automatic drinkers are ideal for the supply of clean fresh water, but they should be checked regularly to see if they are functioning normally and are free from contamination. There is also the potential for them to leak or overflow creating wet bedding or floors and adding moisture to the environment – not ideal for the control of respiratory disease. If there are more than 20 calves in the group there should be at least two water sources (35) to prevent competition for resources.

A frequent complaint from farmers and a reason water is often withheld is that the calves drink too much water and do not drink their milk. This could be because they have mild/sub-clinical gastrointestinal issues and are self-correcting their dehydration, or it could be a learnt behaviour that they think is its milk. A useful tip which applies to individually/paired housed calves with two bucket spaces at the front of the pen is to put the milk bucket in place of the starter ration bucket at feeding time and not in the place of the water bucket, hopefully this way they will learn to see it is a food replacement, not a water replacement.

Drinking water can help with rumen development as the oesophageal groove does not close when drinking water, so it enters the rumen. Here it helps to support the development of rumen microbial populations and rumen development. Water is essential to improve starter ration intake, with 5 L of water needing to be drunk for every 1 kg of starter consumed (35). It is also important if calves are fed high concentrations of CMR to allow correction of high osmolality.

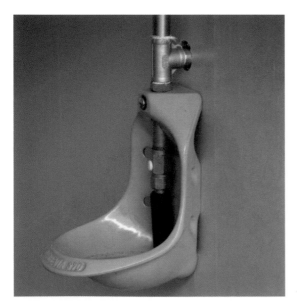

FIGURE 5.24 A small automatic water drinker.

REFERENCES

1. Silva AG, Huber JT, DeGregorio RM. Influence of substituting two types of soybean protein for milk protein on gain and utilisation of milk replacers in calves. J Dairy Sci 1986 Jan 1;69(1):172–80.

2. Nousianinen J. A high quality skim milk-whey-based milk replacer for calves. In: XXIII International Dairy Congress; 1990.

3. Maynou G, Bach A, Terré M. Feeding of waste milk to Holstein calves affects antimicrobial resistance of Escherichia coli and Pasteurella multocida isolated from fecal and nasal swabs. J Dairy Sci 2017 Apr 1;100(4):2682–94.

4. Kargar S, Roshan M, Ghoreishi SM, Akhlaghi A, Kanani M, Abedi Shams-Abadi AR, Ghaffari MH. Extended colostrum feeding for 2 weeks improves growth performance and reduces the susceptibility

to diarrhea and pneumonia in neonatal Holstein dairy calves. J Dairy Sci 2020 Sep 1;103(9):8130–42.

5. Timonen AAE, Autio T, Pohjanvirta T, Häkkinen L, Katholm J, Petersen A, et al. Dynamics of the within-herd prevalence of Mycoplasma bovis intramammary infection in endemically infected dairy herds. Vet Microbiol 2020 Mar 1;242:108608.

6. Cooper R, Watson I. A guide to feeding and assessment of calf milk replacer. Livestock 2013;18(6):216–22.

7. Stabel JR. On-farm batch pasteurization destroys Mycobacterium paratuberculosis in waste milk. J Dairy Sci 2001 Feb 1;84(2):524–7.

8. Stabel JR, Hurd S, Calvente L, Rosenbusch RF. Destruction of Mycobacterium paratuberculosis, Salmonella spp., and Mycoplasma spp. in raw milk by a commercial on-farm high-temperature, short-time pasteurizer. J Dairy Sci 2004 Jul 1;87(7):2177–83.

9. Elizondo-Salazar JA, Jones CM, Heinrichs AJ. Evaluation of calf milk pasteurization systems on 6 Pennsylvania dairy farms. J Dairy Sci 2010 Nov 1;93(11):5509–13.

10. Todd CG, Leslie KE, Millman ST, Bielmann V, Anderson NG, Sargeant JM, DeVries TJ. Clinical trial on the effects of a free-access acidified milk replacer feeding program on the health and growth of dairy replacement heifers and veal calves. J Dairy Sci 2017 Jan 1;100(1):713–25.

11. Jones C, Heinrichs J. Feeding acidified milk to calves. Penntate Extensions 2014. Available from: https://extension.psu.edu/feeding-acidified-milk-to-calves.

12. Teagasc. Feeding yoghurt milk is good for calves. Agriland; 2014. Available from: https://www.agri-land.ie/farming-news/feeding-yoghurt-milk-good-calves/.

13. National Research Council. Nutrient requirements of dairy cattle. National Academies Press; 2001.

14. Heinrichs AJ, Wells SJ, Losinger WC. A study of the use of milk replacers for dairy calves in the United States. J Dairy Sci 1995 Dec 1;78(12):2831–7.

15. Quigley J, Note C. Egg proteins in milk replacer-# 75; 2001. Available from: http://www.calfnotes.com.

16. Rauba J, Heins BJ, Chester-Jones H, Diaz HL, Ziegler D, Linn J, Broadwater N. Relationships between protein and energy consumed from milk replacer and starter and calf growth and first-lactation production of Holstein dairy cows. J Dairy Sci 2019 Jan 1;102(1):301–10.

17. Bascom SA, James RE, Mcgilliard ML, Van Amburgh M. Influence of dietary fat and protein on body composition of jersey bull calves. J Dairy Sci 2007 Dec 1;90(12):5600–9.

18. Hof G. An investigation into the extent to which various dietary components, particularly lactose, are related to the incidence of diarrhoea in milk-fed calves [Internet]; 1980. Available from: https://library.wur.nl/WebQuery/wurpubs/73586.

19. Berends H, van Laar H, Leal LN, Gerrits WJJ, Martín-Tereso J. Effects of exchanging lactose for fat in milk replacer on ad libitum feed intake and growth performance in dairy calves. J Dairy Sci 2020 May 1;103(5):4275–87.

20. Hill TM, Bateman HG, Aldrich JM, Schlotterbeck RL. Effects of fat concentration of a high-protein milk replacer on calf performance. J Dairy Sci 2009 Oct 1;92(10):5147–53.

21. National Research Council. Nutrient requirements of dairy cattle. 7th ed. National Academies Press; 2001.

22. Maynard LA, Norris LC. A system of rearing dairy calves with limited use of milk. J Dairy Sci 1923;6(5):483–99.

23. Knauer WA, Godden SM, McGuirk SM, Sorg J. Randomized clinical trial of the effect of a fixed or increasing milk allowance in the first 2 weeks of life on health and performance of dairy calves. J Dairy Sci 2018 Sep 1;101(9):8100–9.

24. Schäff CT, Gruse J, Maciej J, Pfuhl R, Zitnan R, Rajsky M, Hammon HM. Effects of feeding unlimited amounts of milk replacer for the first 5 weeks of age on rumen and small intestinal growth and development in dairy calves. J Dairy Sci 2018 Jan 1;101(1):783–93.

25. Sejrsen K, Huber JT, Tucker HA, Akers RM. Influence of nutrition on mammary development in pre and postpubertal heifers ~.

26. Molenaar AJ, Maclean PH, Gilmour ML, Draganova IG, Symes CW, Margerison JK, McMahon CD. Effect of whole-milk allowance on liveweight gain and growth of parenchyma and fat pads in the mammary glands of dairy heifers at weaning. J Dairy Sci 2020;103(6):5061–9.

27. Ellingsen K, Mejdell CM, Ottesen N, Larsen S, Grøndahl AM. The effect of large milk meals on

digestive physiology and behaviour in dairy calves. Physiol Behav 2016 Feb 1;154:169–74.

28. Ellingsen K, Mejdell CM, Ottesen N, Larsen S, Grøndahl AM. The effect of large milk meals on digestive physiology and behaviour in dairy calves. Physiol Behav 2016 Feb 1;154:169–74.

29. Garthwaite BD, Drackley JK, McCoy GC, Jaster EH. Whole milk and oral rehydration solution for calves with diarrhea of spontaneous origin. J Dairy Sci 1994 Mar 1;77(3):835–43.

30. Wise GH, Anderson GW. Factors affecting the passage of liquids into the rumen of the dairy calf. I. Method of administering liquids: Drinking from Open Pail versus sucking through a rubber nipple. J Dairy Sci 1939 Sep 1;22(9):697–705.

31. Appleby MC, Weary DM, Chua B. Performance and feeding behaviour of calves on ad libitum milk from artificial teats. Appl Anim Behav Sci 2001 Nov 5;74(3):191–201.

32. Cameron EZ. Is suckling behaviour a useful predictor of milk intake? A review. Anim Behav 1998 Sep 1;56(3):521–32.

33. De Paula Vieira A, Guesdon V, de Passillé AM, von Keyserlingk MAG, Weary DM. Behavioural indicators of hunger in dairy calves. Appl Anim Behav Sci 2008 Feb 1;109(2–4):180–9.

34. Sutherland MA, Lowe GL, Huddart FJ, Waas JR, Stewart M. Measurement of dairy calf behavior prior to onset of clinical disease and in response to disbudding using automated calf feeders and accelerometers. J Dairy Sci 2018 Sep 1;101(9):8208–16.

35. Cooke JS, earing focus: Bloat in young calves. Vet Irel J 2018;8(1):23–5.

36. Jorgensen MW, Adams-Progar A, De Passillé AM, Rushen J, Salfer JA, Endres MI. Mortality and health treatment rates of dairy calves in automated milk feeding systems in the Upper Midwest of the United States. J Dairy Sci 2017 Nov;100(11):9186–93. Available from: http://10.0.12.96/jds.2017–13198.

37. Medrano-Galarza C, LeBlanc SJ, DeVries TJ, Jones-Bitton A, Rushen J, Marie de Passillé A, et al. Effect of age of introduction to an automated milk feeder on calf learning and performance and labor requirements. J Dairy Sci 2018 Oct 1;101(10):9371–84.

38. Bach A, Ahedo J, Ferrer A. Optimizing weaning strategies of dairy replacement calves. J Dairy Sci 2010 Jan 1;93(1):413–9.

39. Hosseini SH, Mirzaei-Alamouti H, Vazirigohar M, Mahjoubi E, Rezamand P. Effects of whole milk feeding rate and straw level of starter feed on performance, rumen fermentation, blood metabolites, structural growth, and feeding behavior of Holstein calves. Anim Feed Sci Technol 2019 Aug 1;255. 114238.

40. Jasper J, Weary DM. Effects of ad libitum milk intake on dairy calves. J Dairy Sci 2002 Nov 1;85(11): 3054–8.

41. Xiao J, Alugongo GM, Li J, Wang Y, Li S, Cao Z. Review: How forage feeding early in life influences the growth rate, ruminal environment, and the establishment of feeding behavior in pre-weaned calves [Internet]. Animals (Basel). MDPI A./G. 2020;10(2):188.

42. Grove-White D. Rumen healthcare in the dairy cow. In Pract 2004;26(2):88–95.

43. Bach A. Effective forage and starter feeding strategies for preweaned calves. WCDS advances in dairy technology 2014.

44. Castells L, Bach A, Araujo G, Montoro C, Terré M. Effect of different forage sources on performance and feeding behavior of Holstein calves. J Dairy Sci 2012 Jan;95(1):286–93.

45. Kertz AF, Reutzel LF, Mahoney JH. Ad libitum water intake by neonatal calves and its relationship to calf starter intake, weight gain, feces score, and season. J Dairy Sci 1984 Dec 1;67(12):2964–9.

Chapter 6

Monitoring growth and the weaning period

Nicola Blackie and Claire Wathes

CHAPTER CONTENTS

The effectiveness of a farm's current management system can be evaluated by monitoring factors such as morbidity, mortality and calf growth rates. Growth rates can give a real-time indicator of calf health, and it is also important to know how well a calf has grown prior to making the decision to wean them. Weaning is a stressful time for a calf, but signals the progression to a ruminant and therefore a change in their management. Getting weaning correct is key to a smooth transition from liquid to solid feed, and allows the calf to sustain its growth rates in the most efficient manner possible.

MONITORING GROWTH

Consistently good growth rates are extremely important when rearing dairy heifers as this enables them to achieve their full genetic potential. The optimum age at first calving (AFC) in terms of their future milk yield, fertility and longevity is around 24 months (1, 2). The most important of these measures with respect to profitability are life-time yield (LTY) and milk produced per day of life (Figure 6.1).

Achieving first calving by 24 months of age also significantly reduces rearing costs. A UK based study completed in 2016 calculated that the cost of rearing a heifer increases by £2.87 per day for every day increase in AFC over 24 months (3). Most adult cows only start to generate an overall profit for the herd about halfway through their second lactation. To reach the breakeven point they have to earn back their own rearing costs from birth.

Heifers should reach their AFC at about 90% of mature bodyweight with sufficient skeletal growth,

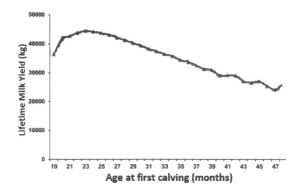

FIGURE 6.1 Relationship between AFC and lifetime milk yield (LTY). Data were derived from 169,443 Holstein heifers joining the UK milking herd between 1996–1998. The peak LTY values were achieved by heifers calving at around 24 months of age, whereas those calving for the first time at 36 months produced on average 6400 kg less milk in their lifetimes.

but without excess body condition as this helps to reduce the risk of dystocia (see Chapter 2). The rate of growth during the rearing period has a direct effect on AFC (4, 5). Growth is at its most efficient in the first 2 months of life, so high growth rates should be targeted during milk feeding. Body size is a major determinant of the age at which an animal reaches puberty (6). Conception rates are improved if heifers have experienced at least one complete oestrous cycle before breeding begins, as this ensures that the reproductive tract is sufficiently mature. In order to achieve an average AFC of 24 months, services must start from about 13.5 months. This requires that all heifers should reach puberty by 1 year of age. Younger heifers also have better fertility, providing another benefit for good early growth. One UK study found that when Holstein-Friesian heifers received a first service at 13 to 14 months of age their conception rate was 84%, compared with only 51% for those not served for the first time until 17 months (7).

The main determinant of growth rate is the feed intake, but it is also influenced by genotype and disease, notably being slowed by episodes of respiratory disease or diarrhoea (8). Aspects of the housing and environment are also influential – for example, the extent to which groups of calves are mixed and seasonal variations in temperature. On farm studies have shown considerable variations in growth rates not only between farms, but also between animals on the same farm (5, 8). It is therefore important to identify the animals that are underperforming at an early stage so that remedial action can be taken. This requires that individual growth rates are monitored routinely.

Benefits of monitoring growth rate

- Achieve target weight/height for breeding.
- Maximise growth efficiency cost effectively.
- Identify underperforming and sick calves.
- Identify problems within your system (e.g. suboptimal environment).
- Helps to decide which heifers to keep for breeding and the most profitable time point to sell or slaughter the remainder.

In summary, it is not possible to manage something reliably unless it has been measured. Monitoring growth from birth can guide continual management improvements so that every heifer is in calf by 15 months of age. Regular weighing helps to ensure that the input of resources, in particular feed, are optimised to ensure that profits are maximised. This is key to running a successful and profitable business.

How to monitor growth

There are a number of ways to monitor growth. This should be undertaken at regular intervals between birth and first calving, but for convenience the precise timing can often be combined with other tasks, such as vaccination or worming. This also facilitates accurate dosing of any medications that are size-dependent. The following ages/stages are ideal.

- Birthweight – to create a baseline figure. If this is not possible, an average of 40 kg for Holstein-Friesian (HF) calves may be used.
- Weaning – to check that they are ready to be weaned.
- 1–2 weeks post-weaning – to assess the extent of any post-weaning growth check.
- 6 months of age – to allow time for remedial action before breeding.
- Pre-breeding – to ensure that an adequate size has been achieved.

It is often useful to record additional information at the same time. For example, when the birth weight is recorded then details of the calving process and colostrum intake can also be added. It does not matter which method is used to monitor growth as long as regular measurements are taken using the same method each time. This allows benchmarking of the herd performance between groups.

A growth rate can only be calculated when at least two measurements of the same animal have been made. The average daily gain (ADG) is then calculated by subtracting the earliest recording from the later recording and dividing by the number of days between. For example, if a calf has a birth weight of 40 kg, and weighs 80 kg when weaned at 8 weeks of age, the ADG in weight is: (80 – 40) / 56. This works out as an ADG of 0.71 kg/day during the pre-weaned period.

Measuring weight

This can be done using either weigh scales or a weigh band. The aim should be for the whole process to be as quick and easy as possible and to avoid stressing the animals. Done calmly, it will provide good training for handling in later life.

Electronic scales are the most accurate. These should be calibrated using a known weight, such as a feed bag, before each session. Newer electronic animal weigh scales can be equipped with a radio-frequency identification (RFID) antenna, which enables the weights to be recorded and stored automatically.

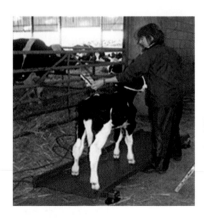

FIGURE 6.2 Weighing a young calf on a metal platform supported by load bars.

Load bars

Load bars are at the cheaper end of the spectrum but are both accurate and readily portable (e.g. to a field location for older animals). They need to be set up on a level surface with a strong, non-slip platform for the animal to stand on, or an existing crush can be used. Younger calves can be halter led (Figure 6.2), but older ones will require a race, which can be made using hurdles.

Calf weigh scales

Specially designed calf weigh units are available. These should have a low entry height, non-slip flooring and doors at each end which can easily be opened and closed from one position. Other possible features are wheels for portability and an integrated battery to ensure a reliable power supply.

Automatic scales associated with automatic milk feeders

Automatic electronic half-body animal scales can be integrated into the feeding box. The calf stands its front legs on the scales while feeding and its weight is then logged automatically. This system has two key advantages. First, it provides a daily reading of weight, allowing accurate assessment of ADGs and rapid identification of any animal that is losing weight, possibly due to diarrhoea. Second, it has the capacity to allocate the calf with an individualised quantity of milk, based on its needs. The feeder can be programmed to wean calves on the basis of their individual weight development. These aids facilitate health management and optimisation of milk provision.

Weigh bands

Weigh bands are the cheapest way of recording approximate calf weights (Figure 6.3). The tape is placed around the chest of the calf just behind the front leg and shoulder blade: it must be flat against the skin and held at a consistent tightness ensuring it is not twisted. The calf should also have its head level with its back – having the head lower to the ground can artificially increase the apparent weight of the calf. This is the easiest and quickest way to weigh pre-weaned calves that are

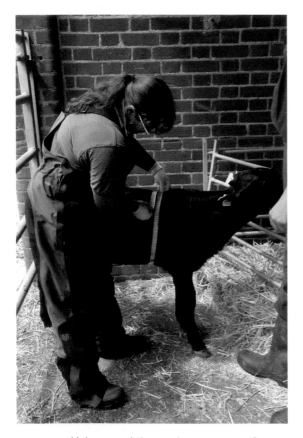

FIGURE 6.3 Using a weigh tape in a young calf.

being kept in individual or small group pens as it avoids the need to take them out of their housing. Providing the procedure is performed carefully, then the estimated weight in young calves is highly correlated with the actual weight ($r^2 = 0.9$ (8)). The method becomes less suitable post-weaning as the animals are usually kept in larger pens and it becomes increasingly hard to perform reliably and safely as they become stronger and more active.

Measuring height

Height is another useful measurement to take, either in addition to or instead of weight (Figure 6.4). Having both enables the farmer to calculate the ponderal index (PI). This determines the relationship between body mass and skeletal size, providing a measure of leanness and showing whether weight and height gain are proportional. In human medicine the PI is widely used to assess children's growth. In calves it is defined as weight (kg) / height (m)^3 (9). Some calves which are poorly grown pre-weaning may later put on extra weight, mainly as fat. This results in short, fat animals, which may meet the weight targets for breeding but have insufficient skeletal growth, making them prone to issues around calving.

For calves in individual pens' height can be measured with reasonable accuracy using a metal tape measure. Alternatively, a measuring stick is placed across the withers or rump while the animal is standing on a flat surface, in the absence of any underfoot bedding material (Figure 6.5). For older animals, it is possible to obtain a reasonably reliable assessment by walking them past fixed height markers on the wall of the building, or by using the bars on a race.

Pelvic measurements

Pelvic measurements are another useful tool to measure growth. These should be performed by a vet on a single occasion as part of a pre-breeding check a few weeks prior to service (Figure 6.6). A

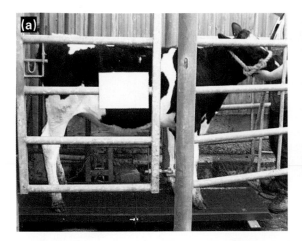
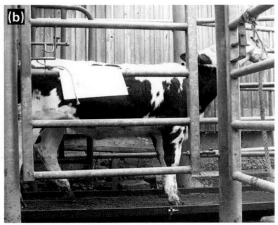

FIGURE 6.4 Measuring 6-month-old heifer calves on the same farm: the animal in (a) has good bone growth, but that in (b) is much shorter, equivalent to one fewer bar on the side of the crush.

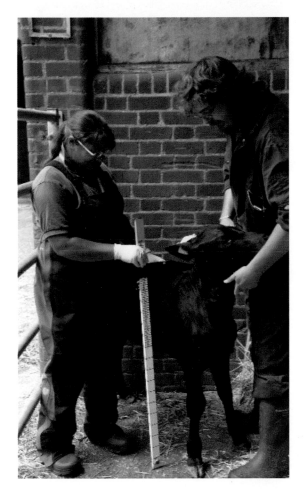

FIGURE 6.5 Using a height stick across the withers on a pre-weaned calf.

sliding calliper device is inserted into the rectum. The width and height of the pelvis are measured and multiplied together to give the pelvic cross-sectional area. The measurement then needs to be adjusted for weight and age. The pelvic area is a useful predictor of the likelihood of future calving problems and may be used to inform which heifers to breed from and the best choice of semen.

The reproductive tract can be examined at the same time to check the ovaries and uterus and assess whether puberty has occurred (Table 6.1) (10). This will also identify any freemartins that are still present.

What to do with the growth measurements

In order to be useful, the growth measurements need to be imported into a spreadsheet to facilitate subsequent analysis. Depending on the setup used, this may happen automatically or require transfer from another device. Many farms now use electronic identification (EID) tags. These enable the operator to identify an individual animal accurately and quickly, and eliminates the need to enter ear tag numbers manually. Growth records can be analysed using Excel, avoiding the purchase of specialist software.

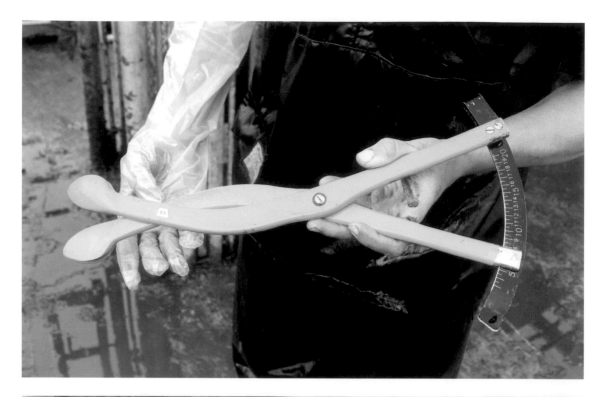

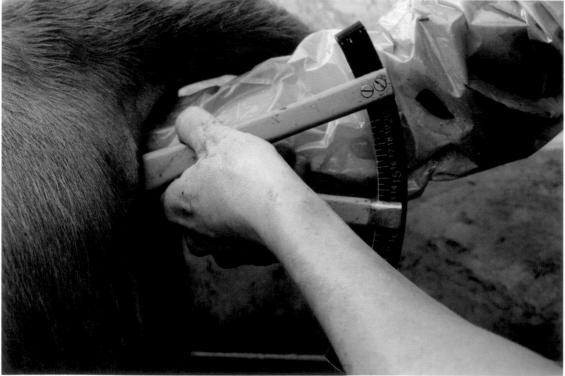

FIGURE 6.6 Calipers used for pelvic measurements. Photos by kind permission of Aly Balsom.

TABLE 6.1 Use of reproductive tract scoring to assess whether heifers are ready for breeding (RTS 4 or 5). CL indicates a corpus luteum.

Reproductive tract score	Follicle size	Uterine horn diameter and tone
1	None	<20 mm, no tone
2	8 mm	20–25 mm, no tone
3	8–10 mm	25–30 mm, slight tone
4	>10 mm, may have CL	30 mm, good tone
5	>10 mm +CL	>30 mm, good tone, erect

TABLE 6.2 Calculations of target weight gains at different ages for a herd of Holstein cows with a mature bodyweight of 680 kg and a mature shoulder height of 145 cm.

Age in months	Stage	Ideal % of mature weight	Ideal % of mature height	Optimum weight (kg)	Optimum height (cm)	Target growth rate (kg/d)
0	Birth			40	78	
3	Post-weaning	17	63	115	91	0.82
6[a]		28	74	190	107	0.82
14	Breeding	55	87	374	126	0.76
24	Calving	90	96	612	139	0.78

Note: [a]Knowing the size accurately at 6 months of age allows time before breeding to take remedial action for any underperforming calves.

The first important step is to calculate the target growth rates (Table 6.2). These will depend on the breed and type, so it is necessary to establish the normal adult size for the cows in the herd. This requires measuring several adult cows (lactations ≥3) at different stages in their lactation to obtain an average. Once this is done, the target weights (or heights) to be reached at key stage are calculated, based on the optimum percentage of adult size. It is then easy to establish how much needs to be gained per day to reach this stage.

It is worth noting that in pre-weaning calves, although feed conversion efficiency is high in the first few weeks of life, in practice growth rates are often low, even with very good management and care, as the calf settles into its feeding behaviours and routines (Figure 6.7). This must be remembered if more frequent weights are taken as results may appear disappointing. However, if measurements of growth are just taken at birth and weaning, the average figure will be easier to interpret.

Decision making using growth data

For the average Holstein heifer to calve at 24 months, she needs to be growing at an average of 0.78 kg/day throughout the entire rearing period. If growth rates are too low then a nutritionist or vet should be consulted for advice. Young animals convert feed into growth most efficiently during the first 2 months of their life, but growth rates will vary according to the energy and protein

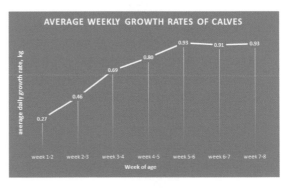

FIGURE 6.7 An example of weekly growth rates achieved by calves in the first few weeks of life.

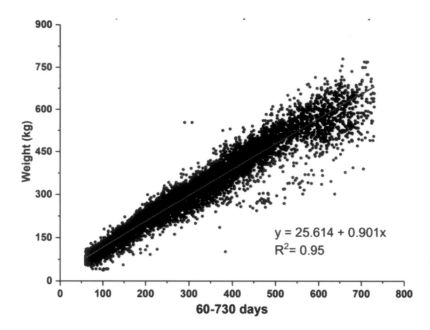

$$y = 25.614 + 0.901x$$
$$R^2 = 0.95$$

60-730 days

FIGURE 6.8 Plot of individual weight measurements from a single herd of Holstein heifers showing a linear increase between weaning and calving.

contents of the milk and the volume and frequency with which it is supplied (see Chapter 5). Weaning is another important time which may result in a growth check if not well managed. Overall it is important to maximise weight gain without creating over-fat heifers and to minimise the size variation within the group.

In terms of analysis, at its simplest, individual size measurements at different ages can be plotted (Figure 6.8). This will show the overall growth rate and identify any outlying animals, mainly those which are too small for their age. There is, however, some evidence that overfed animals may also be less fertile possibly due to poor oocyte quality in over-fat heifers, although the reason(s) remains to be determined conclusively (2). These plots can also be used to compare growth rates between different stages of development in the same batch of heifers. For example, weight increases are often low in the first 3 weeks of life (11), or may reduce significantly if animals are outwintered with insufficient forage availability. It is also possible to make comparisons between batches and use this to assess, for example, a change in feeding regime or housing system.

It should be noted that the pattern of growth differs for weight and height (Figure 6.9). The weight

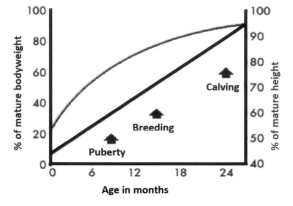

FIGURE 6.9 Target growth for specific time points in a heifer's life.

increase should remain approximately linear from pre-weaning until calving. In contrast, height is mainly influenced by elongation of the long bones due to the formation of new cartilage at the epiphyseal plates (also known as growth plates). The cartilage then becomes ossified, resulting in new bone development. This process is most rapid during early to mid-puberty, when the pubertal growth spurt is occurring. The growth velocity then slows down and will cease altogether once all the growth plates have fused. The important consequence of this is that deficiencies in bone growth before puberty cannot be compensated for in older animals.

WEANING

It is well documented that a calf's rumen develops over time, slowly taking over the role of the abomasum where digestion of milk occurs in the pre-ruminant. The reticulorumen makes up 64% of the stomach volume by 4 weeks of age and increases to 75% at 12 weeks – in an adult cow the reticulorumen volume is 87% (12). Concentrate feed and fibrous feed stuffs are key to helping develop the rumen. Concentrate (starter) feed drives epithelial development of the rumen and the fibrous feeds stretch the rumen and so promote muscularity and volume. Therefore, when considering this transition from pre-ruminant to a fully functioning ruminant, we need to consider the age at which the calf is weaned and whether the rumen is functioning sufficiently at that stage. It has been shown that significant changes in rumen and intestinal microbiota occur at weaning (13), but interestingly these changes are independent of the weaning method used. The age at which calves start to ruminate also varies, but studies have shown that most calves start ruminating from 2 weeks of age (14, 15).

When we consider the gastrointestinal physiology of a young calf, we should consider what the gold standard should be. The most natural calf rearing situation is seen in a suckler beef calf. These calves have much higher growth rates and later weaning at 6–7 months of age than that which is practised on dairy farms. Indeed, early studies showed that under natural conditions calves are weaned between 8.8 and 11.3 months of age and before that suckle around five times a day for approximately 9 minutes at a time (16). Other studies have confirmed the suckling frequency in beef animals of being around five times a day with a duration of 9–12 minutes per bout (17–19). Calves fed by a cow will consume up to 12 L/day across several meals and would be weaned gradually (20). Calves on automatic feeders given ad lib milk follow a similar intake amount (21, 22) and pattern with around 4–9 meals a day (22–24). Therefore, we do need to take this into account when it comes to weaning calves, particularly those on high milk levels.

METHODS OF WEANING

Abrupt weaning (removal of milk feeding either with very few days or no prior reduction in volume) should be avoided as it is very stressful to the calves (25) and does not prepare them for a diet based solely on solid feeds (26, 27). In addition, abruptly weaned calves have a higher incidence of cross suckling straight after weaning which may lead to development of blind quarters in heifers (30).

Step/gradual versus abrupt

Step or gradual weaning can be defined as reducing the milk intakes of the calves over a period of time (Figure 6.10). Step weaning allows the gastrointestinal tract to adjust better to the change in diet, resulting in improved diet digestibility after weaning (29) as the rumen is better able to utilise the fibre and concentrate diet more efficiently. Post-weaning growth rates are also higher in calves which are step weaned (28) compared with abrupt weaning.

There is a huge range in the length of the period and the size of the 'steps' in this process, with too short a period (<7 days) having a negative impact on performance and concentrate intakes. In one study where calves drinking 12 L milk/day, they were gradually weaned over 4, 10, 22 days. They found that gradually weaning over 10 days was most favourable in terms of weight gains (although it should be noted these calves were weaned relatively early at 6 weeks of age) (31). In the authors' experience, weaning over a 14-day (2-week) period works well.

When feeding calves manually, the volumes fed should be gradually reduced, with an example

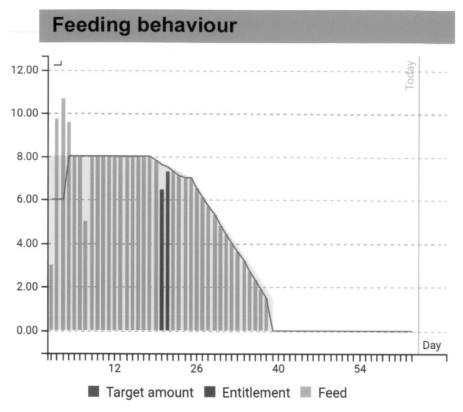

FIGURE 6.10 Computerised calf feeder weaning plan for a calf showing a gradual reduction in milk allowance.

scheme given in Table 6.3. This process can be more gradual in automatic milk feeding systems where the computer is able to manipulate milk volumes in smaller increments than is possible to do by hand feeding.

Dilution weaning

In ad lib milk feeding systems that are not controlled by a computer, weaning by reducing volume is not possible as this will just result in some calves not having access to milk while others can still drink large volumes. Weaning in these systems can be done by diluting the milk (21). This has been proven to work, with one study showing that calves fed whole milk diluted with water prior to weaning ate twice as much concentrates prior to weaning than calves fed un-diluted milk (25). The reduction

in energy that is consumed in diluted milk leads the calf to have an unfulfilled appetite, and so encourages the calves to increase the amount of concentrate they eat. Similar to the step weaning method described above, the dilution of the milk should be gradually decreased over a 2-week period, so at the end of weaning the calves will only be offered water through the teats.

Methods of reducing milk intake to ease weaning transition:
- reduce the amount of milk offered over time
- reduce the number of feeds/day
- dilute the milk replacer with water and offer same volume with reduced milk powder.

TABLE 6.3 An example manual feeding programme for weaning calves over a 14 day period. The second column gives an example feeding scheme for twice daily manual feeding, which reduces the milk volume fed. The third column gives an example on reducing the calf milk replacer (CMR) concentration fed in ad-lib systems where control of volumes consumed is difficult.

Days into weaning programme	Volume fed in AM and PM (L) in a manual feeding system.	Concentration of CMR fed in ad lib system (g/L)
−1	4, 4	150
1	3, 3	130
2	3, 3	130
3	2.5, 2.5	110
4	2.5, 2.5	110
5	2, 2	110
6	2, 2	90
7	1.5, 1.5	90
8	1.5, 1.5	80
9	1, 1	80
10	1, 1	60
11	1, 0	60
12	1, 0	40
13	0.5, 0	40
14	0.5, 0	0

WHEN TO WEAN

Historically farmers used to wean calves off milk at a very young age (6 weeks) age, without any regard for the biological development of the rumen. Growth is most efficient in the milk fed phase, therefore investing more at this stage is likely to pay off with improved growth and potential milk production in lactation. In studies where calves fed high levels of milk (stepped up to 8.5 L/day) and were weaned at 75 days (10.7 weeks) compared with 60 days (8.5 weeks), they showed improved concentrate intakes and weight gains through weaning (32). Weaning later (8 weeks) in comparison to early weaning (6 weeks) has also been shown to create a more gradual shift in the gut microbiota which is beneficial for a healthy rumen (33).

Weaning correctly has positive benefits to the calves, particularly in terms of maintaining stable growth rates and a healthy immune status. Calves have been shown to start eating concentrate feed (at least 40 g/day) at around 36 days of age (34),

however, this can range from 18 to 75 days of age depending on the system. Similarly, calves reached 200 g/day concentrate intake at an average 55 days of age with a range of 23–82 days of age (35). This demonstrates that calves require time to reach concentrate intakes that are capable of meeting their nutritional intakes (which is approximately 1.5–2 kg per day), and will influence when it is appropriate to wean these calves.

Traditional targets for calves to be off milk is for them to be consuming at least 1 kg of concentrate/day for 3 consecutive days. There are multiple studies that have looked at the ages that this might happen when the calves were fed on high levels of milk (12 L/head/day) prior to weaning. They found that calves who were required to consume at least 1.4 kg/day of concentrates for 3 consecutive days were 76 days of age (range: 58–94 days) by the time they were able to do this (35, 36). Delaying weaning from 47 days to 89 days of age for calves on 12 L/day milk resulted in less behavioural indicators of hunger at weaning (38). In another study, calves were fed less milk (6 L/day) and weaned according to concentrate consumption on an individual basis; calves were 65 days of age when milk feeding was stopped (39). These data would suggest that a minimum age would be 8 weeks, with 10 weeks or older being preferable for calves to be fully weaned and off milk. It is also very evident that there is a lot of individual variation and so weaning age should be flexible where possible. In terms of a target concentrate intake for calves to be consuming prior to milk feeding being stopped, it is now recommended that a target of 1.5 – 2 kg of concentrates should be consumed for 3 consecutive days.

ACIDOSIS

There is a considerable volume of work looking at whether calves can develop acidosis. Acidosis in the adult ruminant is well documented and sub-acute ruminal acidosis (SARA) is thought to occur when the rumen pH level is below 5.8 for at least 6 hours per day. In adult cattle, 11–26% of cows suffer from SARA (40–42). There is now evidence that would suggest that this can occur in young calves as well.

Inappropriate weaning techniques can result in very low rumen pH levels. This occurs when the calf ingests excess levels of concentrate, resulting in high levels of short chain fatty acids in the rumen. If weaning occurs at too young an age prior to the rumen becoming fully developed, or if weaning occurs over too short a period of time, the rapid increase in concentrate ingestion results in this acidotic state. This is turn can increase the risk of frothy bloat, as well as being associated with development of a leaky rumen and intestines which can result in systemic inflammation from endotoxins entering the blood stream from the rumen.

Fibre can help to improve the rumen pH level by promoting saliva production that will buffer the rumen content. The provision of hay has also been shown to improve rumen conditions over the weaning transition, with increased hay intake leading to a higher and thus beneficial rumen pH (43).

MAXIMISING CONCENTRATE (STARTER) FEED INTAKE PRIOR TO WEANING

Maximising concentrate intake prior to weaning is important to a smooth weaning transition. A recent study compared gradual and abrupt weaning alongside concentrate intake. Where calves had low concentrate intake prior to weaning, gradual weaning did not improve performance. Therefore, maximising concentrate intake prior to weaning is key. Calves with high concentrate intakes at 5 weeks of age maintained this advantage through weaning and had higher overall weight gains. In this study, gradually weaned calves did spend more time eating concentrate; however, this did not equate to increased intake of concentrate (44). This is in agreement with a further study that also found that pre-weaning concentrate intake could predict a successful weaning transition – this is more evident when calves are fed low levels of milk (45).

One of the challenges when it comes to maximising concentrate intake is with calves that are consuming high levels of milk prior to weaning. This requires a more gradual change between milk and concentrate. Automatic feeders can be useful in this situation as calves can be fed on a curve of increasing milk over time before reaching a peak and then gradually reducing prior to weaning. Gradually reducing milk provisions can help to encourage calves to consume more concentrates. Also, as already discussed, the age of the calves will have an impact on concentrate intake.

Other ways to encourage calves to consume concentrate may be to place small amounts in the bottom of the bucket (if bucket fed) or to offer feeds with novel textures.

A study looked at where the calves were offered concentrates within their pen when fed on an automatic milk feeding system. When concentrates

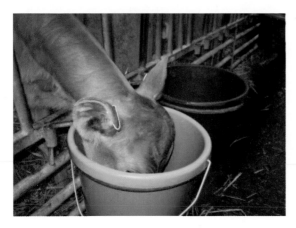

FIGURE 6.11 Calf investigating bucket after milk feed.

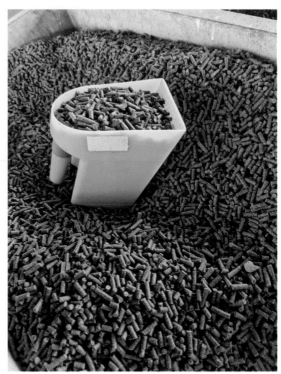

FIGURE 6.12 Calibrated feed scoop that provides a known quantity of concentrate feed to help monitor feed intakes.

were fed next to the milk feeder, there was increased concentrate and water intake compared to when the concentrate was at the back of the pen (46). Anecdotally, calves on restricted milk feeding often look for more food when they have consumed their milk, and so placing the concentrate close to where the milk feeding takes place is likely to improve intakes and thus weaning performance. Be aware that calves that are 'slow learners' when taught to use automatic feeders have been shown to wean later when based on concentrate intake (36).

Concentrate feed composition should remain the same through the process of weaning as this will likely result in a smoother transition as the feed is familiar to the calves. Individually housed calves can have worse neophobic reactions and so vigilance should be exercised. Feed quality should be maintained after weaning, with evidence that poor energy density in rations pre-weaning leads to increased incidence of cross sucking in calves (47).

Measuring starter feed intake

Historical advice was that a calf should be consuming at least 1 kg of concentrate feed per day prior to weaning, but this level is actually quite low in terms of being able to deliver the energy requirements of the calf. A better recommendation is that 1.5–2.0 kg intake per day is preferred for weaning criteria. Measuring this can be done in a number of ways such as physically weighing the feed, or by using a calibrated scoop/bucket (Figure 6.12).

A novel method is to evaluate circulating β-hydroxybutyrate (BHB) levels in the blood; this was shown to have promise as a pen-side test to predict a 3-day average concentrate intake of 1 kg/day when blood levels exceeded 0.2 mmol/L (48). With group housed calves it is particularly important to assess whether every calf in the group is getting sufficient concentrate. Testing BHB levels could be undertaken to assess whether calves are ready for weaning or as a cross-sectional retrospective sample to check rumen function after weaning and therefore assess the ease of transition.

Fibrous foods

As mentioned in Chapter 5, forage should be available to calves prior to weaning. This can be in the form of good quality straw or hay. A review showed that forage availability has variable effects on calf concentrate intakes (49), but where calves were fed high levels of milk (20% of birthweight), offering chopped hay resulted in improved ruminal conditions (higher pH) (50). These calves also consumed more DM (concentrate and hay) than calves which were not provided with hay (50). This effect was also seen in another study in which calves were offered concentrate plus chopped hay and ate more solid feed in the week prior to weaning than those offered concentrates alone (51). These calves also tended to have an increased weight gain at weaning.

There is increased interest in 'blended' diets for calves, with chopped hay or straw being incorporated alongside concentrate feeds for older calves around the time of weaning (Figure 6.13). Care

should be taken to use dust-extracted chopped forage or consider the inclusion of molasses to limit dust.

Whatever the source of fibre provided, it should remain the same over the weaning period to reduce nutritional stress to the calf. If a new fibre source is to be fed in the post-weaning phase, this should either be introduced prior to the weaning period, or be introduced a month or more after weaning once the calf has acclimatised to a purely solid feed diet.

FACTORS THAT MIGHT INFLUENCE THE WEANING TRANSITION

Housing prior to weaning

Prior interaction with other calves may influence the calves' behaviour over weaning. Social

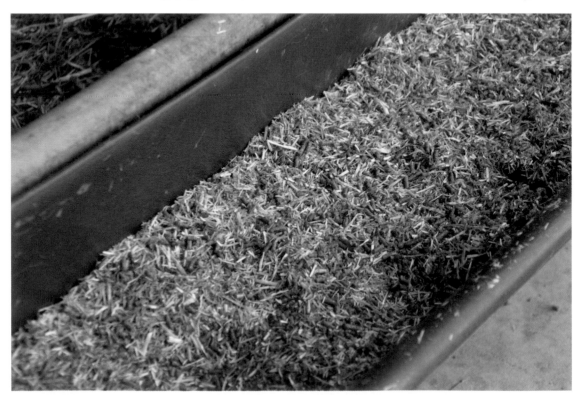

FIGURE 6.13 Trough containing finely chopped straw mixed with the concentrate.

facilitation of behaviour undoubtedly occurs and this can also positively influence welfare. Pair housing has been shown to ease the transition over weaning (52), with less vocalisations at weaning (53) and increased feed intakes and meal number in the week prior to weaning (54) from pair housed calves compared with individually housed calves. Pair housed calves have also been shown to have greater concentrate intake during the weaning period compared to individually housed calves (52, 54, 55). Calves form lasting relationships at an early age (less than 3.5 months of age) (56). Therefore, it may be beneficial to allow them to mix before this age. In addition, a study has shown that housing calves with an older (weaned) companion results in a smoother weaning transition with improved growth rates and influenced feeding behaviour positively (57) compared with calves housed with just similarly aged calves. However, this could have disease impacts with mixing of calves of different ages so care should be taken with this approach.

What time of day to wean/move?

In many situations, mixing animals or changing routines seems to cause least disruption if done in the evening rather than the morning. This is the case with mixing heifers into the milking herd, for example (58). Calves feed significantly fewer times in the dark (23) compared to the light, therefore removing the evening meal may be more natural when weaning. Moving and transport is a stressful experience for the calves, as is the weaning process itself (as shown by increased levels of cortisol indicating stress (59, 60)). It is therefore best if calves are fully weaned and left in their pen for at least 1 week prior to moving them. Castration or dis-budding should also not be done at the same time as weaning as this will compound the stress effect.

Mixing calves

Calves may experience disruption when they are mixed. However, this has been shown to be less of an impact than is seen in adult cattle (60). A study following individual calves mixed into an established group of calves on an automatic feeder found that calves showed alterations in their feeding behaviour on the day of mixing, however, this did not affect milk intake (27). As previously mentioned, calves that have been housed in pairs or small groups are likely to find mixing less stressful than those housed individually prior to weaning. Providing areas for the calves to get away from others in group situations may also help. This can be as simple as dividers on the feeder or bales within the pen (Figure 6.14). The provision of enrichment articles can also help to divert the calves' focus. Hanging balls or brushes are popular with calves, just ensure they are robust and easy to clean.

DRINKING WATER

Drinking water is a legal requirement for calves and should be freely available. This is especially important over the weaning period (35, 62) and after weaning (62–64) when calves will drink more, potentially compensating for the removal of milk. This is more evident in calves fed high amounts of milk pre-weaning.

Water intake is shown to correlate with concentrate intake and thus weight gains (65). Calves show reduced weight gains and had a 31% reduction in concentrate intake when they were not offered water (66). There is also evidence that offering water from birth compared to day 17 improves the richness of the gut microbiota (63) and leads to higher bodyweights at 5 months of age (62).

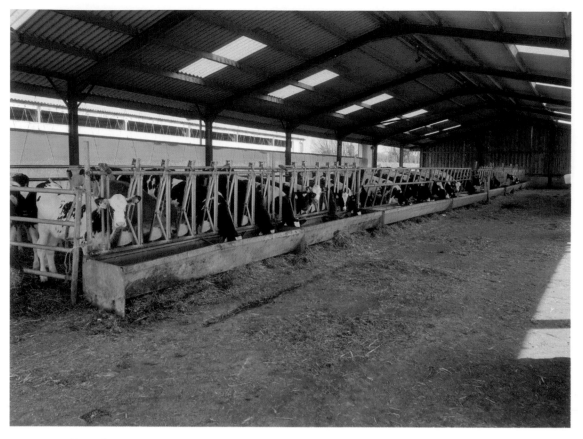

FIGURE 6.14 Use of locking head yokes for feeding weaned calves can help reduce competition and bullying over food.

Hints and tips

- Check that calves are consuming at least 1.5–2 kg of concentrate per day for at least 3 consecutive days prior to weaning.
- Offer appropriate fibrous feeds.
- Consider weaning later (10–12 weeks of age) if your system allows.
- Avoid any growth check – it is possible to wean calves without any loss in growth rate.
- Consider your housing method prior to weaning as this might impact the weaning transition.
- Minimise weaning stress.

- Provide the calves with a comfortable and enriched environment throughout.
- Ensure sufficient clean water is available at the correct height.
- Be flexible – calves will vary a lot!

REFERENCES

1. Bach A. Associations between several aspects of heifer development and dairy cow survivability to second lactation. J Dairy Sci 2011 Feb;94(2):1052–7.
2. Wathes DC, Pollott GE, Johnson KF, Richardson H, Cooke JS. Heifer fertility and carry over consequences for life time production in dairy and beef cattle. Animal 2014;8(suppl. 1):91–104.

3. Boulton AC, Rushton J, Wathes DC. An empirical analysis of the cost of rearing dairy heifers from birth to first calving and the time taken to repay these costs. Animal 2017;11(8):1372–80.

4. Heinrichs AJ. Raising dairy replacements to meet the needs of the 21st century. J Dairy Sci 1993;76(10):3179–87.

5. Brickell JS, McGowan MM, Pfeiffer DU, Wathes DC. Mortality in Holstein-Friesian calves and replacement heifers, in relation to body weight and I.G.F.-I concentration, on 19 farms in England. Animal 2009;3(8):1175–82.

6. Macdonald KA, Penno JW, Bryant AM, Roche JR. Effect of feeding level pre- and post-puberty and body weight at first calving on growth, milk production, and fertility in grazing dairy cows. J Dairy Sci 2005;88(9):3363–75.

7. Cooke JS, Wathes DC. Rearing heifer calves for optimum lifelong production. PhD thesis. 2014.

8. Johnson KF, Chancellor N, Burn CC, Wathes DC. Analysis of pre-weaning feeding policies and other risk factors influencing growth rates in calves on 11 commercial dairy farms. Animal 2018 Jul 1;12(7):1413–23.

9. Swali A, Wathes DC. Influence of primiparity on size at birth, growth, the somatotrophic axis and fertility in dairy heifers. Anim Reprod Sci 2007 Nov;102(1–2):122–36.

10. Holm L, Jensen MB, Jeppesen LL. Calves' motivation for access to two different types of social contact measured by operant conditioning. Appl Anim Behav Sci 2002 Nov 1;79(3):175–94.

11. Bazeley KJ, Barrett DC, Williams PD, Reyher KK. Measuring the growth rate of UK dairy heifers to improve future productivity. Vet J 2016 Jun 1;212: 9–14.

12. Huber JT. Development of the digestive and metabolic apparatus of the calf. J Dairy Sci 1969 Aug 1;52(8):1303–15.

13. Meale SJ, Li S, Azevedo P, Derakhshani H, Plaizier JC, Khafipour E, et al. Development of ruminal and fecal microbiomes are affected by weaning but not weaning strategy in dairy calves. Front Microbiol 2016;7(MAY).

14. Swanson EW, Harris JD. Development of rumination in the young calf. J Dairy Sci 1958 Dec 1;41(12):1768–76.

15. Lopreiato V, Minuti A, Cappelli FP, Vailati-Riboni M, Britti D, Trevisi E, Morittu VM. Daily rumination pattern recorded by an automatic rumination-monitoring system in pre-weaned calves fed whole bulk milk and ad libitum calf starter. Livest Sci 2018 Jun 1;212:127–30.

16. Reinhardt V, Reinhardt A. Natural sucking performance and age of weaning in zebu cattle (Bos indicus). J Agric Sci 1981;96(2):309–12.

17. Lewandrowski NM, Hurnik JF. Nursing and cross-nursing behavior of beef cattle in confinement. Can J Anim Sci 1983 Dec 1;63(4):849–53.

18. Kour H, Patison KP, Corbet NJ, Swain DL. Validation of accelerometer use to measure suckling behaviour in Northern Australian beef calves. Appl Anim Behav Sci 2018 May 1;202:1–6.

19. Alvarez-Rodriguez J, Palacio J, Casasús I, Revilla R, Sanz A. Performance and nursing behaviour of beef cows with different types of calf management. Animal 2009 Jun;3(6):871–8.

20. Khan MA, Weary DM, von Keyserlingk MA. Invited review: Effects of milk ration on solid feed intake, weaning, and performance in dairy heifers. J Dairy Sci 2011;94(3):1071–81.

21. Jasper J, Weary DM. Effects of ad libitum milk intake on dairy calves. J Dairy Sci 2002 Nov 1;85(11):3054–8.

22. Miller-Cushon EK, Bergeron R, Leslie KE, DeVries TJ. Effect of milk feeding level on development of feeding behavior in dairy calves. J Dairy Sci 2013 Jan 1;96(1):551–64.

23. Senn M, Gross-Lüem S, Leuenberger H, Langhans W. Meal patterns and meal-induced metabolic changes in calves fed milk ad lib. Physiol Behav 2000 Jul 15;70(1–2):189–95.

24. Rosenberger K, Costa JIIC, Neave IIW, von Keyserlingk MAG, Weary DM. The effect of milk allowance on behavior and weight gains in dairy calves. J Dairy Sci 2017 Jan 1;100(1):504–12.

25. Jasper J, Budzynska M, Weary DM. Weaning distress in dairy calves: Acute behavioural responses by limit-fed calves. Appl Anim Behav Sci 2008 Mar;110(1–2):136–43.

26. Klopp RN, Suarez-Mena FX, Dennis TS, Hill TM, Schlotterbeck RL, Lascano GJ. Effects of feeding different amounts of milk replacer on growth performance and nutrient digestibility in Holstein calves to 2 months of age using different weaning strategies. J Dairy Sci 2019 Dec 1;102(12): 11040–50.

27. O'Driscoll K, Von Keyserlingk MAG, Weary DM. Effects of mixing on drinking and competitive behavior of dairy calves. J Dairy Sci 2006;89(1):229–33.

28. Steele MA, Doelman JH, Leal LN, Soberon F, Carson M, Metcalf JA. Abrupt weaning reduces postweaning growth and is associated with alterations in gastrointestinal markers of development in dairy calves fed an elevated plane of nutrition during the preweaning period. J Dairy Sci 2017 Jul 1;100(7):5390–9.

29. Dennis TS, Suarez-Mena FX, Hill TM, Quigley JD, Schlotterbeck RL, Hulbert L. Effect of milk replacer feeding rate, age at weaning, and method of reducing milk replacer to weaning on digestion, performance, rumination, and activity in dairy calves to 4 months of age. J Dairy Sci 2018 Jan 1;101(1):268–78.

30. Nielsen PP, Jensen MB, Lidfors L. Milk allowance and weaning method affect the use of a computer controlled milk feeder and the development of cross-sucking in dairy calves. Appl Anim Behav Sci 2008 Feb 1;109(2–4):223–37.

31. Sweeney BC, Rushen J, Weary DM, de Passillé AM. Duration of weaning, starter intake, and weight gain of dairy calves fed large amounts of milk. J Dairy Sci 2010 Jan;93(1):148–52.

32. Mirzaei M, Dadkhah N, Baghbanzadeh-Nobari B, Agha-Tehrani A, Eshraghi M, Imani M, et al. Effects of preweaning total plane of milk intake and weaning age on intake, growth performance, and blood metabolites of dairy calves. J Dairy Sci 2018 May 1;101(5):4212–20.

33. Meale SJ, Li SC, Azevedo P, Derakhshani H, DeVries TJ, Plaizier JC, et al. Weaning age influences the severity of gastrointestinal microbiome shifts in dairy calves [Sci. Rep.] [Internet]. Sci Rep 2017 Mar 15;7(1):1–13.

34. Neave HW, Costa JHC, Weary DM, von Keyserlingk MAG. Personality is associated with feeding behavior and performance in dairy calves. J Dairy Sci 2018 Aug 1;101(8):7437–49.

35. de Passillé AM, Rushen J. Using automated feeders to wean calves fed large amounts of milk according to their ability to eat solid feed. J Dairy Sci 2016 May 1;99(5):3578–83.

36. Neave HW, Costa JHC, Benetton JB, Weary DM, von Keyserlingk MAG. Individual characteristics in early life relate to variability in weaning age, feeding behavior, and weight gain of dairy calves automatically weaned based on solid feed intake. J Dairy Sci 2019 Nov 1;102(11):10250–65.

37. Benetton JB, Neave HW, Costa JHC, von Keyserlingk MAG, Weary DM. Automatic weaning based on individual solid feed intake: Effects on behavior and performance of dairy calves. J Dairy Sci 2019 Jun 1;102(6):5475–91.

38. De Passillé AM, Borderas TF, Rushen J. Weaning age of calves fed a high milk allowance by automated feeders: Effects on feed, water, and energy intake, behavioral signs of hunger, and weight gains. J Dairy Sci 2011 Mar;94(3):1401–8.

39. Roth BA, Hillmann E, Stauffacher M, Keil NM. Improved weaning reduces cross-sucking and may improve weight gain in dairy calves. Appl Anim Behav Sci 2008 Jun;111(3–4):251–61.

40. Garrett E, Nordlund K, Goodger W, Oetzel G. A cross-sectional field study investigating the effect of periparturient dietary management on ruminal ph in early lactation dairy cows. undefined. 1997.

41. Oetzel G, Nordlund K, Garrett E. Effect of ruminal ph and stage of lactation on ruminal lactate concentration in dairy cows. undefined. 1999.

42. Kleen JL, Upgang L, Rehage J. Prevalence and consequences of subacute ruminal acidosis in German dairy herds [Internet]. Acta Vet Scand 2013;55:48.

43. Laarman AH, Oba M. Short communication: Effect of calf starter on rumen pH of Holstein dairy calves at weaning. J Dairy Sci 2011 Nov;94(11):5661–4.

44. Bittar CMM, Gallo MP, Silva JT, de Paula MR, Poczynek M, Mourão GB. Gradual weaning does not improve performance for calves with low starter intake at the beginning of the weaning process. J Dairy Sci 2020 May 1;103(5):4672–80.

45. Haisan J, Steele MA, Ambrose DJ, Oba M. Effects of amount of milk fed, and starter intake, on performance of group-housed dairy heifers during the weaning transition. Appl Anim Sci 2019 Feb 1;35(1):88–93.

46. Parsons SD, Steele MA, Leslie KE, Renaud DL, DeVries TJ. Investigation of weaning strategy and solid feed location for dairy calves individually fed with an automated milk feeding system. J Dairy Sci 2020 Jul 1;103(7):6533–56.

47. Keil NM, Langhans W. The development of intersucking in dairy calves around weaning. Appl Anim Behav Sci 2001 Jun 1;72(4):295–308.

48. Deelen SM, Leslie KE, Steele MA, Eckert E, Brown HE, DeVries TJ. Validation of a calf-side β-hydroxybutyrate test and its utility for estimation of starter intake in dairy calves around weaning. J Dairy Sci 2016 Sep 1;99(9):7624–33.

49. Suarez-Mena FX, Hill TM, Jones CM, Heinrichs AJ. REVIEW: Effect of forage provision on feed intake in dairy calves. Prof Anim Sci 2016;32(4):383–8.

50. Khan MA, Weary DM, Von Keyserlingk MAG. Hay intake improves performance and rumen development of calves fed higher quantities of milk. J Dairy Sci 2011 Jul;94(7):3547–53.

51. Horvath KC, Miller-Cushon EK. Evaluating effects of providing hay on behavioral development and performance of group-housed dairy calves. J Dairy Sci 2019 Nov 1;102(11):10411–22.

52. Overvest MA, Crossley RE, Miller-Cushon EK, DeVries TJ. Social housing influences the behavior and feed intake of dairy calves during weaning. J Dairy Sci 2018 Sep 1;101(9):8123–34.

53. De Paula Vieira A, von Keyserlingk MAG, Weary DM. Effects of pair versus single housing on performance and behavior of dairy calves before and after weaning from milk. J Dairy Sci 2010 Jul 1;93(7):3079–85.

54. Miller-Cushon EK, DeVries TJ. Effect of social housing on the development of feeding behavior and social feeding preferences of dairy calves. J Dairy Sci 2016 Feb 1;99(2):1406–17.

55. Costa JHC, Meagher RK, von Keyserlingk MAG, Weary DM. Early pair housing increases solid feed intake and weight gains in dairy calves. J Dairy Sci 2015 Sep 1;98(9):6381–6.

56. Raussi S, Niskanen S, Siivonen J, Hänninen L, Hepola H, Jauhiainen L, Veissier I. The formation of preferential relationships at early age in cattle. Behav Processes 2010 Jul 1;84(3):726–31.

57. De Paula Vieira A, von Keyserlingk MAG, Weary DM. Presence of an older weaned companion influences feeding behavior and improves performance of dairy calves before and after weaning from milk. J Dairy Sci 2012 Jun;95(6):3218–24.

58. Boyle AR, Ferris CP, O'Connell NE. Are there benefits in introducing dairy heifers to the main dairy herd in the evening rather than the morning? J Dairy Sci 2012 Jul 1;95(7):3650–61.

59. Black RA, Whitlock BK, Krawczel PD. Effect of maternal exercise on calf dry matter intake, weight gain, behavior, and cortisol concentrations at disbudding and weaning. J Dairy Sci 2017 Sep 1;100(9):7390–400.

60. Veissier I, Caré S, Pomiès D. Suckling, weaning, and the development of oral behaviours in dairy calves. Appl Anim Behav Sci 2013 Jul 1;147(1–2):11–8.

61. Cantor MC, Pertuisel CH, Costa JHC [Technical Note]. Technical note: Estimating body weight of dairy calves with a partial-weight scale attached to an automated milk feeder. J Dairy Sci 2020 Feb 1;103(2):1914–9.

62. Wickramasinghe HKJP, Kramer AJ, Appuhamy JADRN. Drinking water intake of newborn dairy calves and its effects on feed intake, growth performance, health status, and nutrient digestibility. J Dairy Sci 2019 Jan 1;102(1):377–87.

63. Wickramasinghe HKJP, Anast JM, Schmitz-Esser S, Serão NVL, Appuhamy JADRN. Beginning to offer drinking water at birth increases the species richness and the abundance of Faecalibacterium and Bifidobacterium in the gut of preweaned dairy calves. J Dairy Sci 2020 May 1;103(5):4262–74.

64. Hepola HP, Hänninen LT, Raussi SM, Pursiainen PA, Aarnikoivu AM, Saloniemi HS. Effects of providing water from a bucket or a nipple on the performance and behavior of calves fed ad libitum volumes of acidified milk replacer. J Dairy Sci 2008;91(4):1486–96.

65. Thickett WS, Cuthbert NH, Brigstocke TDA, Lindeman MA, Wilson PN. The management of calves on an early-weaning system: The relationship of voluntary water intake to dry feed intake and live-weight gain to 5 weeks. Anim Sci 1981;33(1): 25–30.

66. Kertz AF, Reutzel LF, Mahoney JH. Ad libitum water intake by neonatal calves and its relationship to calf starter intake, weight gain, feces score, and season. J Dairy Sci 1984 Dec 1;67(12):2964–9.

Chapter 7

Care of the post-weaning calf

Sophie Mahendran and Claire Wathes

CHAPTER CONTENTS

The post-weaning period follows the transition from milk feeding all the way up to first service of heifers, but it is often partially forgotten about. Maximising labour efficiency may lead to sacrifices in optimal management strategies for these heifers, resulting in reductions to growth rates and extending the period prior to first service and pregnancy. The estimated cost of rearing heifers from weaning to conception is £1.65 per day, and if this period is mismanaged, it can extend the age at first calving (AFC), resulting in an additional cost of £2.87 per day for each day over 24 months old (1).

NUTRITION OF THE POST-WEANING CALF

Maintaining average daily growth rates in the region of 0.8 kg/day is important to reach a service weight equivalent to ~65% of mature bodyweight by 14 months of age. In addition, correct nutrition will help achieve the most beneficial body composition to optimise a heifer's future milk production capabilities aiming for mainly muscular growth and minimising adipose gain. Heifers that calve down with too low a bodyweight will divert more energy towards their own growth requirements at the expense of milk production (2).

The metabolisable energy (ME) maintenance requirement for weaned heifers is 98 kcal/kg$^{0.75}$ of live bodyweight (2), with suggested nutrient requirements shown in Table 7.1. Initially, a large proportion of this energy (and protein) is used for growth of the gastrointestinal tract as they adapt to a solid feed and roughage diet (3). This is most evident in the rumen, which increases from 30% to >70% of the total capacity of the gut (4). There is also a change in liver metabolism post-weaning, with a decrease in glucose supply from a milk diet resulting in an increase in glucogenic processes in the liver (3).

Calves' energy requirements post-weaning increase in relation to their growing body size. It is common for smaller enterprises to feed concentrates (ad lib or rationed) along with a good quality

TABLE 7.1 Dry matter and crude protein intakes for youngstock of different bodyweights (5).

	Bodyweight (kg)				
	100	**150**	**200**	**250**	**300**
Maximum dry matter intake (kg/day)	3.1	4.2	5.2	6.2	7.1
Percentage of crude protein required (%)	19	16	14.2	13.2	12.5

forage, such as hay – both of these should have been available to the calf prior to weaning to enable the rumen to adapt to these feed stuffs (6). In these scenarios, it is best to feed concentrates ad lib for 4–8 weeks after weaning to ensure sufficient energy intakes after the transition to a completely solid feed diet (7), especially as the rumen is not fully developed until 12 weeks of age (Figure 7.1). You can then teach the youngstock to eat competitively when their ration is reduced to 3–4 kg/head/day. It can also be helpful to transition the calves from a concentrate feed of 18% crude protein (CP), down to a 16% CP formulation over this period. Addition

of maize silage to the diet may also be helpful, but as this is a high energy feed, care must be taken to avoid excess weight gain.

Larger farms may elect to feed a total mixed ration (TMR), but the overall cost of this is much higher, and requires a proper feed face (Figure 7.2). Suggested feed space is given in Table 7.2.

As the heifer matures towards puberty, more of this energy gets laid down as fat. Care must be taken to prevent excess energy intakes, leading to increased fat deposition in the body. Historically, research in this area had suggested high growth rates prior to puberty would lead to

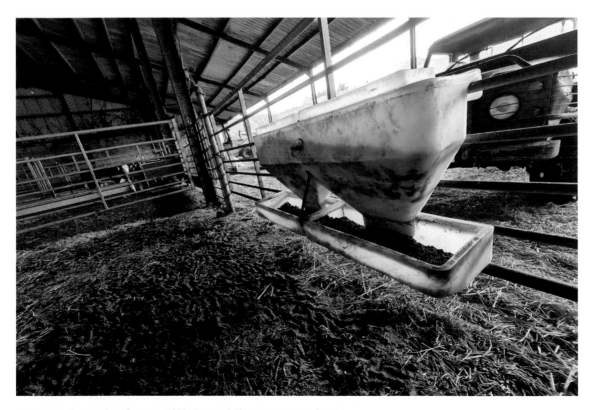

FIGURE 7.1 Example of a small Wydale ad lib concentrate feeder.

TABLE 7.2 Suggested space at the feed face dependent on animal size (8).

Weight of the youngstock (kg)	Width per animal at the feed face or trough (m)
<100	0.30
100–199	0.35
200–299	0.40
300	0.50

fatty infiltration in the mammary gland, resulting in a negative effect on milk yields upon maturity of the animal (9, 10). More recent work has identified that mammary gland development is closely linked to age, time to puberty and hormone profiles (11, 12), with enhanced feeding during the pre-weaning but not post-weaning periods leading to increased mammary parenchyma (13). Therefore, the current recommendation is to aim for intensive feeding during the pre-weaning period to accelerate growth up to weaning, followed by controlled growth up until puberty (6).

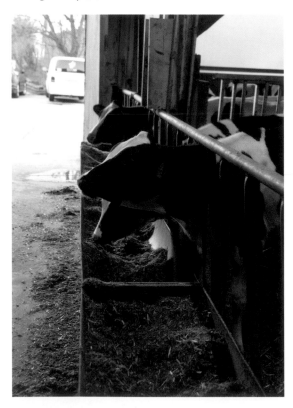

FIGURE 7.2 Weaned calves being fed a TMR from troughs.

Grazing of post-weaning calves

Many calves will be turned out onto pasture to graze after weaning. Grazing can help to reduce rearing costs by an estimated £6.06 per animal (14) due to savings on housing and associated bedding, and reducing the need to feed preserved forages. However, careful management of the pasture is required to ensure sufficient intakes of high-quality grass, otherwise calves will struggle to maintain adequate and consistent growth rates. Grass sward heights are recommended to be 5–6 cm in the spring, 7–8 cm in the summer, and 9–10 cm in the autumn to ensure adequate intakes (7). The calculated required dry matter (DM) intakes of grass are shown in Table 7.3.

The transition of calves to a grazing system does need some careful consideration in terms of the development of foraging skills, new dietary habits and adaptation of the rumen to a grass diet (16). In suckler herds, the calf will learn to graze from their dam, and to recognise nutritious plants that are suitable to eat (17) (Figure 7.3). When the calf is separated, they must learn how to graze from their conspecifics (other members of the group), which can slow the ingestion of food. Including a couple of older animals with prior grazing knowledge in a group of youngstock when they are first put onto pasture can help with social facilitation and learning how to graze (16). Heifer calves may also be outwintered on pasture or on root vegetable grazing, but this will also require adequate feed supplementation to maintain growth.

Selection of low risk pastures for the first grazing season of youngstock can help minimise exposure to high worm burdens. High risk pastures are permanent pastures that were grazed by first year

TABLE 7.3 The calculated dry matter intake of grass per day required by heifers to maintain daily growth of 0.8 kg/day (15).

Energy values for grass (MJ/kg)	Bodyweight (kg)				
	100	150	200	250	300
12	2.3	2.8	3.3	3.8	4.3
11.5	2.3	3.0	3.5	4.0	4.4
11	2.5	3.1	3.6	4.2	4.6
10.5	2.6	3.2	3.9	4.4	4.9
10	2.7	3.4	4.0	4.6	5.1
9.5	2.8	3.6	4.2	4.8	5.4
9	3.0	3.8	4.4	5.1	5.7

calves either in the same or previous year. Medium risk pastures were previously grazed by adult cattle, and low risk pastures are new leys, silage aftermaths or pastures grazed by sheep.

Calves at pasture may need supplementation (usually by concentrate feeds or boluses) to ensure adequate vitamin and mineral levels (trace elements) are achieved. These are important for catalysing

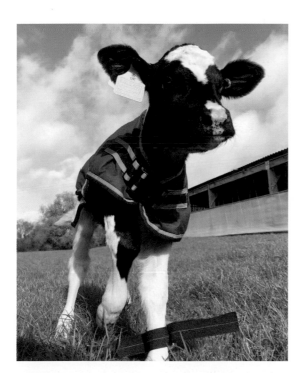

FIGURE 7.3 In natural settings, calves will learn to graze from observing their dam, but this is replaced by peer learning in all-calf groups.

biochemical reactions in tissues; low levels in the diet resulting in a transition from depletion, deficiency, dysfunction to disorders seen as clinically abnormal animals (18). The important trace elements and the effects of deficiencies include the following.

- Copper – used in the body for haemoglobin synthesis, enzyme systems, pigment, disease resistance and fertility. Copper interacts with sulphur, iron and molybdenum to reduce its absorption. Deficiencies cause anaemia, poor growth and depigmentation of hair.
- Selenium – forms a component of glutathione peroxidase (an antioxidant). Deficiencies linked with low levels of vitamin E cause myopathies (white muscle disease), potentially with sudden death.
- Zinc – forms a component of enzymes and is involved in the immune system. Absorption is reduced by phytate, which is found in unensilaged maize. Deficiencies can cause parakeratosis, poor growth and reduced appetite.
- Cobalt – used in the rumen to synthesise B12. Most forage contains plenty of cobalt from the soil. Deficiency causes poor growth rates, with thin poor quality hair coats.
- Iodine – used to produce thyroid hormones, and affects the immune system. Levels are lowest in spring grass, and can also be lowered by ingestion of goitrogens from brassicas and legumes. Deficiencies are implicated in poor fertility and poor growth rates.

TABLE 7.4 Minimum and suggested lying areas per calf in loose housing.

Size of calf (kg)	Minimum area (m²)	Recommended area (m²)
100–149	1.5	4.0
150–199	2.0	5.0
>200	3.0	6.0

HOUSING OF THE POST-WEANING CALF

It is best to delay movement of calves immediately after weaning as this is a stressful period when they are at an increased risk of developing disease (6). Many calves will be housed in large groups in loose straw yards during the post-weaning period (Figure 7.4). This provides the most comfortable housing type, but there should ideally be a concrete feed passage ~2 m wide, that is easily scraped on a daily basis (or a minimum of three times per week). Minimum lying space is given in Table 7.4

(8). These sheds should provide the same environmental condition as the pre-weaning shed, with good ventilation and lighting still important.

The provision of concrete is important to allow pre-conditioning of the feet to concrete (19). This pre-conditioning can reduce the likelihood of development of claw horn lesions, with research showing that heifers exercised on concrete have increased digital cushion thickness in their feet (20). This should have a protective effect against them developing lameness when they enter the milking herd (21).

In order to ensure a smooth transition into the

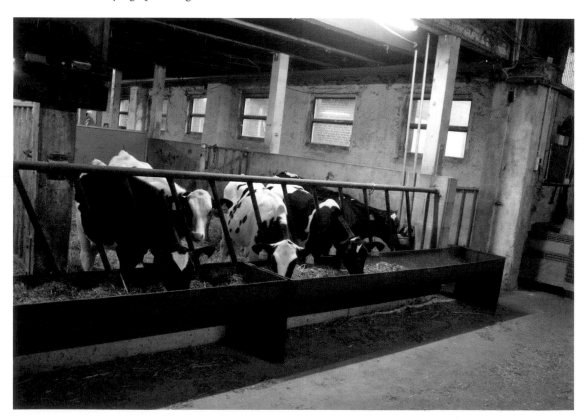

FIGURE 7.4 A large loose straw pen with a feed barrier for housing post-weaning calves.

TABLE 7.5 Suggested cubicle dimensions for different sizes of heifers.

Heifer weight (kg)	150	200	300	400	500
Width (m)	0.6	0.7	0.85	0.95	1.10
Length (m)	1.6	1.7	1.95	2.15	2.4

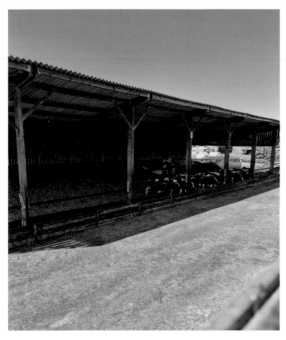

FIGURE 7.5 A typical straw yard set-up that enables a concrete strip to be left in front of the feed barrier to help adaptation of the feet to hard standing.

milking herd it can be helpful to train heifers to use a cubicle, which reduces excessive standing times at the vulnerable period for lameness development when they join the milking herd (22). Housing in cubicles is very common on the continent, where provision of grazing is much more limited. Suggested dimensions for cubicles are in Table 7.5 (8).

ENDOPARASITES

Ostertagia ostertagi

The most common nematode (round worm) that affects calves is *Ostertagia ostertagi*, with the syndrome sometimes referred to as parasitic gastroenteritis (PGE). This condition leads to reduced growth rates and weight loss, reduced feed intakes (23), diarrhoea and, in severe cases, hypoalbuminaemia due to loss of protein through the intestines.

Pasture that has previously been grazed by other cattle will be contaminated with overwintered eggs and larvae, which the calves will ingest when grazing. The level of pasture contamination with *Ostertagia* appears to be increasing, with one study indicating a threefold increase in pasture burden over a 30-year period (24).

The lifecycle of *Ostertagia* is demonstrated in Figure 7.6. Type I *Ostertagia* is the direct lifecycle that occurs during the summer grazing period, with wet summers producing earlier peaks in the levels of infective L3 larvae on pasture. *Ostertagia* larvae develop into adults in the gastric glands of the abomasum. This causes damage to the abomasal wall, and reduces its production of hydrochloric acid (HCl). This gives a rise in abomasal pH level from 2.0 up to 7.0, which reduces the cleavage of pepsinogen into pepsin (as it requires an acidic environment) (7). The pepsinogen then enters the blood, so serum pepsinogen levels can be checked as a diagnostic indicator. A sample from seven different animals should be taken, and if the average serum pepsinogen level is >2.6 units of tyrosine, the group should be treated (25). The more usual method of diagnosing endoparasite burdens is made through faecal egg counts (FECs), with a count of >200 eggs per gram indicating anthelmintic treatment is required.

Cattle immunity against *Ostertagia* develops slowly over the first grazing season, only after long and repeated exposure to parasites on pasture. This natural immunity is then boosted in the second grazing season to give a non-sterile immunity (26).

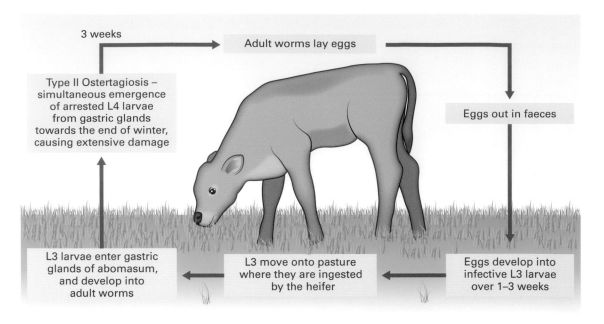

FIGURE 7.6 The lifecycle of *Ostertagia*.

At the end of the grazing season, Type II *Ostertagia* can occur, when there is arrested development of L4 larvae (hypobiosis) to allow them to overwinter in the calf, so improving the nematodes' survival. Late in the winter or the following spring, there is simultaneous emergence of the adult worms from the abomasum. This can cause severe clinical signs with diarrhoea and weight loss, although this tends to only affect a small proportion of the group. This also causes contamination of the pasture for other grazing cattle.

Treatment of *Ostertagia* worm burdens is through the use of anthelmintics. Type I *Ostertagia* should be managed by anthelmintic treatment in the early part of the grazing season (the first 3–4 weeks), with use of narrow spectrum levamisole being appropriate (27). This can be done in conjunction with FECs to assess worm burdens, or by regular monitoring of daily liveweight gain to identify reduction in performance that might indicate a worm burden (28). Other control measures to reduce risks associated with PGE include turning heifers out to grass when greater than 6 months old, and also limiting access to permanent pasture as these remain contaminated with L3 larvae. Type II Ostertagia is treated at housing with either a benzimadazole or macrocyclic lactones (ML) which are effective against arrested larvae.

Other nematodes that can infect calves are *Cooperia oncophora* (the main contributor to raised FECs in youngstock), *Trichostrongylus axei*, *Capillaria bovis*, *Oesophagostomum radiatum* and *Trichuris globulosa*.

Lungworm

Lungworm in calves (sometime called husk) produces a parasitic bronchitis caused by *Dictyocaulus viviparous*. The lifecycle of lungworm is slightly different to other nematodes in that the adult worms develop in the lungs of the calf (Figure 7.7). Here, the adults lay oocytes that already contain fully developed L1 larvae that hatch and migrate up the trachea, being swallowed by the animal and being passed out in faeces onto the pasture. This means that diagnosis has to be made via a specific type of FEC – a faecal Baerman flotation test. This enables detection of L1 larvae that are excreted in the faeces. Lungworm ELISAs

How to carry out faecal egg counts

- Collect individual animal faecal samples directly from the anus (or very fresh from the ground). If you want to do a pooled sample, still collect individual samples, and weigh out an equal amount from each sample to pool together.
- To make the saturated salt solution, fill a bottle with water and add enough salt until no more dissolves and you see salt collecting in the bottom of the bottle (roughly 3/4 of a cup of salt to a pint of water).
- Homogenise the faecal sample so it has an even consistency.
- Weigh out 2 g of faeces into a cup, and add 28 mL of the saturated salt solution. Mix well.
- Pour the solution through a sieve and into another cup – this removes the large organic matter. Press as much liquid out as possible using a spoon.
- Immediately fill both chambers of a McMaster slide with this fluid using a pipette/syringe.
- Look at the slide under the microscope using 10× magnification. Count eggs in both chambers of the slide. It may help to let the slide rest for 5 minutes to let the eggs float to the surface if you are having difficulty seeing any.
- To calculate the egg burden:

  total egg count (chamber 1 + chamber 2) × 50 = eggs per gram
  (multiplying by 50 is the factor to adjust for the ratio of faeces to fluid)
  200 eggs/gram is considered a significant level that requires treatment.

are also available, but care with interpretation is needed as it only indicates exposure as opposed to active infection.

Types of anthelmintic (wormer)

There are three main groups of anthelmintic available (15).
1 Benzimidazoles (BZ) – white drench, broad-spectrum effective against nematodes and some tapeworms.
2 Levamisol (LV) – yellow drench, very short acting, with a low toxic dose.
3 Macrocyclic lactones (ML) – clear drench:
   a these products have a persistent action due to storage in fat
   b available as pour-on products that provide ease of application
   c have activity against ectoparasites such as lice and mites.

Resistance to anthelmintics in cattle is relatively uncommon in the UK, with many suspected cases being a result of treatment failures due to causes other than resistance. Development of anthelmintic resistance can be slowed by only treating animals with anthelmintics when necessary, maintaining an *in refugia* population of worms within untreated cattle, and placing treated cattle back out on pre-grazed pasture after treatment to dilute the population of resistant worms that survived treatment with anthelmintics. Post-treatment FECs can be carried out if there is a suspicion of anthelmintic resistance, for example, 7 days after LV treatment, 10–14 days after BZ and 14–16 days after a ML treatment.

Survival of L1 larvae on pasture is very weather dependent, requiring warm and wet conditions for development into L3 larvae. The infective L3 larvae can then be ingested directly from pasture, or can be distributed around pasture by an association with *Pilobolus* fungi. The infective dose of L3 larvae is relatively small compared to other nematodes (7).

Clinical signs that develop in infected youngstock include coughing but with no raised temperature, weight loss and poor growth (due to damage caused by immature worms migrating from the

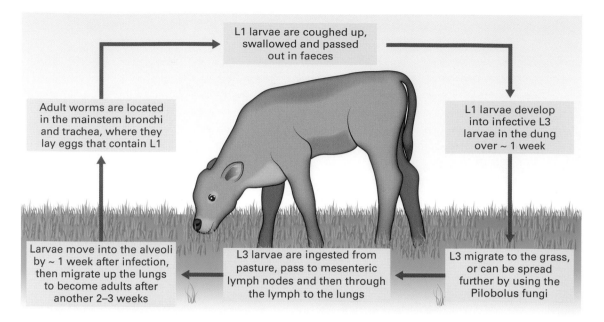

FIGURE 7.7 Lifecycle of lungworm.

intestines, via the lymphatics and blood to the lungs). Heavy worm burdens can be fatal.

It is important that youngstock develop immunity to lungworm, through controlled exposure to the parasite, or by vaccination. Using slow-release anthelmintic boluses prior to turnout can prevent development of immunity, resulting in a high risk during the second grazing season. Vaccination with a product that contains an irradiated larvae (Huskvac) must be administered prior to the start of the grazing season to allow the calves' own immune system to be stimulated (15).

Treatment for lungworm is through the use of any of the anthelmintic groups. However, care must be taken if there are clinical signs, as killing large numbers of worms within the lungs causes large inflammatory responses, and so should be administered with NSAIDs or steroid at the same time.

Liver fluke

Liver fluke infection is caused by the trematode *Fasciola hepatica*. Cattle tend to develop a chronic form of the infestation, with burdens causing reduced growth rates, weight loss and occasionally hypoalbuminaemia and anaemia.

The liver fluke lifecycle is shown in Figure 7.8, with a relatively long lifecycle of ~18 weeks. The condition arises in warm and wet conditions, with the optimum temperature for the whole lifecycle being above 10°C over the whole 24-hour period (7). The lifecycle also requires the presence of the mud snail *Galba truncatula* (which inhabits wet ground in the summer) for development of miracidium into cercaria stages. Once metacercariae have been ingested from pasture, they migrate from the small intestine, through the abdomen to the liver. Here, the immature fluke migrate through the liver, causing fibrosis which results in economic losses from rejection of livers at slaughter. Final development into a mature adult fluke occurs in the small bile ducts.

Liver fluke is also known to make cattle more susceptible to developing other diseases such as those caused by *Salmonella* Dublin and *Clostrium novyi* by creating anaerobic areas in the liver.

Liver fluke can be diagnosed by FECs, antibody ELISA detection in serum (although antibodies can persist for up to 7 months after exposure), and also the faecal copro-antigen ELISA (26). If animals are

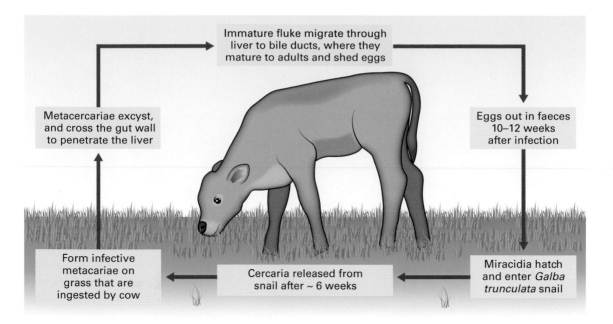

FIGURE 7.8 Lifecycle of liver fluke.

sent to the abattoir, reports can give an indication of the level of liver damage and presence of fluke. This valuable information can build a picture of whether fluke are an issue on a farm, and how effective any control programmes currently are.

Control of liver fluke is mainly through the use of flukicides. Timing of treatments depends on the weather conditions and the products used (due to the range of effectiveness on different fluke stages). Flukicides effective against immature fluke (<6-weeks old) can be used to treat cattle at housing, and other products should be used 4–6 weeks post housing (26).

Tips to ensure the effective use of anthelmintics and flukicides

There are separate flukicides available for use in cattle:

1 triclabendazole – effective on fluke from 2 days
2 nitroxynil – effective on fluke from 7 weeks
3 oxyclozanide – effective on fluke from 10 weeks
4 closantel – only available in combination with ivermectin wormer, Effective on fluke from 6 weeks.

- Use the correct type of product (active ingredient), and apply in the correct method (e.g. ensure the dosing gun used is calibrated and working accurately).
- Ensure the product is stored correctly to avoid inactivation (usually a cool place), and do not use after the use by date.
- Treat with the correct dose rate to avoid insufficient treatment (e.g. get accurate weights of the youngstock, or dose for the heaviest animal in the group).
- Do not apply topical pour-on products when the weather is bad (i.e. heavy rain).
- Reduce pasture contamination and infectious pressures by using pasture rotations, grazing silage aftermath and putting down new leys each year to reduce permanent pastures.
- Keep cattle off pasture for 24–48 hours after treatment with anthelmintics to reduce contamination of the pasture.

Coccidiosis

Coccidia are single cell parasites that affect the gastrointestinal tract. The main genus of Coccidia

Lifecycle of Coccidia

Internal phase in the calf
- Ingestion of sporulated oocyst – these are ubiquitous in the environment.
- In the asexual phase, once oocysts are in the small intestine, sporozoites are released from the oocyst, and enter enterocytes where they multiply to form merozoites. The infected enterocytes then rupture. Calves get clinical signs prior to shedding in high infectious states due to the intestinal damage at this stage.
- In the sexual phase in the large intestine, the merozoites differentiate into male and female gametocytes, which produce oocysts that pass out of the calf in faeces.

External phase in the environment
- The oocyst has to undergo sporulation outside the host in the environment in order to become infective. This process is temperature dependent, taking between 1–5 days at 20°C.

The pre-patent period differs between pathogenic species of Coccidia, with the time from oocyst ingestion to oocyst excretion varying from 10 to 20 days. Once sporulated, the oocysts are resistant to most disinfectants. In conjunction with their ability to multiply rapidly in the host (1:24 million), this can create very high infectious pressures. Disinfectants that are active against coccidia include:
- Kilcox: 4% for 4 hours contact time
- Keracox: 4% for 2 hours
- Bio-00-cyst: 3% for 2 hours
- Interkokask: 2% for 24 hours
- Neopredisan: 4% for 4 hours.

that affect youngstock are *Eimeria*, with the four main pathogenic species being *Eimeria bovis*, *E. zuernii*, *E. auburnensis* and *E. alabamensis* (29). While Coccidia infections usually occur during housing, *E. alabamensis* does survive on pasture.

Coccidiosis can cause both subclinical and clinical disease. Subclinical signs include a decreased appetite and poor growth following from intestinal damage, and clinical signs include diarrhoea, abdominal pain, acute weight loss, straining to defecate and a rectal prolapse (30). Nervous coccidiosis has been reported in North America, which is thought to be caused by *Eimeria*-related neurotoxins and electrolyte imbalances, resulting in neurological symptoms such as seizures and nystagmus (31).

Diagnosis of coccidiosis is via clinical signs. It can be confirmed by a FEC ($\geq$5000 oocysts/g), ideally from multiple animals in the group, but it must be remembered that early on in the disease course there may be few oocysts being shed. Speciation of the oocysts can be helpful to identify pathogenic species, but requires submission to specialist laboratories. If youngstock die, histological samples of the intestines, as well as mucosal scrapings, can be taken.

Coccidiosis should be considered a herd level infection due to naïve youngstock shedding very high numbers of oocysts into the environment, leading to faecal–oral transmission (31). This means that treatment of animals is generally done at the group level, although targeted treatment for those showing clinical signs is possible. Table 7.6 gives some common ionophores.

Treatment of animals prophylactically should not be done from birth as you want to expose susceptible animals to ingestion of low doses of oocysts to allow an immune response to develop without clinical signs. Instead, metaphylactic usage of ionophores after infection (usually ~14 days after exposure) should be done in high risk groups (31).

Prevention of high infective levels of coccidial oocysts in the environment is through excellent

TABLE 7.6 Common ionophores

Ionophore and product name	Mode of action	Method of administration	Location of action	Duration of action
Diclazuril (e.g. Vecoxan)	Coccidiocide – kills the coccidia	Oral drench	Acts in the small and large intestine	2 hours, so likely to need a second treatment
Toltrazuril (e.g. Baycox)	Coccidiocide	Oral drench	Acts in the small and large intestine	2.5 days May be used for prevention, with blanket treatment of the cohort ~10 days after exposure (not done immediately as you want them to have some exposure to stimulate an immune response)
Decoquinate (e.g. Deccox)	Coccidiostat – inhibits development of the internal stages of the coccidia	Given in-feed (mixed with concentrates)	Acts in the small intestine with no effect in the large intestine	Feed for 28 days Can be used as a treatment (1.0 mg/kg), or preventatively (0.5 mg/kg)

hygiene and low stocking densities. For housed animals, regular mucking out and disinfection of sheds (every 4–6 weeks), cleaning of equipment and not feeding from the ground are important. For grazing animals, ensuring a reasonable stocking density to prevent excess faecal contamination of the grass and poaching of high through-put areas is important. Youngstock develop immunity following infection, but this is quite specific to the species of coccidia that they were infected with, providing little cross-protection and leaving animal vulnerable to reinfections with other species (31).

HEIFER BREEDING: FIRST SERVICE

The future of dairy heifer calves reared on farm is to become replacement animals for the milking herd. These animals need to join the herd with the ability to achieve their full lifetime potential for milk production. To reach this end target, heifers must grow sufficiently to reach puberty in good

time, become pregnant and then carry a calf to term (Figure 7.9).

There is substantial evidence that the optimum AFC in terms of maximising future performance and economic returns is between 23 and 24 months (32–34). Seasonally calving herds also require an AFC close to 2 years in order to maintain their annual calving pattern. Few dairy herds, however, currently meet this target. In order to achieve it, the heifer rearing process up to the point of breeding needs to have maintained consistently good growth rates and health, as discussed earlier in this book. Heifer fertility must also be excellent. Continued growth during the first pregnancy should ensure that heifers are sufficiently grown to calve without difficulty and then go on to achieve a good first lactation milk yield. In practice the target is to calve at 90–95% of mature BW, and it is also essential that their frame size is sufficient (see Chapter 2). As heifers age, the rate of growth of bone and lean body tissue like muscle begins to slow, and rates of adipose/fat deposition increases, so care must also be taken to prevent over-conditioning and production of fat heifers.

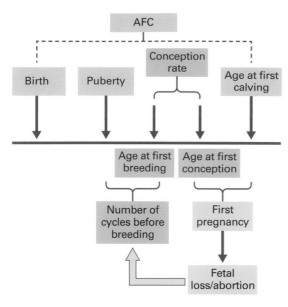

FIGURE 7.9 Schematic showing the key reproductive events for a dairy heifer. The goal is to achieve an AFC of about 24 months. The key determinants are shown in red. Puberty should occur in sufficient time to allow at least one complete oestrous cycle before breeding begins. The conception rate then determines the age at conception. The length of the first pregnancy is fixed unless the heifer suffers from fetal loss or abortion, in which case the breeding cycle must begin again.

Puberty

Puberty is reached when a heifer first ovulates a potentially fertile oocyte and also shows visible signs of oestrus, followed by regular oestrous cycles (35). The reproductive tract and ovaries both undergo rapid development in the last few months before puberty, driven by a rise in secretion of the pituitary hormone follicle stimulating hormone (FSH) and an increase in luteinising hormone (LH) pulsatility (36). Ovarian oestradiol production increases and finally triggers an LH surge that causes the dominant follicle to ovulate (37). The first ovulation is, however, often a silent heat with no signs of bulling (34). The reproductive tract continues to develop post-pubertally under the influence of the steroid hormones oestradiol and progesterone produced by the ovary, and there is evidence that

the likelihood of conception improves over the first few oestrous cycles (38). Ideally, a heifer, therefore, needs to have had at least one full oestrous cycle prior to being served to ensure the highest level of fertility. The recommendation in dairy herds is for puberty to occur by 12 months of age and in seasonal herds heifers should reach puberty at least 4–6 weeks before the start of the designated breeding period.

The age at which dairy heifers reach puberty is, however, variable. It generally occurs at between 7 to 14 months (39) but is highly dependent on bodyweight, and hence the growth rate up until that point (Figure 7.10) (36, 40). Different cattle breeds typically reach puberty at a different proportion of mature bodyweight, with figures ranging from 55% to 65% (41) and a moderate heritability of 0.40 (42). In Holstein heifers it is suggested that they should have achieved 55% to 60% of their mature bodyweight at first service, which is generally about 375 kg (43). Heifers with a suboptimal growth rate due to insufficient nutrition and/or disease will not reach puberty until after the time when they should have been bred, so inevitably causing a delay in AFC (Figure 7.10).

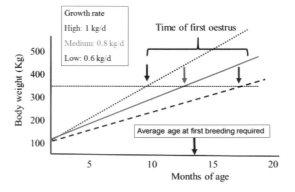

FIGURE 7.10 The relationships between growth rates, weight and age at first oestrus in Holstein heifers. In this example, the average weight at puberty is about 350 kg (horizontal line). The age at which this is reached will be around 10 months for heifers growing at 1 kg/d, 13 months for a growth rate of 0.8 kg/d but not until 17 months if the growth rate is only 0.6 kg/d. This is not until after the ideal age at first breeding, which is 13.5 months.

Management of breeding

The age at conception is determined by a combination of the age at first breeding and the conception rate (Figure 7.9). As gestation length is fixed, these two measurements determine the AFC. Heifers should be the most fertile animals on the farm, with two UK surveys reporting first service conception rates of 67% (44, 45). Another UK study comparing two methods of synchronisation and fixed time AI reported conception rates of 55–60% (46). This is in accord with an analysis of conception rates in the USA, which found that the highest rates of 56% were achieved in Holstein heifers aged 15–16 months at breeding, with lower success in both younger and older animals (47). The rate declined to only 42% in those aged 25–26 months. This reduced fertility in the older animal again emphasises the need to have a robust system in place to ensure that all animals grow well and are served in a timely fashion.

Apart from the requirement that heifers have reached puberty, the conception rate is influenced by all the same factors which affect adult cows. These include heat detection, management of the insemination process and environmental issues, such as heat stress. Details of insemination practice (e.g. use of oestrous synchronisation, handling of straws) are outside the scope of this book. With heifers it is, however, particularly important to remember that they are less accustomed than cows to being handled, so setting up the race appropriately and maintaining a calm environment are both necessary for optimum results when using AI. Around the service period they should be maintained on the same diet and managed without alteration for 6 weeks both prior to and after service to avoid stress-induced early embryonic loss (6). Another issue to remember for animals which fail to conceive is the possibility that they may be freemartins (see Chapter 1). It should be noted that conception rates to first service will never be 100% however good the management, with an average of 1.4 services per conception (and a range of 1 to 5 services) (44). As the gestation length is approximately 9 months, the herd as a whole needs to achieve an average age at conception of 15 months if the average AFC is going to be 24 months. In practice this means that the service period needs to start at around 13.5 months of age.

A UK-based survey of breeding practices on 101 farms found that 20% used entirely natural service on their replacement heifers, with a further 50% of farms running them with a sweeper bull after an initial number of inseminations had failed (45) (Figure 7.11). This would often be from a beef breed. Heifers should have the best genetics on the farm, and hence are the best animals to focus on for the most rapid improvement in herd genetics. Using bulls is considered an easy option as it requires relatively low intensity management, but this is actually a wasted opportunity. Utilising sexed semen, ideally with genomic testing, will allow selection of the best semen to suit the evolving needs of the herd, thereby generating the most rapid supply of the next generation of high achieving heifers. This aspect was discussed in Chapter 1. Another consideration when using a bull is that his fertility, soundness and disease status also need to be confirmed before his introduction to the herd.

Pregnancy loss and disease

Potential diseases to which heifers are exposed have already been covered (see Chapter 1). Apart from adverse effects on growth rate, for animals of breeding age these may impact directly on fertility through reduced conception rates, fetal mortality and abortion. Abortion is reported to occur in around 4–5% of dairy heifers and has a major impact on their AFC, as they then have to be rebred (Figure 7.9) (44, 48). Heifer abortion also increases the likelihood of culling by 2.7-fold in their eventual first lactation (48). There are many bacterial, viral, protozoan and fungal pathogens that can reduce cattle fertility and so potentially affect breeding heifers (49). Specific studies on heifers are limited, but *Neospora caninum* is particularly

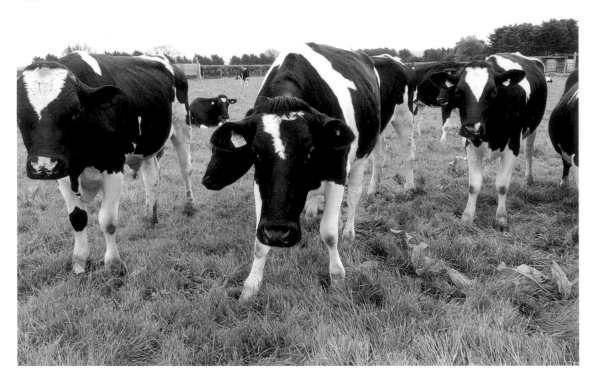

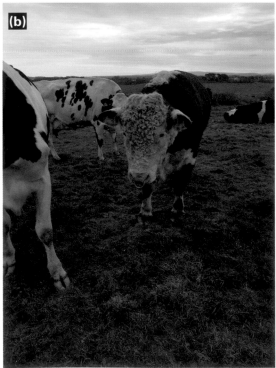

FIGURE 7.11 Bulling heifers in a field with (a) a young Holstein-Friesian breeding bull for natural service or (b) an easy breeding beef bull such as a Hereford, often used for serving heifers that do not hold to artificial insemination.

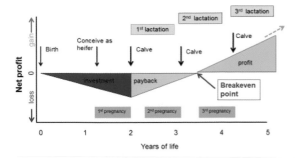

FIGURE 7.12 Diagrammatic representation of the economic costs of rearing a dairy heifer. The time until first calving can be considered as an investment phase. Income generation begins at the start of the first lactation, but the payback period generally extends until around the middle of the second lactation. It is only after this that the individual animal starts to generate a profit for the farm. Any animal which dies or has to be culled before the breakeven point is reached will generate a net loss.

known to be associated with fetal losses and abortions in this age group (50, 51).

Economics

Any delay in AFC prolongs the length of the rearing phase and inevitably increases its costs. Furthermore, dairy heifers do not start to repay the investment cost in their production until they start milk production (Figure 7.12), with an estimated breakeven point being reached at 530 ± 293 days for UK herds (1). Management decisions on key reproduction events and grazing policy have the greatest impact on the time taken for heifers to start making a profit for the farm, with an increase in the mean cost of rearing of £2.26 for each extra day in age at conception and of £2.87 for each extra day in AFC (1, 45).

REFERENCES

1. Boulton AC, Rushton J, Wathes DC. An empirical analysis of the cost of rearing dairy heifers from birth to first calving and the time taken to repay these costs. Animal 2017;11(8):1372–80.

2. Van Amburgh ME, Soberon F, Meyer MJ, Molano RA. Symposium review: Integration of postweaning nutrient requirements and supply with composition of growth and mammary development in modern dairy heifers. J Dairy Sci 2019;102(4):3692–705.

3. Baldwin RL, McLeod KR, Klotz JL, Heitmann RN. Rumen development, intestinal growth and hepatic metabolism in the pre and postweaning ruminant*. J Dairy Sci 2004;87:E55–65.

4. Warner RG, Flatt WP, Loosli JK. Dietary Factors Influencing Development of Ruminant Stomach. J Agric Food Chem 1956;4(9):788–92.

5. National Research Council. Nutrient requirements of dairy cattle. 7th ed. National Academies Press; 2001.

6. Drew B. Targets for rearing dairy heifers – Weaning to calving. In Pract 1998 Jan 1;20(1):35–8.

7. Green MJ, Bradley AJ. Dairy herd health; 2012.

8. AHDB. Youngstock and heifers [Internet]. Dairy housing: A best practice guide. 2015.

9. Swanson EW. Effect of rapid growth with fattening of dairy heifers on their lactational ability. J Dairy Sci 1960;43(3):377–87.

10. Sejrsen K, Huber JT, Tucker HA, Akers RM. Influence of nutrition on mammary development in pre and postpubertal heifers. J Dairy Sci 1982; 65(5):793–800.

11. Meyer M. Developmental, nutritional, and hormonal regulation of mammary growth, steroid receptor gene expression and chemical composition of retained tissues; J Dairy Sci 2005; 89(11):4298–4304.

12. Meyer MJ, Capuco AV, Ross DA, Lintault LM, Van Amburgh ME. Developmental and nutritional regulation of the prepubertal bovine mammary gland: II. Epithelial cell proliferation, parenchymal accretion rate, and allometric growth. J Dairy Sci 2006 Nov 1;89(11):4298–304.

13. Soberon F, Van Amburgh ME. Effects of preweaning nutrient intake in the developing mammary parenchymal tissue. J Dairy Sci 2017 Jun 1;100(6):4996–5004.

14. Boulton A. An economic analysis of heifer rearing and breeding selection in Great Britain – An empirical analysis. PhD Thesis, Royal Veterinary College; 2014.

15. Sherwin V, Remnant J. Weaning and postweaning management of dairy replacement heifers. In Pract 2018 Dec 1;40(10):449–56.

16. Arrazola A, Dicker K, Vasseur E, Bergeron R. The effect of early housing and companion experience on the grazing and ruminating behaviour of naïve heifers on pasture. Appl Anim Behav Sci 2020 Apr 1;226. 104993.

17. Velázquez-Martínez M, López-Ortiz S, Hernández-Mendo O, Díaz-Rivera P, Pérez-Elizalde S, Gallegos-Sánchez J. Foraging behavior of heifers with or without social models in an unfamiliar site containing high plant diversity. Livest Sci 2010;131(1): 73–82.

18. Suttle N. Assessing the needs of cattle for trace elements. In Pract 2004 Nov 1;26(10):553–61.

19. Webster AJF. Effects of housing and two forage diets on the development of claw horn lesions in dairy cows at first calving and in first lactation. Vet J 2001 Jul 1;162(1):56–65.

20. Hirst WM, Murray RD, Ward WR, French NP. A mixed-effects time-to-event analysis of the relationship between first-lactation lameness and subsequent lameness in dairy cows in the UK. Prev Vet Med 2002 Jul 25;54(3):191–201.

21. Gard JA, Taylor DR, Wilhite DR, Rodning SP, Schnuelle ML, Sanders RK, et al. Effect of exercise and environmental terrain on development of the digital cushion and bony structures of the bovine foot. Am J Vet Res 2015 Mar 1;76(3):246–52.

22. Logue DN. Effect of cubicle training dairy heifers before first calving on the subsequent behaviour and hoof health. In: 13th International symposium and 5th conference on lameness in ruminants. Maribor, Slovenia; 2004.

23. Forbes AB, Huckle CA, Gibb MJ, Rook AJ, Nuthall R. Evaluation of the effects of nematode parasitism on grazing behaviour, herbage intake and growth in young grazing cattle. Vet Parasitol 2000 Jun 10;90(1–2):111–8.

24. Fox MT, Hutchinson M, Riddle A, Forbes AB. Epidemiology of subclinical dairy cow nematode infections on five farms in England in 2002 and a comparison with results from 1978 to 1979. Vet Parasitol 2007 May 31;146(3–4):294–301.

25. Charlier J, Dorny P, Levecke B, Demeler J, von Samson-Himmelstjerna G, Höglund J, Vercruysse J. Serum pepsinogen levels to monitor gastrointestinal nematode infections in cattle revisited. Res Vet Sci 2011 Jun 1;90(3):451–6.

26. Taylor MA. Sustainable worm control strategies for cattle: A technical manual for veterinary surgeons and advisors. Control of Worms Sustainably, COWS.

27. Taylor M. Use of anthelmintics in cattle. In Pract 2000;22(6):290–304.

28. Höglund J, Morrison DA, Charlier J, Dimander SO, Larsson A. Assessing the feasibility of targeted selective treatments for gastrointestinal nematodes in first-season grazing cattle based on mid-season daily weight gains. Vet Parasitol 2009 Sep 16;164(1):80–8.

29. Stromberg BE, Moon RD. Parasite control in calves and growing heifers. Vet Clin North Am Food Anim Pract. Elsevier 2008;24(1):105–16.

30. Keeton STN, Navarre CB. Coccidiosis in large and small ruminants. Vet Clin North Am Food Anim Pract. W. B. Saunders 2018;34(1):201–8.

31. Bangoura B, Bardsley KD. Ruminant coccidiosis. Vet Clin North Am Food Anim Pract 2020;36(1):187–203.

32. Pirlo G, Miglior F, Speroni M. Effect of age at first calving on production traits and on difference between milk yield returns and rearing costs in Italian Holsteins. J Dairy Sci 2000 Mar 1;83(3):603–8.

33. Ettema JF, Santos JEP. Impact of age at calving on lactation, reproduction, health, and income in first-parity Holsteins on commercial farms. J Dairy Sci 2004 Aug 1;87(8):2730–42.

34. Wathes DC, Pollott GE, Johnson KF, Richardson H, Cooke JS. Heifer fertility and carry over consequences for life time production in dairy and beef cattle. Animal 2014;8(suppl. 1):91–104.

35. Perry GA. Physiology and endocrinology symposium: Harnessing basic knowledge of factors controlling puberty to improve synchronisation of estrus and fertility in heifers. J Anim Sci 2012 Apr;90(4):1172–82.

36. Gasser CL. Joint Alpharma-beef species symposium: Considerations on puberty in replacement beef heifers. J Anim Sci 2013 Mar;91(3):1336–40.

37. Day ML, Imakawa K, Wolfe PL, Kittok RJ, Kinder JE. Endocrine mechanisms of puberty in heifers. Role of hypothalamo-pituitary estradiol receptors in the negative feedback of estradiol on luteinizing hormone secretion. Biol Reprod 1987;37(5):1054–65.

38. Byerley DJ, Staigmiller RB, Berardinelli JG, Short RE. Pregnancy rates of beef heifers bred either on puberal or third estrus. J Anim Sci 1987;65(3): 645–50.

39. Taylor V. The growth hormone (GH) and insulin-like growth factor axis in relation to fertility in high yielding dairy cows. University of London; 2001.

40. Archbold H, Shalloo L, Kennedy E, Pierce KM, Buckley F. Influence of age, body weight and body condition score before mating start date on the pubertal rate of maiden Holstein-Friesian heifers and implications for subsequent cow performance and profitability. Animal 2012 Jul;6(7):1143–51.

41. Larson RL. Heifer development: Reproduction and nutrition. Vet Clin North Am Food Anim Pract. Elsevier 2007;23(1):53–68.

42. Laster DB, Smith GM, Cundiff LV, Gregory KE. Characterisation of biological types of cattle (Cycle II) II. Postweaning growth and puberty of Heifers1. J Anim Sci 1979 Mar 1;48(3):500–8.

43. Margerison J, Downey N. Guidelines for optimal dairy heifer rearing and herd performance. In: Garnsworthy PC (ed.) Calf and heifer rearing: principles of rearing the modern dairy heifer from calf to calving. Nottingham University Press; 2005. p. 307–38.

44. Brickell JS, McGowan MM, Wathes DC. Effect of management factors and blood metabolites during the rearing period on growth in dairy heifers on UK farms. Domest Anim Endocrinol 2009 Feb 1;36(2):67–81.

45. Boulton AC, Rushton J, Wathes DC. A Study of Dairy Heifer Rearing Practices from Birth to Weaning and Their Associated Costs on U.K. Dairy Farms. Open J Anim Sci 2015;05(2):185–97.

46. Walsh JP, Coates A, Lima F, Smith R, Oikonomou G. Randomised clinical trial evaluating the effect of different timing and number of fixed timed artificial inseminations, following a seven-day progesterone-based protocol, on pregnancy outcomes in UK dairy heifers. Vet Rec 2017;181(22):595–9.

47. Kuhn MT, Hutchison JL, Wiggans GR. Characterization of Holstein heifer fertility in the United States. J Dairy Sci 2006;89(12):4907–20.

48. Bach A. Associations between several aspects of heifer development and dairy cow survivability to second lactation. J Dairy Sci 2011 Feb;94(2):1052–7.

49. Givens MD, Marley MSD. Infectious causes of embryonic and fetal mortality. Theriogenology 2008 Aug 1;70(3):270–85.

50. Davison HC, French NP, Trees AJ. Herd-specific and age-specific seroprevalence of Neospora caninum in 14 British dairy herds. Vet Rec 1999 May 15;144(20):547–50.

51. Brickell JS, McGowan MM, Wathes DC. Association between Neospora caninum seropositivity and perinatal mortality in dairy heifers at first calving. Vet Rec 2010 Jul 17;167(3):82–5.

Chapter 8

Calf health management

Sophie Mahendran and Richard Booth

CHAPTER CONTENTS

Maintaining the best health in your calves is important to ensure welfare and productivity are not compromised, as well as keeping the rearing process as simple and stress free as possible. The common calf health management procedures in the UK are described in this chapter, along with common infectious diseases that will likely be encountered.

Although it is important to reduce the challenges faced by a calf, following the best practice rearing methods described in this book should produce resilient calves, meaning that the calf has the ability to recover after a challenge (usually a disease). Resilience is an active phenomenon, and is affected by many factors both innate to the calf and from its environment. Establishing the level of calf resilience can be done through assessment of the overall performance of the calf in the face of challenges (Table 8.1), and so record keeping is vital to informed decision making and data analysis on farm, in addition to the legal requirement for recording individual drug treatments with volume administered and batch number. While the use of paper records is still allowed, it is much more appropriate to use computerised record-keeping software. Mobile devices, such as tablets, are commonplace and mobile apps are now available through a number of companies

TABLE 8.1 Key performance indicators for monitoring calf health on farm.

Area to monitor	Target (%)
Stillbirth rate	<5
Perinatal mortality rate (within first 2 hours)	<5
Pre-weaning mortality rate (from 24-hours old to weaning)	<5
Calf mortality rate, 1–6 months of age	<3.5
Calf mortality rate, 6 months of age to breeding age	<4
Incidence of navel ill	<5
Incidence of diarrhoea	<10
Incidence of BRD	<15

(e.g. Total Dairy), with the ability to directly enter treatments as they are given, but also to look up the history of animals to help with decisions about future treatments and management changes (Figure 8.1).

Some of the significant events in a calf's life are detailed in Figure 8.2, with each of these posing a challenge to its health and welfare.

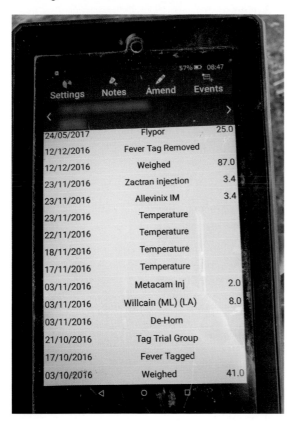

FIGURE 8.1 An example of on farm software on a tablet device that can be used to keep records.

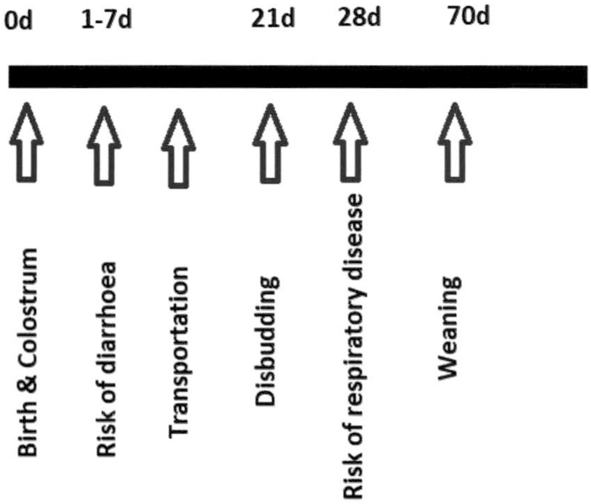

0d   1-7d   21d   28d   70d

Birth & Colostrum • Risk of diarrhoea • Transportation • Disbudding • Risk of respiratory disease • Weaning

FIGURE 8.2 Some of the significant events in the early life of a calf.

TRANSPORTATION AND SALE OF CALVES

Many dairy farms will sell their beef calves at an early age, helping to free up space and reduce the use of resources that may be required for rearing of replacement heifers. Some dairies will also send their heifers away to specialist rearing units, only returning to the main dairy when they are due to calve for the first time. In addition to following the relevant legislation, it must be remembered that very young calves are incredibly vulnerable to the stress and disease risk caused by transport, especially if they are moved through collection points that bring them into contact with animals from other farms. As a minimum, the relevant legislation for calf transport (Box 8.1) and sale at market (Box 8.2) in the UK should be noted and followed.

> **Box 8.1** UK Legislation for calf transport – Welfare of Animals (Transport) Order 1997
>
> Newborn animals in which the navel has not completely healed shall not be considered fit for transport.

> **Box 8.2** UK Legislation for selling calves at market – Welfare of Animals at Markets Order 1990
>
> - No person shall bring to a market a calf which is less than 7-days old or which has an unhealed navel.
> - No person shall bring to a market a calf which has been brought to a market on more than one occasion in the previous 28 days.
> - It shall be the duty of the owner of any calf in a market on any day, to remove it from the market within 4 hours of the time when the last sale by auction of a calf has taken place on that day.

Regardless of the minimum legislative requirements, some milk contracts are now also restricting the age at which calves can be moved off farm. Farms under tuberculosis (TB) restriction further complicate calf movements where movement is prohibited unless to a designated approved finishing facility (AFU).

When transporting calves, it is important that the trailer is completely clean (i.e. no faecal contamination from other cattle) to reduce the risk of faeco-oral transmission of infectious disease. If transporting calves any significant distance (i.e. outside of the farm) the trailer must be well bedded with straw to provide a safe and comfortable lying area.

DISBUDDING OF CALVES

Disbudding involves the removal of the horn bud prior to its attachment to the skull (which happens at around 2 months of age). After this time, the procedure is referred to as dehorning, which is considered more painful and harder to carry out than disbudding. The timing of disbudding is important, as it is a stressful event that has been shown to reduce growth rates in the subsequent few days. Avoid carrying it out at the same time as other management changes (such as if calves move pens or groups) and also avoid weaning time as this is already a stressful period for the calf.

There are some legal points to note around the act of disbudding and these surround the requirement to use local anaesthesia and observing the upper age limit for chemical cauterisation.

> **UK Legislation for calf disbudding – Protection of Animals (Anaesthetics) Act 1954**
>
> - It is an offence to disbud calves without the use of an anaesthetic other than when chemical cauterisation is used.
> - Chemical cauterisation may only be used during the first week of life.

Disbudding methods

There are several disbudding methods.

Chemical cauterisation

This involves the application of an alkaline caustic paste that destroys the germinal tissue of the horn bud. Legally this can only be done within the first week of life. Use of these products should be discouraged, but where they are used, great care is required to minimise any spread of the paste onto the surrounding skin. It should also only be used in calves housed in single pens to avoid the risk of calves rubbing against each other or licking the paste off.

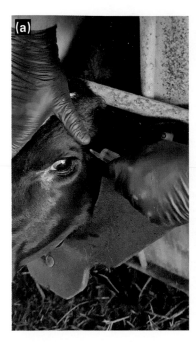
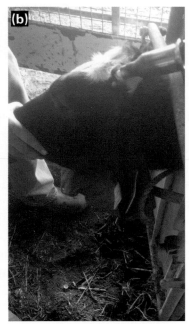
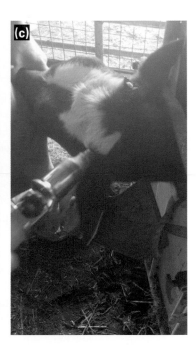

FIGURE 8.3 (a) Local anaesthetic being injected for a corneal block and (b and c) a hot iron being used to disbud a calf.

Hot iron disbudding

This is the most commonly used technique for disbudding, and must be done in conjunction with the use of anaesthetic. The aim of disbudding is to destroy the germinal epithelium around the peripheral base of the bud, preventing it from growing into a horn (Figure 8.3).

There are many brands of handheld gas devices available, and these are quick and easy to use. There are also electric devices that can be used in very young calves that only have very small buds.

Local anaesthesia for disbudding

The most common technique is to utilise local anaesthetic (e.g. procaine) in a perineural corneal nerve block (anywhere between 3–10 mL depending on the size of the buds). This blocks a branch of the lacrimal nerve, which is from the ophthalmic division of the trigeminal nerve, and innervates the horn corium and skin around the base of the horn. In addition to local anaesthetic, a NSAID should be given to these calves.

The correct location for the corneal block is underneath the lateral ridge of the frontal bone, which is located halfway between the lateral canthus of the eye and the horn bud. A suitably sized needle (e.g. 18 g 1" needle) is then inserted up to a depth of 1 cm, either perpendicular to the skin or angled towards the horn bud. Draw back on the needle to ensure there is no blood (if there is, just reposition the needle), and inject the local anaesthetic. After the needle is withdrawn, give the area a vigorous massage to disperse the anaesthetic around the nerve, and leave it for ~10 minutes to take effect. Signs of an effective nerve block include ptosis (droopy eye lid), and a complete lack of sensation around the base of the horn bud (which can be assessed by pricking with a needle). If the calf is still responsive, additional local anaesthetic can be applied in the same area.

Calf restraint for disbudding

Restraint of calves for disbudding can be by manual restraint or through the use of a calf crush (Figure 8.4). It is also possible to use systemic sedatives (e.g. xylazine) to knock down calves prior to disbudding. This technique is popular in Europe, and removes the stress of handling of these calves due to their recumbency. However, it does require the presence of a vet, and local anaesthetic and NSAIDs are still required. There is also additional risk inherent with the use of sedatives, and although complications are uncommon, the farmer should still be made aware of them.

Breeding of polled (hornless cattle) is increasing. There are already several polled mutations, but these are mostly in beef breeds (1). There is current work underway to try to introduce polled genes into high genetic merit dairy bulls, but this currently achieved using gene-editing, which is illegal in the UK (2).

CASTRATION OF CALVES

Removal of testicles makes male calves easier and safer to manage and to group house without the risk of unwanted pregnancies. Again, there are several methods of castrating that can be used, but regardless of the technique, local anaesthesia and NSAID pain relief must be administered with ALL techniques to minimise compromise of welfare. The reduced average daily live weight gain and potential weight loss associated with castration increases with the age at which it is done. This means that castration should be done as early as reasonably possible, avoiding other stressful events such as weaning. Prior to castration, ensure that both testicles are present, and if the animal is a cryptorchid (only has one testicle), do not remove the one palpable testicle – males with a retained testicle can still be fertile.

There are some legal points to note around castrating calves concerning who is able to carry out the castrations, the need to use local anaesthesia and the upper age limit for rubber ringing.

UK Legislation for calf castration – Protection of Animals (Anaesthetics) Act 1954

- It is an offence to castrate calves over 2 months of age without use of an anaesthetic.
- Use of a rubber ring to restrict the flow of blood to the scrotum, is only permitted without an anaesthetic if the device is applied during the first week of life.

Veterinary Surgeons Act 1966

- Only a veterinary surgeon may castrate a calf which has reached the age of 2 months.

Rubber ringing

Application of a rubber ring/elastration to constrict blood flow to the testicles and scrotum can only be done before 7 days of age. This technique is associated with chronic pain and prolonged healing times, and multiple rings should never be applied to the same animal (3). Care must be taken to ensure that both testicles are trapped below the ring for successful neutering. Ensure the scrotal wound is visually assessed regularly to monitor healing, and to check for signs of infection or abscess formation, with the scrotal skin taking up to 3 weeks to slough off.

Surgical castration

Surgical castration involves the physical removal of the testicles (two techniques are described here). Whichever technique is used, it is important that the calf is housed in a very clean environment with high hygiene standards due to the higher risks of infection, with prophylactic antibiotic usage sometimes being appropriate. When applying local anaesthetic, injecting directly into the stroma of

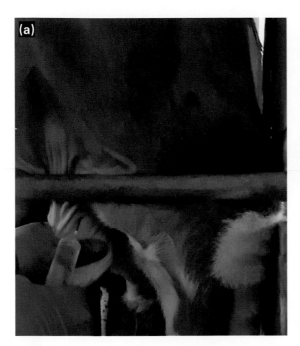

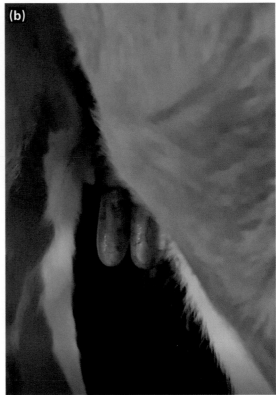

FIGURE 8.4 (a) Injection of local anaesthetic into the area around the spermatic cord should result in loss of cremaster muscle action, (b) resulting in the testicles hanging out of the scrotum once the base of the scrotum has been removed.

the testicles should be avoided as the vaginal tunic is inelastic, leading to pain as the testicles distend. Instead, inject local anaesthesia around the spermatic cord at the neck of the scrotum (~10 mL per side) along with some subcutaneously in the base of the scrotum (Figure 8.4). Leave the local anaesthetic for ~10 minutes to take effect.

The two techniques for surgical castration are (i) open (incise through the vaginal tunic so peritoneal cavity is open) and (ii) closed (no incision through the vaginal tunic). Both methods risk wound infection occurring, and care must be taken as to the time of year this is carried out to avoid the risk of myiasis occurring from fly larvae. Restrain the calf either manually or within a calf crush – having someone to tail jack the calf is helpful (hold the tail straight up) to encourage the animal to stand still, but this must not be done with excessive pressure or force. Ensure that the scrotum is clean prior to surgery, with clipping of the hair unnecessary. If the scrotum appears visually clean, do not attempt

to wash it as this increases the risk of wicking of bacteria up into the wound.

Incision into the scrotum can be done via two 'J' shaped incisions through the skin on each side of the scrotum, or in smaller calves, complete removal of the base of the scrotum (scrotal ablation) (Figure 8.4b). Each testicle is then grasped in turn and extended down, with any attached fascia stripped back up proximally. In smaller calves, the spermatic cord can then be twisted a dozen times to aid with haemostasis, and then firm downward pressure applied to remove the testicle and part of the spermatic cord. Ligation of the spermatic cord in smaller calves is not necessary, but in larger calves (>3 months old), it may be appropriate to use ligatures or emasculators to crush the spermatic cord and reduce the risk of haemorrhage. In larger calves, a Henderson castration tool may also be used (Figure 8.5), which is a clamp in an electrical drill that rotates until the testicle comes away.

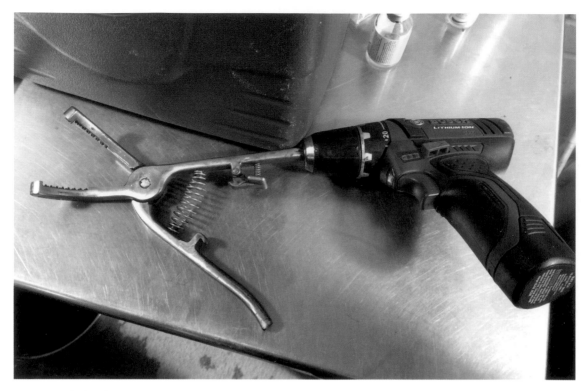

FIGURE 8.5 A Henderson castration tool.

Emasculators

Emasculators are an instrument that combine both a crushing and cutting zone, and is often favoured for use in surgical castration of older or larger bull calves where there is a higher risk of excessive bleeding occurring. The emasculator is applied to one spermatic cord at a time, making sure that there is minimal tension applied to the cord. The emasculator crushes the spermatic cord proximally, and cuts the cord distally (so it is important that you put the emasculator on in the correct orientation of nut-to-nut). The emasculator should be left in place to crush the cord for 3–5 minutes (depending on the size of the spermatic cord), and on removal the testicle will fall away.

Burdizzos

Bloodless castration can be done using burdizzos. This method has the least risk of infections or secondary complications as it does not broach the skin, but it also has the highest likelihood of failure. For this method you still need to block the spermatic cord and the skin at the neck of the scrotum, prior to crushing the spermatic cord through the scrotal skin. The burdizzo is applied for 10 seconds per site, and this is done at four sites staggered at the scrotal neck to allow maintenance of scrotal skin blood supply. If the spermatic cord is not fully crushed, the animal will remain fertile.

SUPERNUMERARY TEAT REMOVAL

Supernumerary teats are additional teats attached to the udder (often on the posterior of the udder), which may be functional (attached to the mammary gland and so can express milk) or non-functional (not able to express milk). Depending on the location of the teat, they may interfere with milking in the adult animal, or if connected to the actual gland, they may be a risk factor for mastitis development. However, most supernumerary teats go on to cause NO problems with milk production in the lactating animal, and so removal is often unnecessary.

There are some legal points to note around removal of supernumerary teats concerning who is able to carry the procedure out and the need to use local anaesthesia.

> ### UK Legislation for calf supernumerary teat removal – Veterinary Surgeons Act 1966
>
> - Only a veterinary surgeon may remove a supernumerary teat from a calf which has reached 3 months of age.

> ### Protection of Animals (Anaesthetics) Act 1954
>
> - It is an offence to remove a supernumerary teat from a calf which has reached 3 months of age without the use of an anaesthetic.

If the decision is made to remove a supernumerary teat, this should be done at an early age. Local anaesthetic must be applied to the base of the teat, and NSAID pain relief given. The teat can then be removed either using a sharp pair of scissors or a scalpel blade and the wound either stitched or left to heal by secondary intention (wound is left open to **heal by granulation, contraction, and epithelialization**).

INFECTIOUS CALF DISEASES

Calves are highly susceptible to infectious diseases due to their poorly developed immune system, and the immune-compromising effect that stressful events, such as transport, mixing, disbudding, castration and weaning, can have on them. Stress has a negative impact on the hypothalamic–pituitary–adrenal axis, resulting in the secretion of glucocorticoids that impair leucocyte function and down regulate neutrophils.

Many of the diseases described below can be prevented or alleviated by management strategies, with buy-in from all members of staff being critical for sustainability and longevity of improvements. Colostrum has a crucial role to play in development of a healthy calf (see Chapter 3), as does adequate nutrition which is needed to fuel the immune system (see Chapter 5).

Calf navel disease

The navel is the area where the umbilical cord attached the calf to the dam in the uterus, allowing transport of nutrients and oxygen during gestation. The umbilical cord is made up of several structures, including the umbilical veins and arteries, the amniotic membrane and the urachus.

At birth the umbilical cord ruptures, leaving what is best thought of as an open wound with direct connections to the blood, liver and bladder of the calf. If this umbilical region is contaminated with dirt and faecal material, bacteria can quickly penetrate into the calf's body, resulting in both systemic and more localised infections (Figure 8.6). In order to prevent this from occurring, disinfection of the navel with a 10% iodine solution (either spray or ideally a dip cup) should be done as soon after birth as possible, and ideally a total of three times (once when you check the sex of the calf, once when you feed the calf colostrum, and once when you move the calf from the calving pen to the calf shed). The iodine has both a disinfectant ability as well as being a drying agent to help the

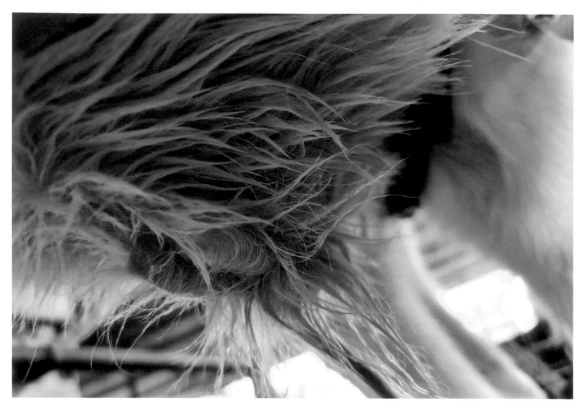

FIGURE 8.6 An enlarged navel with the surrounding hair appearing wet and discoloured.

umbilical stump regress. There are other products available to use on the navel, such as chlorhexidine based solutions, but iodine is relatively inexpensive and effective.

Infections of the navel area can create four different conditions (Table 8.2).

All of these conditions cause inflammation and potential infection of the umbilical structure, usually with a mix of bacterial environmental bacteria (*Escherichia coli*, *Staphylococcus* spp.,

Trueperella pyogenes, *Fusobacterium necrophorum*). These infections can lead to a systemic bacteraemia, with infection often spreading to joints (joint ill), as well as occasionally to the brain and eyes, along with infrequent development of generalised septicaemia.

Common clinical findings in a calf affected by any of the umbilical conditions includes being anorexic, dull, depressed and they may be pyrexic (≥39.5°C). Care must be taken to differentiate these

TABLE 8.2 Four different conditions that can develop due to infections of the umbilical area.

Condition	Description
Omphalitis	Inflammation of the external aspects of the umbilicus.
Omphalophlebitis	Inflammation of the umbilical veins, which can extend from the umbilicus to the liver.
Omphaloarteritis	Inflammation of the umbilical arteries, which can extend from the umbilicus to the internal iliac arteries.
Urachitis	Inflammation of the urachus, which can extend from the umbilicus to the bladder.

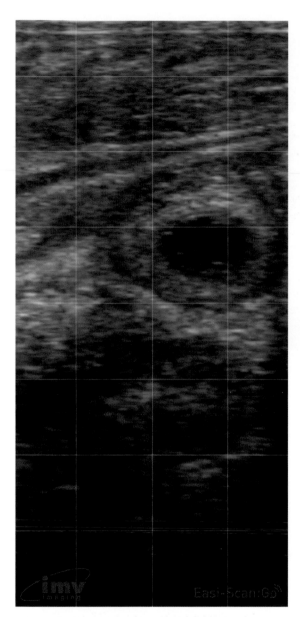

FIGURE 8.7 An ultrasound image of an infected umbilicus showing an area of fluid within the remaining cord remnants.

umbilical conditions with other differential diagnoses, which include a patent urachus or an umbilical hernia. Diagnostic investigation through the use of careful palpation and ultrasound can help to distinguish the specific condition (Figure 8.7), although many superficial infections will respond to antibiotics, such as amoxicillin or oxytetracycline, along

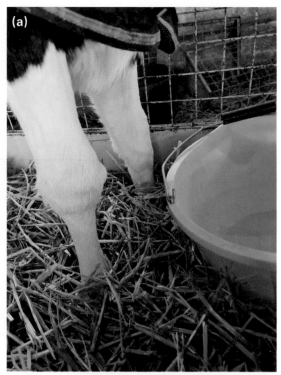

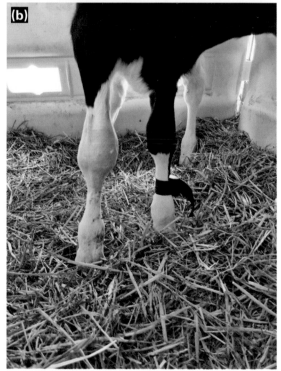

FIGURE 8.8 Calves displaying swollen front knees associated with joint ill.

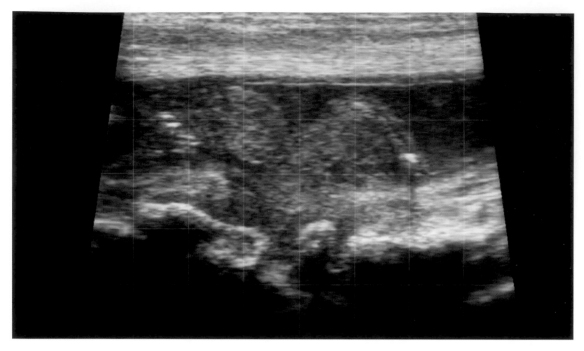

FIGURE 8.9 Ultrasound of a knee with joint ill. There is increased fluid present containing hyperechoic material (likely pus) and an uneven joint surface.

with NSAIDs. If an abscess is present in the umbilical region, this may be lanced with a scalpel, and the area lavaged to remove as much pus and debris as possible. More extensive infections may require surgical resection or removal of infected remnants.

Joint ill

Joint ill is properly referred to as septic arthritis, and it usually occurs secondary to poor navel care and poor colostrum management. One or more joints can be affected, with the knees, hock and stifles being common sites (Figure 8.8). Calves present as lame, often with swelling of the joints involved, and heat on palpation. This is a very painful condition, so calves may be reluctant to move around, with reduced feed consumption and growth rates. Further investigations into the severity of the joint infection can be performed via radiography of the affected joint, or by ultrasound (Figure 8.9).

Treatment is generally with an extended course

(2–4 weeks) of antimicrobials such as a beta-lactam antibiotic, in conjunction with pain relief via NSAIDs. In some cases, joint flushing may be attempted, but this often has limited success in the field.

Calf diphtheria

Calf diphtheria is also known as oral necrobacillosis, and is caused by the ubiquitous bacteria *F. necrophorum*. The disease can present itself in two forms (necrotic stomatitis and necrotic laryngitis), with the former being a much more common presentation (Table 8.3).

A predisposing condition for this disease is damage to the mucosa, which allows entry and establishment of the bacteria. This can be caused by erupting teeth, damaged and roughened feeding equipment, poor quality prickly forage or a concurrent upper respiratory tract infection that causes coughing and ulceration to the mouth

TABLE 8.3 Comparison of the different forms of calf diphtheria.

Necrotic stomatitis	Necrotic laryngitis
Necrotic ulceration of the cheek	Necrotic ulceration of the larynx
Foul smelling breathe, an external swelling usually on the mandible (Figure 10)	Difficulty breathing and a cough, calf may be pyrexic and can lead to aspiration pneumonia
Treat with beta-lactam or oxytetracycline antimicrobial and NSAID for 5 days	Treat with an extended course of antimicrobial (such as a beta lactam) and NSAID for 2-3 weeks. If severe breathing difficulty, may need tracheotomy.
Good prognosis	Guarded prognosis

and larynx mucosa. The biggest management risk factor is unhygienic environmental conditions, with dirty milk feeding equipment being used for a large number of calves acting as a classic source of infection.

Calf diarrhoea

Calf diarrhoea (often referred to as scour), is the most common calf disease with between 20–75%

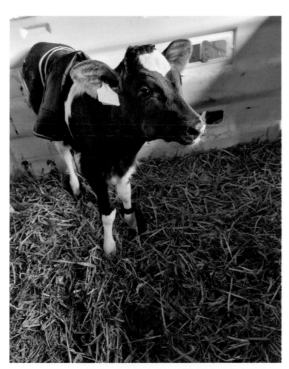

FIGURE 8.10 A calf with a classic lump visible on the lower mandible, indicative of diphtheria

morbidity found on some farms (4), and up to a 57% mortality rate (5). It is a multifactorial disease, involving aspects of both the calf, environment and pathogen, which combine together to cause sickness. This means that a holistic approach to managing diarrhoea outbreaks on farm is needed, both to control the disease within the current cohort, and to prevent spread to new and arriving youngstock.

There are two main sets of causes of diarrhoea; non-infectious (sometimes referred to as nutritional scour) and infectious causes (Table 8.4).

Diagnostic testing can be helpful to identify the cause of the diarrhoea, and is mainly focused on ELISA tests that can be done on farm for rapid results. Faecal samples can also be collected and sent to commercial laboratories for pathogen identification via culture, polymerase chain reaction (PCR) and microscopy for protozoal oocysts. This can be an important step for informing specific treatment protocols and management strategies.

Effects of diarrhoea on the calf

Physiologically, there are two types of diarrhoea that can occur; hypersecretory and malabsorptive. Hypersecretory diarrhoea commonly occurs with *E. coli* infections due to dysfunction of small intestinal cell metabolism. This leads to a net secretion of the electrolytes chloride, sodium and water into the intestinal lumen, which overwhelms the absorptive capacity of the large intestine and results in increased fluid content of the faeces (6). Malabsorptive diarrhoea is caused by villi atrophy, resulting in an inability to absorb electrolytes and

TABLE 8.4 Infectious and non-infectious causes of calf diarrhoea.

Non-infectious causes of diarrhoea	Infectious causes of diarrhoea
Hygiene of the milk mixing and drinking equipment	Bacteria: *E. coli*, *Salmonella enterica* subsp. *enterica* (*Salmonella* Dublin), *Clostridium perfringens*
Milk powder mixing concentration – high concentrations (>18%), especially in young calves can cause intestinal osmotic problems	Viruses: rotavirus, coronavirus, norovirus
Milk powder mixing temperature – mixing milk powder at low temperatures <40°c will not allow fat to dissolve	Protozoa: *Cryptosporidium parvum*, coccidiosis (*Eimeria* spp.)
Irregular feeding times – calves like regular mealtimes, with irregularity causing stress	
If using an automatic feeding machine, check calibration of mixer and dispenser	

water out of the intestinal lumen. Irrespective of the cause of the diarrhoea, it results in dehydration and metabolic acidosis from either electrolyte imbalances or D-lactate build-up (7).

Diarrhoea causes damage to the intestinal enterocytes, which impairs their digestive ability. This allows undigested carbohydrates to reach the large intestine, producing an acidic environment and favouring growth of lactic acid-producing gram-positive bacteria. Clinical signs of D-lactataemia include a decreased palpebral reflex, broad-based stance and ataxic movements due to the direct toxic effects on the brain. Signs associated with just a simple dehydration include a reduced suckle reflex, enophthalmos and an increased skin tent.

Calf diarrhoea also causes hyperkalaemia. This is a complicated physiological effect as potassium is actually lost from the body due to dehydration triggering aldosterone release from the pituitary gland, which acts on the kidney to conserve sodium and water, but results in loss of potassium from the body. However, potassium is also used to buffer the high levels of hydrogen ions found in the blood due to acidosis, along with impairment of sodium/potassium ATPase. Overall this results in increased extracellular potassium (i.e. more potassium in the blood stream), resulting in hyperkalaemia. The clinical signs associated with hyperkalaemia are muscular weakness (showing clinically as an inability to stand), and severe dehydration. Calves suffering from hyperkalaemia respond promptly to fluid therapy treatment, unlike calves suffering from D-lactataemia, which takes time to leave the body.

Treatment for diarrhoea

Treatment regimens will depend on the severity of the diarrhoea and the clinical state of the calf. The following is a guide to assessing the dehydration level of a calf(6):

- Mildly dehydrated 6–8%: skin tent duration 1–2 seconds, eyeball recession 2–4 mm
- Moderately dehydrated 8–10%: skin tent duration 2–5 seconds, eyeball recession 4–6 mm
- Severely dehydrated 10–12%: skin tent duration 5–10 seconds, eyeball recession 6–8 mm.

Calves with mild diarrhoea

Mildly affected calves are those who are generally still able to stand and may have a suckle reflex, and clinically are mildly to moderately dehydrated. For these calves the most important component of a treatment plan for calf diarrhoea is the use of oral rehydration therapy (ORT).

The main aims of ORT is to expand the plasma volume, correct electrolyte imbalances, provide

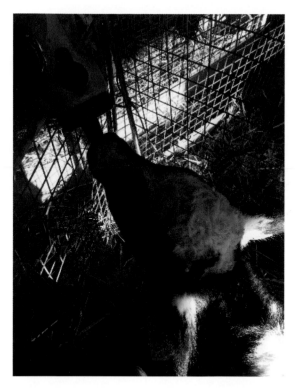

FIGURE 8.11 A calf suckling ORT from a teat bottle.

energy for sodium and water uptake from the small intestine, and to act as an alkalising agent (acetate and propionate which are metabolised to bicarbonate) to address metabolic acidosis (7). ORT solutions can be given via a teat bottle if the calf will suckle (Figure 8.11), or via an oesophageal feeder. Although the latter option is much quicker, the authors strongly encourage taking the time to get calves to suckle, with repeated use of a feeding tube causing irritation to the pharyngeal area, along with calves becoming stressed and resenting future handling. ORT should be given as extra 3 L feeds, thereby increasing fluid intakes as well as addressing electrolyte imbalances. In these mildly affected calves, routine milk feeds should still be offered at normal feeding times, with additional electrolytes given at lunch time and the evening. If calves are not willing to suckle milk feeds, these milk meals can also be replaced by ORT in the short term.

There are also some electrolyte products that can be added directly to milk, which can be useful in situations where the calves are still drinking milk, but have loose faeces and perineal staining but are otherwise bright, alert and responsive. However, calves with diarrhoea will still need EXTRA fluid in the form of additional ORT outside of normal mealtimes to correct dehydration.

Continued provision of milk feeds is vital for supplying energy to the calf. During cases of diarrhoea only part of the intestine is affected – the rest of the intestine is still capable of digesting milk to utilise the energy from it for the body to use, so it is vital that milk feeding continues if the calf will voluntarily drink it. Milk must not be given by oesophageal feeder as it will end up in the rumen, leading to putrefaction and bloating. It is worth noting that calves with diarrhoea may have reduced lactase activity, which is responsible for hydrolysing the lactose in milk to glucose. This means less glucose (and therefore energy) is accessible to the calf from the milk. However, this can be combated by adding lactase to the milk (available in tablet form from chemists) to aid the lactose breakdown. The addition of bicarbonate directly to milk to combat acidosis should also be avoided as this increases abomasal pH levels, thus reducing the protective effect against bacteria entering the intestines.

In addition to ORT, NSAIDs can be useful to reduce gastrointestinal cramping and discomfort, leading to increased voluntary feed intakes and improved calf welfare.

Calves with severe diarrhoea

More severely affected calves are those that are recumbent, or are diagnosed as suffering from metabolic D-lactate acidosis. They may be classed as clinically moderately or severely dehydrated (see definitions of dehydration above), and will require intravenous fluid therapy. The use of Hartmann's solution or 0.9% saline is common, but additional potassium should be avoided as the calf will initially be hyperkalaemic due to the hydrogen/potassium ion exchange that occurs.

Prior to IV fluid administration, the calf must be isolated and the jugular area clipped and cleaned.

Placement of jugular catheters can be challenging in dehydrated calves, so having excellent lighting is important. Lying the calf on a straw bale, and allowing its head to hang down can improve jugular filling. Also using a scalpel blade (after application of local anaesthesia) to cut through the skin and down to visualise the jugular can help. Additionally, use of ultrasound to identify the location of the jugular within the neck can be done in difficult situations. Jugular catheters should be sutured or glued into place, and bandaged to prevent the calf rubbing it out. Fluids should be pre-warmed to body temperature prior to administration to help prevent further cooling of the calf's core body temperature (Figure 8.12).

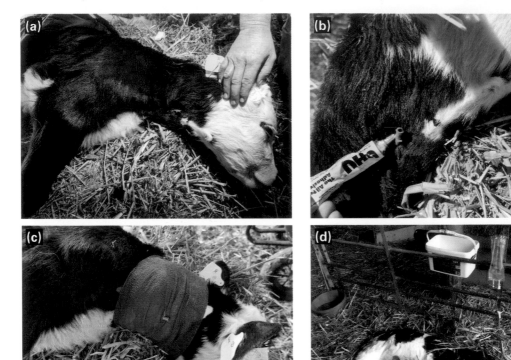

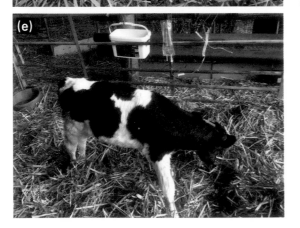

FIGURE 8.12 Series of images showing the steps in providing intravenous fluid therapy. (a) The calf should be restrained in lateral recumbency in an area with good light. The site should be clipped and cleaned prior to insertion of the catheter to reduce the chance of phlebitis. (b) The catheter can be secured in place using super glue, or by stitching it to the skin. (c) The catheter should be bandaged in place to reduce the risk of the catheter being dislodged. (d) The fluid should be pre-warmed in a bucket of hot water before administration. Hanging of the fluid bag at a level that will remain above the calf even when it stands up is needed to ensure good flow of the fluid. (e) Clinical improvement in the condition of the calf can be fairly rapid after intravenous fluid therapy (IVFT), with less severely affected calves able to stand after only 1L of fluid has been administered. Once the calf has become mobile, supervision of the drip line and catheter are needed to prevent kinking or pulling out of the catheter.

Litres of fluid calf needs to receive over a 24-hour period =

(fluid deficit × kg bodyweight) + (maintenance 50 mL/kg/day)

You can also add 100 mL/kg/day to cover ongoing losses from continued diarrhoea.
For example, a 50 kg calf that is 10% dehydrated needs:

(0.1 × 50 kg) + (50 mL × 50 kg) + (100 mL × 50 kg) = 10 L over 24 hours

It is possible to provide a fluid bolus to calves via an 80 mL/kg/hour bolus for up to 30 minutes – practically speaking this usually means opening up the valves on the drip fully and squeezing the bag. The fluid administration can then be slowed down to give one-half of the fluid imbalance over the first 6 hours and the rest over 24 hours.

While the fluid volumes calculated above are manageable in hospitalised settings, controlling this on a farm may be difficult due to lack of supervision and an inability to change fluid bags easily. In the authors' experience, use of a rough calculation whereby the percentage dehydration as bodyweight of the calf is taken to estimate the immediate fluid deficit of the calf works well. For example, a 50 kg calf that is 10% dehydrated will require an approximate 5 L of fluid. This can then be administered from a single fluid bag (1, 3 and 5 L bags are commercially available), and is usually enough to re-perfuse the kidneys and improve the hydration status of the calf back to a point where ORT can then be initiated to correct the remaining deficits.

If a calf is suffering from metabolic acidosis (clinically demonstrated by a decreased palpebral reflex, broad-based stance and ataxic movements), IV fluid therapy with bicarbonate-containing fluids is ideally required. You should aim to correct the acidosis over a 6 to 12 hour period, with caution required if measurement of the acid-base balance and base deficit is not possible (i.e. if you do not

have access to a blood gas machine). Generally, a base deficit of 10 mmol/L is a safe figure to use in calculations for the amount of bicarbonate needed by a calf, with rehydration of the calf allowing the kidneys to further correct any remaining acidosis. If you are in doubt about whether to add bicarbonate to the IV fluids, it is best not to. Rehydration of the calf with isotonic fluids will allow re-perfusion of the kidneys and self-correction of the acid-base imbalance over time, usually with little detriment to the prognosis of the calf.

Amount (mmol) of bicarbonate to give = bodyweight (kg) × base deficit (mmol/L) × 0.5
1 g of sodium bicarbonate = 12 mmol.
For example, a 50 kg calf needs:
50 kg × 10 mmol/L × 0.5 = 250 mmol of bicarbonate
250 mmol ÷ 12 = 21 g of bicarbonate administered over 6 to 12 hours.

Calves often respond well to IV fluids, and if they are able to stand after administration of a couple of litres, they will usually have return of the suckle reflex. Offering them oral fluids is then important, and this can be either milk or ORT. However, care must be taken using NSAID in severely dehydrated calves as repeated treatments of NSAID can lead to abomasal ulceration and possible renal effects (Figure 8.13). Generally, antimicrobial use for diarrhoea in calves is unnecessary. The main exception to this is if *Salmonella* is identified, or if calves are becoming septicaemic, which can happen following severe *E. coli* infections.

Lastly, tender loving care (TLC) is required for calves suffering from diarrhoea. Ensuring they are kept out of drafts, warm and dry is important, so extra bedding and a heat lamp can be useful. If calves have a calf jacket on, ensure that it is not becoming wet and covered in faeces, and if necessary, change it for a clean jacket. Calves with severe scour often get scalding of the skin around the perineum and hind legs, with hair loss and

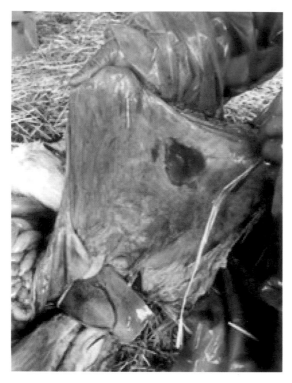

FIGURE 8.13 A post-mortem image of an abomasal ulcer in a calf that had received repeated NSAID treatments due to continued diarrhoea.

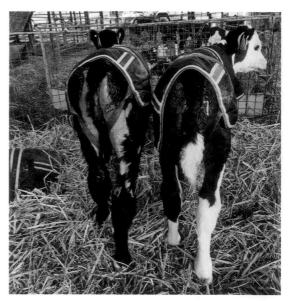

FIGURE 8.14 Comparison of a calf that has had diarrhoea (on the left) and one that has not (on the right). The hair loss can be clearly seen due to scalding of the skin.

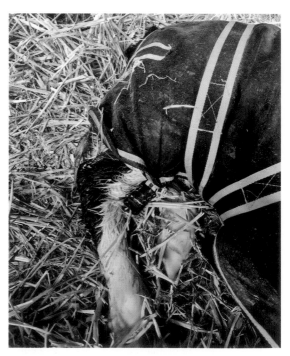

FIGURE 8.15 Faecal staining of the backlegs is common with very watery diarrhoea. These legs should be gently cleaned with warm water to reduce discomfort, skin scalding and risk of fly strike.

sore skin (Figure 8.14). Gently cleaning this area with warm water and cotton wool can reduce the discomfort associated with this, and application of an emolliating cream (e.g. udder cream) can help reduce skin irritation (Figure 8.15). This is especially important in the summer months when the risk of fly strike is quite high – use of topical permethrin pour-ons can be applied to reduce the risk of this occurring.

Prevention strategies

It must be stressed that caring for calves with diarrhoea is time consuming and hard work created by the extra visits to provide fluids and time caring for individuals. This is why it is important to put the extra effort into preventing disease occurring in the first place rather than subsequently trying to fix it. Most cases of diarrhoea will have an infectious component, with the major pathway of transmission for all infectious agents being the faecal-oral route, so housing hygiene is paramount. Rotavirus and coronavirus are shed for 5–7 days from infected calves, and along with *E. coli*, are also shed by adult cows, meaning calving pen hygiene must be addressed. Use of vaccines in the dam for rotavirus, coronavirus and *E. coli* during the dry period will increase protective antibody levels in the colostrum, helping to boost calf immunity to these diarrhoea pathogens. Colostrum management should also be assessed to ensure there is no failure of passive transfer, which could be contributing to an increased risk of disease in the calves (see Chapter 3). If there is a concern over a nutritional cause of the diarrhoea, careful assessment of the milk feeding routine is needed (see Chapter 5).

To reduce the risk of spread of infectious pathogens, ensuring pens are kept clean with ample thick bedding that is topped up daily to reduce contact of the calf with faecal material is important. This is especially critical in the winter to reduce the effect of cold stress. In outdoor hutches, avoid bedding the outside run areas unless they are situated under a roof – straw that is rained on becomes a reservoir for bacteria and protozoa, creating a dirty area that is unlikely to dry out in damp climates. Hygiene in group pens around busy areas such as the feeder and water trough are also important (Figure 8.16). Build-up of manure both on the floor and on feeding equipment increases the risk of faeco-oral transmission, and again must be cleaned as frequently as possible.

Isolation of sick individuals is very helpful for reducing the spread of disease, and this is important when dealing with *Cryptosporidium* spp. due to the ability of the oocysts to survive in the environment for many months in warm, moist conditions. Thorough cleaning (ideally at higher temperatures, such as with steam) and disinfection of a pen following housing of sick calves is needed, with disinfectants containing hydrogen peroxide, formaldehyde or amine-based products (e.g. Kenocox) being effective against *Cryptosporidium* oocysts. Halofuginone can be used to minimise

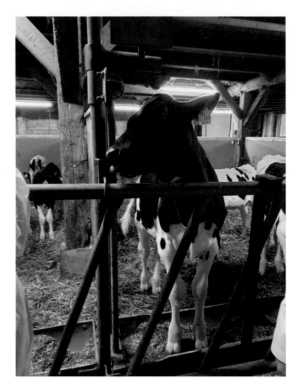

FIGURE 8.16 Feeding systems that allow calves to stand in or easily defecate in are a risk for the spread of pathogen between calves.

group level spread of *Cryptosporidium* spp. It is an oral treatment given for 7 days from birth, but should only be used as cover while management changes are taking place. It should not be used as a long-term solution in lieu of creating a clean environment.

Coccidiosis generally occurs in slightly older calves following ingestion of large quantities of sporulated oocysts from the environment. The coccidian causes damage to the gut mucosa, especially in the large intestine, resulting in blood being seen in the faeces. Predisposing factors are again hygiene related (Figure 8.17), with high stocking densities and faecal contamination in conjunction with stressful events often leading to outbreaks. Oral anti-coccidial treatments of the whole group can also be used (diclazuril at 1 mg/kg or toltrazuril at 20 mg/kg), and it is also possible to provide in-feed treatment with decoquinate at 1 mg/kg for 28 days. However, like halofuginone, this should

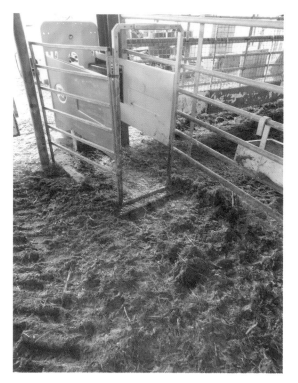

FIGURE 8.17 A build-up of manure around an automatic calf feeder feeding station is a particular risk factor for cryptosporidiosis and coccidiosis.

not be considered a long-term solution, with environmental hygiene improvements required.

Bovine respiratory disease

Bovine respiratory disease (BRD) is more commonly referred to as 'pneumonia', and in youngstock usually affects calves from 2-weeks to 6-months old. However, it is better described as a disease complex due to its mixed aetiology involving many pathogens (viral, bacterial and mycoplasma), with multifactorial interactions between the host, pathogen and environment. BRD is one of the leading causes of reduced productivity in calves and subsequently adult cattle, with each case estimated to cost the farmer ~£45. A prospective cohort study of UK farms found an incidence of 46% of pre-weaned calves affected, with a range of 20–78% between farms (8). The average mortality

rate in calves ranges from 2–8%, with reduced daily growth rates and the associated costs of drug treatments to factor in. Longer term losses are also seen, with heifers that experience four or more episodes of BRD being 1.9 times less likely to finish their first lactation (9).

The anatomy of the respiratory tract in cattle is the main reason cattle are so predisposed to developing respiratory disease. At birth the lungs are still developing and so have poorer protective mechanisms, along with a reduced immune system efficacy. The anatomy of the lungs is such that it has few connections between different lung lobes (of which there are six) meaning there is an increased risk of atelectasis and reduced air flow to an entire lung lobe when there is infection. There are large amounts of connective tissue in the lungs, which increases the resistance that occurs during breathing and increases the risk of pathogens being deposited in the lungs. Cattle also have a small tidal volume : surface area proportional to their body mass, resulting in higher resting respiratory rates, and a relatively poor capillary blood supply to each alveoli for gas exchange.

The respiratory tract has several physiological adaptations to aid in respiratory pathogen trapping and removal, such as nostril hairs acting as a physical barrier to large particles, a mucous lining of the respiratory tract to help trap pathogens and which contains several antimicrobial factors such as lysozymes and IgA, along with cilia that help transfer particulates back along the respiratory tract towards the nares for expulsion. There are also nonspecific immune cells, such as bronchoalveolar macrophages and neutrophils, that have phagocytic functions and can induce release of cytokines (proteins that are secreted by leukocytes to modulate the immune system) such as interleukin (IL)-8, which acts as a chemoattractant for immune cells to sites of inflammation. Some respiratory viruses are able to infect the ciliated respiratory epithelium as well as respiratory immune cells, thereby interfering with their function of bacterial clearance and killing, resulting in increased chances for bacterial infection.

TABLE 8.5 Details of the different infectious agents that can cause BRD.

Viral pathogens	Bacterial pathogens	Parasites
Parainfluenza virus 3 (PI3)	*Mannheimia haemolytica*	*Dictyocaulus viviparous*
Bovine respiratory syncytial virus (BRSV)	*Pasteurella multocida*	
Infectious bovine rhinotracheitis (IBR)	*Histophilus somni*	
Bovine coronavirus		
Bovine viral diarrhoea virus (BVDV)	*Mycoplasma bovis*	

In addition to the purely respiratory pathogens, prior infection with bovine viral diarrhoea virus (BVDV) can create a local and systemic immunosuppression through infection of mononuclear phagocytes, again increasing the risk of concurrent pathogen establishment.

Causes of BRD

There are a multitude of pathogens that can be involved in BRD, often with more than one being present concurrently (Table 8.5).

The respiratory viruses are thought to interfere with the calve's immune system, decreasing its ability to respond to subsequent bacterial infections. Many of the bacterial pathogens are ubiquitous and often found in the nasopharyngeal commensal microflora of healthy animals. These bacteria are capable of forming biofilms and have different virulence factors that enhance the bacteria's ability to invade and colonise the lower respiratory tract, leading to tissue destruction and an inflammatory response.

Risk factors predisposing calves to development of BRD are anything that induces stress (which raises cortisol levels and impedes the immune system), including transport, co-mingling with calves of different ages or calves from different farms, and weaning. In addition to this, environmental conditions such as poor ventilation, reduced air quality (including dust and ammonia), shared air spaces with older animals, cold and wet weather all increase the risk of calves developing respiratory disease. This means that good management and housing can go a long way to reducing the risk of BRD occurring.

Clinical signs of BRD

The earliest physiological response induced by respiratory pathogens is pyrexia ($\geq39.5°C$), which is known to occur prior to development of other clinical signs, such as nasal or ocular discharge and a cough. Changes in behaviour are also early indicators, with calves being slower to feed, spending more time lying down and generally having a quieter demeanour. Having a good stockperson who is able to pick up on these subtle signs is invaluable, with early identification allowing treatments to have much higher success rates.

Carrying out regular systematic checks on calves such as through using the Wisconsin calf scoring system can help to identify calves with disease (Table 8.6). It provides a method to identify and quantify the severity of any clinical signs being displayed by the calf, which can then be used to make treatment decisions and carry out further monitoring on the progress of the calf's condition.

Diagnosis of BRD

Identifying the causative pathogens of a BRD outbreak will help establish the epidemiology of the disease, which, in turn, will inform treatment and vaccine selection. Diagnostics are best performed in animals that have not received antimicrobial therapy, as this can alter the findings.

Deep nasopharyngeal swabs

Deep nasopharyngeal swabs are simple to carry out, and can be used for both bacterial culture and

TABLE 8.6 Description of the modified calf scoring point allocation system for assessing calf health, adapted from the University of Wisconsin-Madison calf health scoring system (10).

Clinical parameter	Points and description			
	0	**1**	**2**	**3**
Nasal discharge	Normal, serous discharge	Small amount of unilateral, cloudy discharge	Bilateral, cloudy or excessive mucus	Copious, bilateral mucopurulent nasal discharge
Ocular discharge	Normal	Mild ocular discharge	Moderate bilateral ocular discharge	Heavy ocular discharge
Mental demeanour	Normal – bright, alert, responsive	Dull but responds to stimulation	Depressed, slow to stand or reluctant to lie down	Unresponsive to stimulation
Cough score	No cough	Induce single cough	Induce repeated coughs or occasional spontaneous cough	Repeated spontaneous coughing
Faecal score	Normal	Semi-formed, pasty	Loose, but stays on top of bedding	Watery, sifts through bedding
Naval score	Normal	Slightly enlarged, not warm or painful	Slightly enlarged with slight pain or moisture	Enlarged with pain, heat or malodorous discharge
Joint score	Normal	Slight swelling, not warm or painful	Swelling with pain or heat, slight lameness	Swelling with severe pain, heat and lameness

viral PCR tests. The swab has a sheath to protect it from contamination when passing through the outer nares, and aims to collect a sample from the nasopharyngeal area. However, there is a risk that pathogens detected in this upper respiratory tract area may not be fully representative of the pathogens in the lower respiratory tract.

Serology

Serology and paired serology are also easy to perform, requiring only jugular blood samples collected in plain vacutainers. Single serology can be used in older animals to establish what pathogens they have been exposed to, and should only be collected after maternally derived antibodies have waned at around 9 months of age. Paired serology can be used in an outbreak to establish active exposure. Two samples are taken from the same animal 2–3 weeks part, with identification of a rising titre

to a pathogen indicating that this pathogen is involved in the BRD outbreak.

Bronchoalveolar lavage and transtracheal lavage

Bronchoalveolar lavage (BAL) and transtracheal lavage (TTL) are both methods of collecting a representative sample from the lower respiratory tract. Both of these techniques aim to introduce 0.9% sterile saline into the lungs, which is then aspirated back. The sample can then be used for PCR and culture and sensitivity tests. These procedures can be tricky to carry out for the inexperienced, and require two people for the restraint and sampling of the calf. In BAL a guarded sterile silicon tube (inner tube 4 mm diameter and 1.5 m long, outer tube 8 mm diameter and 1 m long) with lubrication on the end is passed via the ventral meatus and down through the larynx into the trachea. This procedure requires the calf's head to be slightly raised and extended to aid passage of the tube. Correct positioning of the tube in the trachea will elicit some coughing, and breathing will be identifiable in the tube by condensation being visible or air movements felt at the end of the tube. The inner tube is then extended down into the lungs, and is advanced until resistance is felt, indicating the tube is in a bronchus. 50 mL of sterile saline is then introduced into the lungs, and is withdrawn straight away – it must be noted that you will only aspirate 10–30 mL of fluid back from the lungs. The fluid should have a frothy, slightly opaque appearance.

The procedure for a TTL is similar, but a small incision is made directly through the skin of the neck after application of local anaesthetic, and into the trachea. The guarded sterile tube is then introduced via this hole, and the inner tube is advanced down into the lungs. This helps to avoid any contamination from the upper respiratory tract.

Thoracic ultrasound

Thoracic ultrasound makes use of a linear probe often used for cattle reproductive ultrasound as it is able to fit into the intercostal spaces (ICS) to visualise the surface of the lungs. There is no need to clip the hair from the area as soaking in 70% isopropyl alcohol will create adequate contact for the probe. Both sides of the thorax should be scanned, starting caudally in the 8–9th ICS where the edge of the liver or spleen can be seen, and working cranially to the heart base. The ultrasound is able to visualise the pleural surface (Figure 8.18) and detect lung

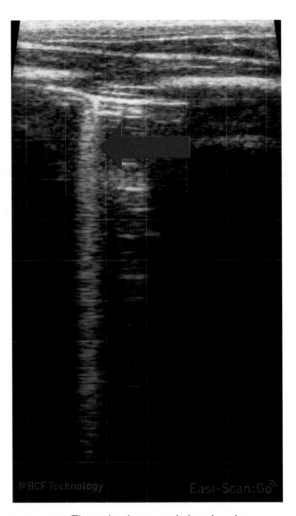

FIGURE 8.19 Thoracic ultrasound showing the presence of a comet tail (B line) from the pleural surface.

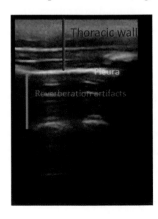

FIGURE 8.18 Normal anatomy of the lungs that can be seen on thoracic ultrasound. In normal aerated lung, reverberation artifacts (A lines) can be seen which is completely normal.

inflammation and consolidation caused by respiratory disease (11). This is seen visually as comet tails (Figure 8.19) or consolidation (Figure 8.20). It is common to see small numbers (three or fewer per image field) of comet tails in healthy lungs, but any consolidation is abnormal. In heifers with consolidation ≥3 cm, it has been demonstrated to lower average daily growth (12) and reduce first lactation milk yields by ~525 kg (13). Lesions that are not superficial cannot be visualised with this imaging modality due to poor travel of ultrasound waves through aerated lung tissue.

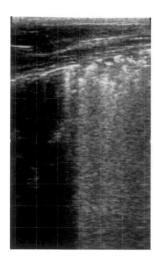

FIGURE 8.20 Thoracic ultrasound demonstrating consolidation of the lungs.

Post-mortem

If calves have died during a BRD outbreak, the findings of a post-mortem can be very helpful to identify the types of pathology occurring, and also to take lung samples for testing. If possible, fresh carcases should be sent to a laboratory for a full post-mortem, but satisfactory results can be achieved via an on farm inspection. Fresh and preserved samples (in formalin) from the trachea, lungs (at the junction between healthy and abnormal tissue) and (if possible) brain should be sampled for histopathology. Swabs of lung tissue from each of the lobes should also be collected for pathogen culture and PCR. This can be done in a sterile manner by first searing the surface of the lung with a hot blade, followed by an incision into the lung and insertion of a swab.

Treatment of BRD

Successful treatment of BRD relies on early identification of affected animals, prompt application of treatments, and careful monitoring to assess disease progression and the requirement for further treatments. Treatment of BRD generally comprises of combined antimicrobial and NSAID drugs. Successful use of diagnostics to identify pathogens, along with establishing antimicrobial sensitivity, can be challenging and expensive with BRD, but

should definitely be used in high prevalence or high mortality situations.

Drug selection should be based on pharmacokinetics (movement and distribution of drugs within the body) and pharmacodynamics (relation between drug concentration and antimicrobial activity) models of action, which assesses the levels reached in lung tissue as well as plasma levels. An example of this is macrolides, which have low plasma levels compared to their minimum inhibitory concentrations (MIC; the lowest concentration of drug that inhibits bacterial growth), but they are able to concentrate in the pulmonary epithelial lining fluid in the lungs, therefore, providing good treatment for respiratory infections. Other considerations to ensure treatment compliance include the length of the course, with single-dose long acting treatments often desirable due to the reduced time commitment, which can be a very important factor for busy stock people.

Many of the antimicrobial classes are considered suitable for use in treating BRD (beta-lactams, macrolides, tetracyclines, florenicol). Florenicol is often considered a suitable first line choice due to its wide spectrum of activity (including against *Histophilus somni* and *Mycobacterium bovis*) and a duration of action of up to 4 days. NSAIDs treatment should also be used to reduce inflammation and improve the demeanour of the calf, thus encouraging feed consumption which is important to provide energy to the immune system. Use of drugs that are more COX-2 specific (COX is an enzyme in the inflammatory pathway that is inhibited by NSAIDs) reduces potential side effects such as gastrointestinal ulceration (e.g. meloxicam). An additional factor to consider is the ease of administration of the NSAID – many drugs are injectable, with some formulations combined with an antimicrobial so that only one injection is required. There are also topical and in-feed products available, with selection of the correct one determined by the management strategies on the farm.

An additional treatment that may benefit some calves is the use of mucolytics, such as bromhexine. Bromhexine is a mucoregulator, which increases the viscosity of secretions improving mobilisation and drainage of mucus, thereby enhancing patency of the airways.

Prevention of BRD

The most important factor in preventing BRD is ensuring calves have a strong and effective immune system, which begins with excellent colostrum management (see Chapter 3) and proper nutritional provision (see Chapter 5). Correct management of the housing environment is the next most important factor for long-term reductions in BRD prevalence. One of the most common areas for improvement is the ventilation of the calf shed, with the overarching aim being to improve air quality (see Chapter 4). This can be achieved by increasing the air inlet area in the sides of the shed or through the use of positive pressure ventilation systems, such as tube fans, to blow air into the shed. Installation of tube fans should only be done following consultation and specific design of a tube with a qualified agricultural engineer who can assess correct tube placement, the size of the fan required and the correct placement of the holes within the tube to ensure consistent air delivery throughout the whole shed (Figure 8.21).

Humidity also has a significant impact on respiratory health in calves and adult cattle. It is recommended humidity levels be kept lower than 70%. However, in the UK, weather in the late autumn, winter and early spring results in often quite high background humidity levels; making it harder to maintain low humidity levels in housing. Shed hygiene is therefore critical; appropriate drainage for urine and milk and maintaining clean and dry bedding will improve the air quality at calf level.

Vaccination can play an important role in control and prevention of BRD, but it must be remembered that this will not prevent disease in the face of overall poor calf management (e.g. poor hygiene and air quality, and insufficient nutrition). Pathogen identification is important to establish the most useful vaccine to use, and also when to implement programmes to provide protection at the most critical time periods. Intra-nasal vaccines can be given from 7 days of age, with a quick onset of mucosal protection after 4 days meaning they can also be used in the face of a BRD outbreak. Depending on the product, systemic vaccines can be given from 2 weeks of age, but the primary course requires a minimum of two injections and the duration of cover is generally only 6 months. When using any vaccine, it must be remembered that proper storage and administration is vital to ensure the efficacy of the product.

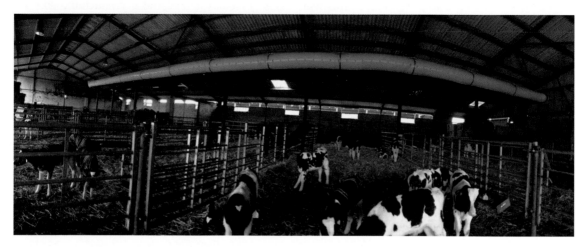

FIGURE 8.21 Positive pressure ventilation tube across the length of a calf shed that otherwise had very poor ventilation.

CONTRACTED TENDONS

Calves can be born with contracted flexor tendons in the front limbs, typically seen as knuckling, and usually affecting the fetlock of the calf. The inability to fully extend the leg affects how well the calf can walk. It can be a uni- or bilateral condition, with varying degrees of severity.

This condition is sometimes seen in association with other congenital abnormalities, such as a cleft palate, arthrogryposis (potentially associated with Schmallenberg virus or bluetongue virus) or dwarfism. However, the most common cause is uterine malpositioning, especially in large calves where the legs have been in a tucked position during foetal development.

Calves that are only mildly affected, and are still able to ambulate relatively well, will only need conservative management. Encouraging the calf to walk around, as well as providing physical therapy in the form of stretching and massaging the limbs into a straight position will help. Ensuring the calf is kept on deep bedding will protect the skin from abrasions if the calf tends to bend forward onto the dorsal skin of the fetlock area.

In more severe cases, splints can be applied to the legs – these are commercially available, and are placed along the back of the leg to maintain an extended position (Figure 8.22). The splint should not be placed above the knee as this will prevent the calf from being able to stand up and lie down unaided, with extended periods in lateral recumbency being a risk factor for respiratory issues. Splints can be uncomfortable for the calf, so ensuring NSAIDs are provided can help. The splints should not be left on for more than 1 week at a time, and care must be taken to ensure no rubs develop.

In extreme cases of contracted tendons, surgical resection of the superficial digital flexor tendon may be required, followed by casting of the limb to provide stability.

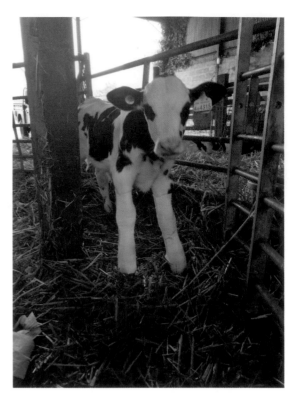

FIGURE 8.22 Calf that had contracted tendons in its front fetlocks with splints on both legs.

DERMATOPHYTOSIS

More commonly referred to as ringworm, dermatophytosis is a fungal infection of the hair shaft and skin caused by *Trichophyton verrucosum*. This is a zoonotic condition, so people in contact with these animals should wear appropriate PPE. It is commonly seen in group housed calves, especially when there are low light levels and moist conditions. The spores of the fungus can survive in the environment and on carrier animals for long periods of time, meaning the same buildings often have recurring problems with infection. Clinical signs include areas of hair loss (often circular) with a crusty appearance (Figure 8.23), which gradually regress over a few months. Heavily affected animals may also experience some reduction in weight gains. There is no specific treatment for those affected, and calves will self-cure. A prophylactic vaccine is available for use on farms that have large numbers of calves

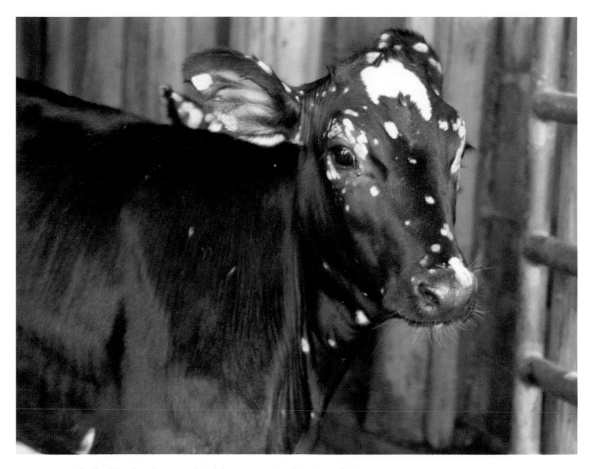

FIGURE 8.23 Calf with classic round hairless areas indicative of ringworm.

affected by the condition. In the authors' experience, high levels of ringworm are often associated with poor housing conditions and may also indicate a problem with nutrition. The immune system of healthy calves should be able to deal with the infection easily, so seeing calves with heavy ringworm burdens indicates that the immune system may not be functioning as optimally as it should.

BLOAT

Rumen bloat in calves can either be caused by free gas or formation of 'froth' in the rumen where gas is trapped in a foam. Bloat is caused by three main mechanisms in calves.

- Milk fermentation in the rumen of young calves. Milk usually enters the rumen due to poor feeding techniques and failure of oesophageal groove closure (see Chapter 5), allowing gas to be produced in the rumen. This can therefore be managed by correcting feeding management.
- Excessive concentrate ingestion in slightly older calves. Calves transitioning from milk onto solid feeds sometimes gorge on concentrates, particularly when they are not available ad libitum. This again allows excessive fermentation and accumulation of gas in the rumen, and can be managed by reducing concentrate intakes and increasing forage ingestion.
- Vagus nerve damage, usually as a consequence of severe pneumonia. The vagus nerve

innervates the forestomachs, but it passes through the thorax of the calf, meaning it can become inflamed during cases of respiratory disease, or even compressed by enlarged lymph nodes, resulting in dysfunction (14). This type of bloat is often more chronic in nature.

Acute bloat in calves may need relieving in an emergency situation. The severest cases can kill calves due to compression of the thorax and caudal vena cava, preventing breathing and return of blood to the heart. Passing a stomach tube into the rumen should allow release of gas but, in an emergency, a rumenotomy may be required. In chronic bloat where there is recurrence of gas accumulation, insertion of a trocar into the rumen will allow continuous release of free gas (Figure 8.24),

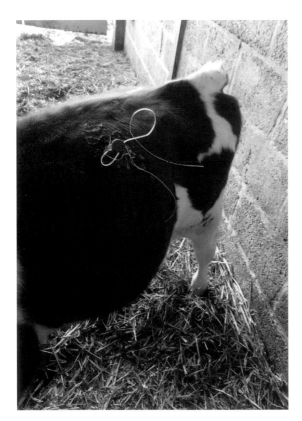

FIGURE 8.24 Calf with a 'Red Devil' rumen trocar in the left paralumbar fossa.

or even creation of a permanent rumen fistula. Any incision into the rumen will lead to contamination of the abdominal cavity, so antimicrobial cover and NSAID treatment will be required to reduce peritonitis.

INFECTIOUS BOVINE KERATOCONJUNCTIVITIS

Infectious bovine keratoconjunctivitis (IBK) is commonly referred to as New Forest eye, and is caused by the bacteria *Moraxella bovis*, which is spread by flies. Calves are usually affected in the summer period when fly numbers are highest, but the risk can be exacerbated by long grass or stalky forages that may cause trauma to the eye. IBK causes ocular ulcers which may affect both eyes and is very painful. The first indication of IBK may be epiphora (runny eyes), often seen with blepharospasm and cloudy corneas.

Treatment of mild cases uses topical antibiotic eye tubes (usually containing cloxacillin) for 3–5 days, along with NSAIDs. In more severe cases, bulbar subconjunctival or subpalpebral injections of antimicrobials with dexamethasone may be used to allow a steady release of antimicrobials over the globe. However, if animals are very fractious, this technique may be difficult, and can be replaced by systemic treatment with antimicrobials such as a tetracycline or florfenicol. If the ulceration is severe, placing a patch of material over the eye will provide some protection (Figure 8.25), or the eyelids may be sutured shut while the ulcer heals.

Management strategies to reduce occurrence include good fly control, including regular application of topical permethrin fly repellent, and use of permethrin coated ear tags to protect the face. Ensuring adequate feed space is also important so that cattle are not forced to have their heads in close proximity; this will help reduce spread within a group.

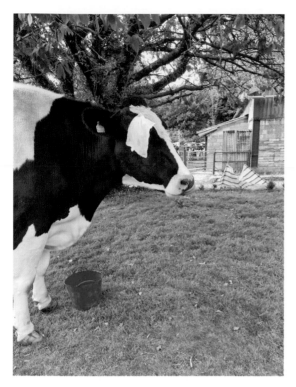

FIGURE 8.25 Material patch covering an eye affected by IBK.

REFERENCES

1. Wiedemar N, Tetens J, Jagannathan V, Menoud A, Neuenschwander S, Bruggmann R, et al. Independent polled mutations leading to complex gene expression differences in cattle. PLOS ONE. Moore S (ed.) 2014 Mar 26;9(3):e93435.

2. Carlson DF, Lancto CA, Zang B, Kim ES, Walton M, Oldeschulte D, et al. Production of hornless dairy cattle from genome-edited cell lines. Nat Biotechnol 2016 May 6;34(5):479–81.

3. Becker J, Doherr MG, Bruckmaier RM, Bodmer M, Zanolari P, Steiner A. Acute and chronic pain in calves after different methods of rubber-ring castration. Vet J 2012 Dec;194(3):380–5.

4. Windeyer MC, Leslie KE, Godden SM, Hodgins DC, Lissemore KD, LeBlanc SJ. Factors associated with morbidity, mortality, and growth of dairy heifer calves up to 3 months of age. Prev Vet Med 2014 Feb 1;113(2):231–40.

5. USDA. Part II: Changes in the U.S. Dairy Cattle industry, 1991–2007. 2007.

6. Smith GW. Treatment of calf diarrhea: Oral fluid therapy. Vet Clin North Am Food Anim Pract 2009;25(1):55–72, vi.

7. Lorenz I, Fagan J, More SJ. Calf health from birth to weaning. II. Management of diarrhoea in pre-weaned calves. Ir Vet J 2011 Sep 14;64(1):9.

8. Johnson KF, Chancellor N, Burn CC, Wathes DC. Prospective cohort study to assess rates of contagious disease in pre-weaned UK dairy heifers: Management practices, passive transfer of immunity and associated calf health. Vet Rec Open 2017 Apr 1;4(1).

9. Bach A. Associations between several aspects of heifer development and dairy cow survivability to second lactation. J Dairy Sci 2011 Feb;94(2):1052–7.

10. McGuirk S. Troubleshooting dairy calf pneumonia problems. In: Proceedings of the twenty fifth annual ACVIM forum. Seattle, WA; 2007.

11. Ollivett TLL, Caswell JLL, Nydam DVV, Duffield T, Leslie KEE, Hewson J, Kelton D. Thoracic ultrasonography and bronchoalveolar lavage fluid analysis in Holstein calves with subclinical lung lesions. J Vet Intern Med 2015 Aug 30;29(6):1728–34.

12. Dunn TR, Ollivett TL, Renaud DL, Leslie KE, LeBlanc SJ, Duffield TF, Kelton DF. The effect of lung consolidation, as determined by ultrasonography, on first-lactation milk production in Holstein dairy calves. J Dairy Sci 2018 Jun 1;101(6):5404–10.

13. Berman J, Francoz D, Dufour S, Buczinski S. Bayesian estimation of sensitivity and specificity of systematic thoracic ultrasound exam for diagnosis of bovine respiratory disease in pre-weaned calves. Prev Vet Med 2019 Jan 1;162:38–45.

14. Trent AM, Ducharme NG, Fubini SL, Steiner A. Surgery of the calf gastrointestinal system. In: Farm Animal Surgery. Elsevier Inc.; 2017. p. 505–18.

Chapter 9

Dairy sourced beef

Benjamin Barber

CHAPTER CONTENTS

This chapter discusses the rearing of calves for either beef or veal, with a focus on specialised rearers that accept Holstein-Friesian entire bull calves of variable health status from multiple dairy sources. Many of the concepts have been discussed in other chapters, but here we relate them specifically to dealing with rearing dairy breed beef calves.

WHY USE DAIRY BULL CALVES FOR BEEF?

Since the collapse of live exports, dairy-bred bull calves have been considered of low value in the UK,

with some being euthanased on farm as unmarketable. The development of an integrated beef supply chain, which redistributes these calves to dedicated rearing units via collection points, has rejuvenated demand for such calves as well as provided a more ethically acceptable solution for producers. More information has been produced on the economics of rearing male dairy calves and the margins involved, which has shown that intensive finishing of these cattle can consistently provide positive net profits.

These factors, alongside a UK industry goal of ending the routine euthanasia of calves and providing them with adequate care, has led to the increased supply of suitable calves and uptake of this model of beef production. Approximately 50% of the UK's beef now originates from the dairy herd. An increase in the number of dairy bull calves entering the beef chain rose by 59% from 2006 to 2015. Despite this, the Agriculture and Horticulture Development Board (AHDB) estimates that each year, of the 390,000 dairy sired bull calves born, 60,000 died or were euthanased on the dairy farm of origin. It should also be noted that while more dairy bull calves are entering the beef chain than previously, an estimated 77,000 of them died in abattoirs before 8 weeks of age (1).

Led by consumers and retailers, many milk processing groups continue to promote strategies and enforce policies that protect dairy-bred bull calves from being euthanased at the dairy source or reared for only a short duration. This includes reviewing breeding strategies that increases the uptake of sexed dairy semen and beef semen that will produce marketable animals, ensuring farms have an outlet for calves in all seasons, as well as encouraging a contingency plan if bovine tuberculosis (TB) movement restrictions are imposed. Farms are also improving the management of dairy-bred bull calves to increase their potential productivity and therefore value in longer term rearing systems.

Intensive beef systems can be an efficient form of farming, conforming to high levels of health and welfare that also provide an outlet for calves from the dairy herd which would not otherwise have had a purpose (Figure 9.1).

SYSTEM SETUP

With the average dairy herd calving all year round and consisting of 125 adult milking cows, it is almost impossible to produce large consistent batches of calves without sourcing from multiple dairies. After being purchased and sorted by the

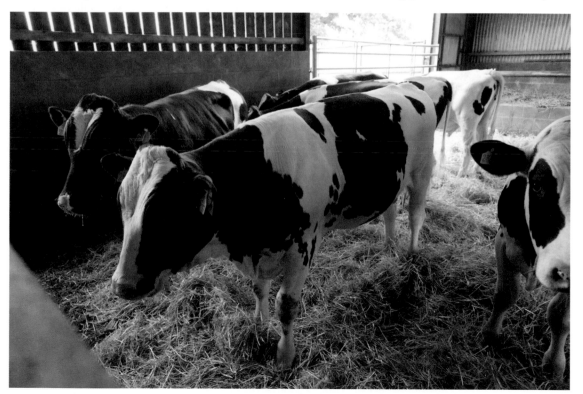

FIGURE 9.1 An example of very clean Holstein-Friesian bulls being housed in a straw yard.

Calves typically 2–6-weeks old, are purchased by the integrated supply chain from multiple dairies with variable health status

↓

Via a collection centre they are sorted based on weight, conformation and breed. A batch of pre-sorted calves is then transported to a specialist rearing unit

↓

On entry to the rearing unit, calves are started on CMR using various feeding methods and eventually weaned at approx. 8–10 weeks of age

↓

When animals have reached ~140 kg BW after being on the unit for 3 months, some rearers will then transport animals onto specific finishing units rather than continue the process themselves

↓

The age and weight at slaughter will depend on the desired product, breed, and performance of that animal
(see Table 9.1)

integrated beef supply chain via a collection centre, calves are transported as a consistent batch to a dedicated rearer with an all-in all-out policy.

Animals are then reared to a certain age and weight based on the desired product, breed, and performance of that animal (Table 9.1).

In the UK, veal production typically refers to rosé veal produced from Holstein-Friesian bulls slaughtered between 8 and 12 months of age. In comparison, most veal on the continent is white veal produced from dairy bulls fed an iron-deficient diet of primarily liquid milk, alongside specially formulated roughage. The lack of iron reduces haemoglobin levels, creating an artificially anaemic state which gives the carcase its paler appearance. In the EU, veal – both white and rosé – is defined as originating from calves that are slaughtered at less than 8 months of age.

WELFARE CONCERNS WITH VEAL PRODUCTION

The product veal has often had negative connotations, with a public perception of deprived, restricted animals fed a diet artificially deficient in iron and solid structure. These historical management conditions were proven to lead to abnormal behaviour, poor gut development and impaired immune function.

In the UK this image is far from the truth with 'veal crates' – wooden crates where animals were kept isolated and physically restricted – having been banned since 1990. Typical rearing systems are now straw-based, light, well ventilated sheds, where social interaction between calves and the ability to exhibit normal behaviours are encouraged

TABLE 9.1 Common examples of UK systems that intensively rear calves sourced from the dairy herd.

Breed	Product	Typical age at slaughter	Typical liveweight at slaughter (kg)	Typical deadweight (kg)	Average DLWG from birth to slaughter (kg)
HF bull	Rosé veal	~11 months	460	235	1.3
HF bull	Beef	~12.5 months	480	245	1.25
HF × BB	Beef	~14 months – finished intensively	620	340	1.4
HF × BB	Beef	>16 months – finished on grass	620	340	1.1

Note: HF, Holstein-Friesian; BB, Belgian Blue.

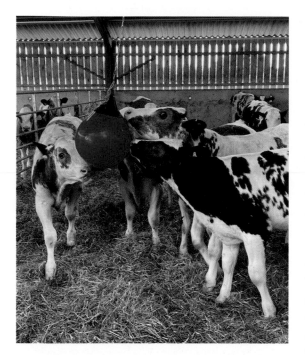

FIGURE 9.2 Enrichment placed in calf pens.

(Figure 9.2). The diet includes forage, concentrates and water, and is fed with the objective of maximising health and performance. There is a requirement for calves under 100 kg to have an unobstructed space allowance of >1.5 m² each, but it is advised to provide significantly more than this when considering potential health and production benefits.

HEALTH

The UK integrated beef supply chain, rearing and finishing calves sourced from the dairy herd, is already operating at a high level, enforcing some of the strictest welfare standards in the world.

A paramount factor in the development of the UK system has been the strong relationship between the supply chain and veterinary health advisors. The focus on areas of management, such as hygiene, building design, feeding advice, cleaning protocols and vaccinations, has resulted in a UK industry that already is one of the lowest users of antibiotics compared to similar systems globally.

The main risk in such operations though is the introductory period for calves entering the rearing unit – an event which contributes to the majority of the disease and production losses that are experienced over the course of the chain.

Calves will often enter the rearing units at a young age – typically between 2–6 weeks of age – having been sourced from dairies with varying types of management and disease status (Figure 9.3). The low relative value of these animals can put them at risk of receiving below the normal standard of care. In particular, the lack of emphasis on optimal colostrum management can place failure of passive transfer (FPT) as a common occurrence. Calves can be transported over long distances, first between the dairy source and a collection centre, and then again from the centre to the rearing unit. On arrival at the rearing unit, it is inevitable that some calves will be subjected to alternative nutrition and feeding methods compared to what they were used to. The variable disease status and protective immunity of each calf will also lead to a rapid swapping of pathogens among the batch. Such a situation has the potential for a relatively large incidence of disease, most notably respiratory disease (pneumonia), the consequence being there is a requirement to treat, often with antimicrobials (2).

There is an increasing awareness of antibiotic use within agriculture and its contribution to the antibiotic resistance of bacteria that pose a threat to human health. While the UK has banned using antibiotics as either growth promoters or in a prophylactic manner, there is still the potential for metaphylactic treatment of large groups based on surpassing individual treatment thresholds. This can be a necessity in order to prevent unacceptable losses and safeguard adequate calf welfare. Even when antibiotics are used responsibly, there is still considerable scope to reduce and refine their use in this high risk introductory period.

There is concern over the intensive use of antimicrobials within well-developed systems that rear calves for veal, and the associated antimicrobial resistance (3). A recent study looking at the

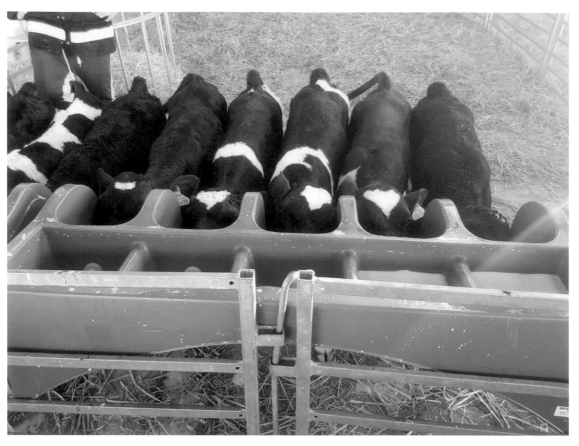

FIGURE 9.3 A group of similarly aged calves showing consistency in size and conformation, indicating good health.

antimicrobial data from 45,001 calves managed by two large, white veal integration companies situated in Belgium, found average antimicrobial usage to be 30.1 (± 10.4) defined daily doses (DDD) per animal per year (4). Another study that looked at 186 calf batches across the French white veal sector found that calves were exposed to an average of 8.55 (± 2.21) antimicrobial courses over the 5 to 6 months of the fattening process, with a range of 2.75 to 15.86 treatments per calf (5). A report by the Netherlands Veterinary Medicines Institute looking at antimicrobial usage in livestock during 2018, found veal farming sectors to have the second highest average DDD at 19.52 per animal per year when compared to other significant livestock sectors (6). When rosé veal starter farmers were focused on, they were found to be of particular

concern with 71% of the 256 farms falling below the 2019 intervention threshold of 67 DDD per animal per year. Whole group oral antibiotic treatments are considered to be the main contribution to these figures (7). The combination of risk factors already discussed as well as the advanced setups that allow one caretaker to look after 2000 calves, can promote a culture of treating the group rather than the individual.

Disconcertingly, strong evidence has been found on these units that points towards the direct relationship between antibiotic use in animals and the transfer of antimicrobial resistant organisms to humans. One study showed that the prevalence of MRSA was 15.9% in persons living and working on a Dutch veal calf rearing unit, which is significantly elevated compared to the estimated <1% prevalence within the general Dutch community (8). This evidence is strengthened by the similar type and antimicrobial susceptibility pattern of the isolates found in both humans and animals within the study.

Distinct differences that are likely to increase the antimicrobial usage within the veal sector of other countries, compared to the UK veal sector, include the following.

- The increased transport times calves are subjected to.
- The increased batch sizes which allow further opportunity for disease spread and reduced individual treatments.
- The reduced age and weight that calves will typically enter the rearing system.
- The increased proportion of calves that are reared as white veal, which is associated with a weakened immune system due to management practices.

Despite this, the UK should not be complacent in its own practices. The industry should continue to apply pressure to reduce antimicrobial usage and review management practices to support this, especially as post 2020 UK industry targets are likely to include calf rearing units as a discrete focus area (9).

RESPIRATORY DISEASE

Respiratory issues are the major cause of mortalities, treatments and animals being rejected within the beef integrated chain. Consequently, they are also the main driver for antimicrobial usage within these systems.

The point that calves enter the rearing system can be a 'perfect storm'. Calves that have a high risk of having a FPT are then transported, mixed and managed differently in one sudden move. If not being checked prior to movement, dairy sources will almost certainly have different health statuses and herd immunity. The result is a rapid spread of primary respiratory pathogens through a group of immuno-compromised calves (10).

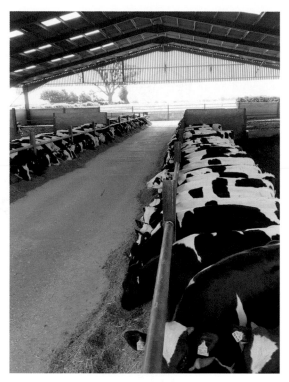

FIGURE 9.4 A large shed housing dairy bulls for finishing. Feed access and ventilation will have been discussed here. Image courtesy of Tudor Farming.

Prevalence

Respiratory disease causes the majority of individual treatments and mortalities seen during the rearing stage of beef integrated systems. There can be considerable variation in the percentage of calves treated for pneumonia between each batch. When mixing calves from different dairy sources, the percentage treated for pneumonia on average rests around 25%, though can range from <10% to >50% of the batch. The factors important in this variation will include aspects of rearer management and parameters of the calves entering the unit – calf factors on entry are described in more detail within this chapter.

Many cases of pneumonia within these systems are also likely to be subclinical and go undetected. One study that looked at the correlation between lung lesions and estimated daily live weight gain

(DLWG) in UK bull beef sourced from the dairy herd, found that of the 645 animals sampled 48% of them had at least one lung lobe showing signs of consolidation (12). Interestingly, animals in this study with three or four lung lobes showing signs of consolidation, were found to have reduced estimated DLWG of 141 g (±38) and 194 g (±45), respectively. The hidden costs of pneumonia are therefore a major concern within these systems.

Pathogens implicated

The common pathogens involved in a respiratory outbreak within these systems would be typical to most cattle farms, the presentation and severity can be markedly different. In the majority of outbreaks multiple pathogens will often be implicated as an inciting cause. If paired serology is performed when pneumonia cases typically peak, approximately 2–3 weeks after entry, simultaneous seroconversion is commonly detected for multiple viruses that are considered primary causes of respiratory disease (11).

Most bacteria that have been described as having the potential to be a primary pathogen in calf pneumonia are ubiquitous and can be found using deep naso-pharyngeal swabs (NPS) and broncho-alveolar lavage (BAL) in both healthy and non-healthy calves during outbreaks. Similarly, it is common to detect more than one species of pathogenic bacterium present, using post-mortem culture and histology (11).

In summary, pneumonia outbreaks that occur soon after entry are most often caused by multiple pathogens, both viral and bacterial. There is also the added fact that each new batch of calves that enter the rearing unit may have an entirely different disease and immune status. This constantly fluctuating cycle can mean that performing standard diagnostics for every pneumonia outbreak can be unjustified unless being done with a clear question or plan in mind. Ideally, protocols on units that rear beef sourced from the dairy herd should assume that all common pneumonia-causing pathogens will be present among every batch that enters.

Motives for investigating the underlying pathogens involved in pneumonia outbreaks include:

- confirmation of vaccination protocol efficacy
- concerns over antimicrobial resistance (which may be in reaction to increasing retreatment rates)
- when specific pathogens are suspected that may lead to changes in management or treatment, some examples include:
  - viral outbreaks where vaccinating with intranasal vaccine may limit spread
  - suspicion of Salmonella involvement
  - suspicion of animals persistently infected (PI) with BVD.

Depending on management protocols already in place, there may be further specific management or treatment procedures that can be implemented based on a successful diagnosis.

First and second line antimicrobial choices are decided upon with the intention of covering for the bacteria most likely to be involved. The antibiotic chosen must reach the required levels within the respiratory tract and be effective against Pasteurellaceae and *Mycoplasma* spp. As a result, most pneumonia protocols consist of oxytetracyclines, florfenicols and macrolides. Fluoroquinolones would also satisfy these criteria but are not advised due to their critical importance within human medicine.

Respiratory vaccines

Vaccine regimes should be designed to be broad-spectrum, providing immunity for both viral and bacterial components.

Intranasal vaccines are often incorporated into vaccine protocols at entry due to their ability to stimulate rapid mucosal immunity within calves as well as overcome any interference from maternally derived antibodies (MDA). Intranasal vaccines are available for bovine herpesvirus 1 (BHV-1), bovine respiratory syncytial virus (BRSV) and parainfluenza virus type 3 (PIV-3), with onset of immunity claimed as being between 4–7 days after administration. By administering on entry, the objective is to achieve immunity prior to the expected peak in pneumonia cases a few weeks later. It is strongly advised that with all prescribed vaccines, farm compliance is periodically checked. Unsatisfactory administration, particularly with intranasal vaccines, can be a common cause for suspected vaccine failure.

Intranasal vaccines can also be used effectively in the face of a viral outbreak. On rearing units where viral vaccine protocols are not being implemented on entry, or where there may be failure of the protocol to control the virus it is expected to immunise against, intranasal vaccines can be used to reduce the shedding and spread among a susceptible population. Care should be given to clinically unwell animals, and only healthy animals vaccinated in this manner.

Bacterial vaccines are also an important component for any vaccine protocol, with vaccines available for immunisation against *Mannheimia haemolytica* and *Histophilus somni*. Although the inactivated vaccines available do not claim onset of immunity until 5–6 weeks after initiating and are at risk of interference from MDA, anecdotally the author has found a reduction in clinical cases which are primarily bacterial in origin, during the first few weeks after starting the primary course. Traditionally, there has been a recognised pattern of respiratory viruses initiating diseases with bacteria arriving second and further exacerbating the problem. However many pneumonia cases appear to be solely bacterial in origin on post-mortem histology, perhaps made possible by other stresses that calves are exposed to.

At the time of writing, *Mycoplasma bovis* vaccines had been developed and were commercially available, but trial work so far has shown them not to be sufficiently efficacious or to have yielded poor results (14).

Diagnostic methods for respiratory disease outbreaks

- Paired serology approx. 2 weeks apart – Correlate seroconversion with treatments to diagnose active presence of pathogenic viruses and *Mycoplasma bovis*. Disadvantages are it takes time to perform and MDA or antibodies produced from vaccine administration on entry can make it difficult to interpret.

- Culture – Specifically required for antimicrobial sensitivity testing. Can be performed on NPS, BAL samples and on tissues from post-mortem. Many studies have shown good correlation between NPS and BAL samples when performed and compared at a group level with multiple calves sampled (13). Considering this, the author prefers to use the less invasive method of NPS when collecting samples for culture from groups of live animals.

- PCR – Can also be performed on NPS, BAL samples and on tissues from post-mortem. This has high sensitivity and is able to detect both viruses and bacteria of significance. However, it will only detect pathogens that are present at the time of sampling.

- Post-mortem – Veterinarians experienced with post-mortems may be able to determine gross pathology indicative of certain disease processes, for example, discrete foci of caseous necrosis in the cranioventral lobes are often indicative of *Mycoplasma bovis* infection. This is also an essential opportunity to rule out other differentials, concurrent diseases and take samples for submission.

- Histology – Lung histology can be useful for determining the original cause of the pneumonia (i.e. viral or bacterial), rather than just determining what the predominant pathogen is at the time of death.

SALMONELLA

A study in England and Wales found that 7.5% of 449 dairies were positive for *Salmonella enterica* subsp. *enterica* serotype Dublin (*S. enterica* Dublin) on culture of pooled faecal samples and slurry (15). Though *S. enterica* Dublin does not commonly circulate among every batch of reared calves, when it does, both the production and zoonotic consequences can be high if not detected early. The disease can present in a variety of ways. Although diarrhoea with pyrexia is typically the most common presenting symptom, many calves do not show diarrhoea at all. The disease can also present as septicaemia, pneumonia and meningitis. In some cases, the first indication to the farmer that Salmonella may be present is when treatment success begins to drop for what were considered to be standard pneumonia cases. *S. enterica* Dublin outbreaks are typically seen at 6–10 weeks of age after calves have been present on the rearing unit for several weeks.

Individual faecal cultures from animals showing clinical signs is the most common approach to testing. Sensitivity is quoted between 60–100% depending on presentation, though is markedly reduced by prior antibiotic treatment and pooled sampling (16). Serology is sensitive at a herd level if testing entire groups but is difficult to interpret in animals under 3 months of age due to poor antibody response and MDA interference – it is therefore not typically advised for rearing units. Screening on entry with faecal culture has poor sensitivity and once again serology is difficult to interpret. Ensuring Salmonella is not brought on to farm is best done by selectively buying from farms that routinely perform their own herd surveillance for the pathogen.

Confirmation of Salmonella disease in a batch of calves will lead to Public Health England being notified, along with revision of the standard treatment protocols. Antimicrobial choices will be revised to reflect a gram-negative bias and should ideally take into consideration antimicrobial culture and sensitivity results. Vaccination against Salmonella strains can also be administered around entry as a preventative, if deemed a significant risk.

INFECTIOUS DISEASE SURVEILLANCE ON ENTRY

Similar to performing diagnostics during pneumonia outbreaks, surveillance of infectious disease on entry needs to be done with a clear question in mind. When purchasing from multiple different sources with each calf batch, determining disease status from each calf will lead to little change in management. Only if a decision is made to change the system and purchase from a small selection of sources consistently, can selective vaccine and management protocols be introduced. In this case, it would certainly be good practice to ascertain dairy source disease status going forward.

Bovine viral diarrhoea virus (BVDV) is perhaps the only exception to this rule. The ability of the virus to produce PI animals that will continuously shed the disease into the environment, means that it is important actions are taken to prevent the introduction of PI animals onto the rearing unit. Practically this leads to animals being blood or tissue sampled for BVD antigen on entry, with PI animals being swiftly removed when found.

DATA ANALYSIS

Meaningful, reliable data is a cornerstone to all forms of efficient intensive farming, and rearing dairy sourced calves for beef is no exception. An extensive amount of data should be available to the veterinarian wishing to understand the rearing unit under their care, the majority of which should be available for analysis as it is a legal requirement to record it.

By capturing a reasonably modest amount of performance data, animal information and treatment data; significant conclusions can be

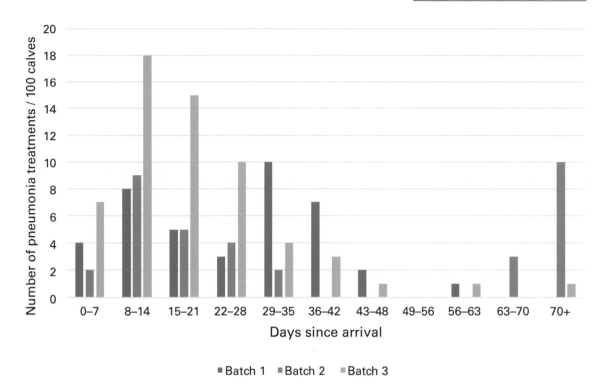

FIGURE 9.5 Number of pneumonia treatments administered compared to the time since arrival at the veal unit.

drawn and decisions made. Further variables can always be included at a later date to provide more context. Figure 9.5–9.7 demonstrate some examples of basic data analysis that can be done on veal rearing units.

Batch 1 (blue bars) in Figure 9.5 shows an increase in the number of treatments around weeks 5 and 6 after entry. Factors to investigate in relation to this include the following.

- Management procedures – are procedures causing unnecessary stress? Is appropriate analgesia being administered for castrations and disbudding?
- Weaning – poorly implemented weaning strategies such as abrupt or very short weaning periods can cause unnecessary stress and nutritional gaps that lead to increased treatment rates. Is >2 kg of concentrate being consumed before milk withdrawal? Are other actions performed alongside weaning, exacerbating problems?

Batch 2 (orange bars) in Figure 9.5 shows an increase in treatments towards the end of the rearing phase, just prior to when many would be transported onto a finisher unit. You would expect animals to be at their most resilient at this point. Factors to investigate in relation to this include the following.

- Stocking density – are animals reaching higher weights but being kept in the same pen? Is the pen area suitable for animals at their heaviest just prior to departure? Are there flow problems within the chain meaning that animals are remaining on farm for too many days?
- Environmental build-up – are intervals between cleaning out too long? Do buildings have poorly designed drainage?
- All-in all-out policy – are additional animals coming on to farm and having contact with the last batch prior to departing? This would lead to another circulation of disease.

Batch 3 (grey bars) in Figure 9.5 shows a more accentuated peak of treatments around the high risk period, 2–3 weeks after entry. Factors to investigate in relation to this include the following.

- Introductory protocol – are electrolytes being provided at the start and efforts made to initiate calves onto milk feeding? Are calves being sorted to ensure suitable stocking and competition?
- Vaccine protocol and efficacy – are viruses being suitably controlled where possible, reducing shedding and spread at this high risk stage?
- Cleaning protocols – poor hygiene of feeding equipment will allow quicker spread of pathogens between animals and poor environmental cleaning between batches will allow build-up to occur, increasing the starting baseline pressure.
- Nutrition – Are the calves' energy requirements being supplied by a clean, consistent milk feed which they are dependent on in the early stages, or are they being under-fed leading to a compromised immune system?

In Figure 9.6 batch 1 shows a typical retreatment rate which you would expect to see. Around 20%

of calves that received an initial first line treatment for pneumonia go on to require the second line treatment after not improving or suffering a relapse later on in the rearing period. A small percentage may then require a third treatment though these calves require individual consideration on whether treatment is in the interest of the calf and integrated chain.

Batch 2 shows a high retreatment rate of 45%. The poor success rate of the initial first line treatment requires investigation, with consideration given to the following.

- Treatment choice – is antibiotic choice appropriate for the pathogenic bacteria you would typically expect to see and being given alongside anti-inflammatory medicines?
- Competency with medicines – are medicines being correctly administered? Type, volume and route of administration should all be checked. Are medicines being stored correctly, administered hygienically and discarded if expired?
- Stockpersonship – delays in treatment after onset of clinical signs significantly reduces

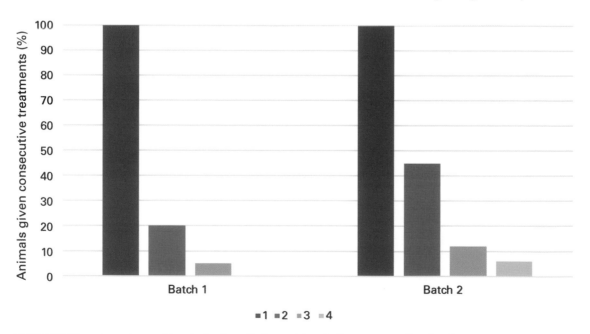

FIGURE 9.6 The percentage of treated calves that requiring further consecutive treatments.

treatment success. Are sick calves being picked out quickly enough? Are all staff members that are responsible for treatments competent and is there clear communication happening within the team?

- Unusual pathogen – presence of BVD PI animals in a batch would lead to increased treatment rates. You might also expect a poor response from Salmonella cases depending on the antibiotic choices being used.

Figure 9.6 shows that there are also a significant number of animals that are being treated three or four times. This may warrant investigation, looking again at the considerations above and the decision-making process for repeat offenders. Pneumonia is a painful condition and we need to act in the best interest of the animal, which may be euthanasia if prognosis is poor. Even if an animal which has been treated several times appears to improve, there is good evidence that DLWGs are significantly reduced for the remainder of its life

and therefore culling may also be the preferred economic choice.

DLWG is one of the most sensitive forms of data available to the veterinarian with the average, spread and percentage of outliers that have not met the target all acting as useful indicators of performance.

Figure 9.7 shows weight gains against seasonality and is just one example of how weight gains might be displayed and reviewed. Many rearers would expect changes in performance with seasonality. Autumn would typically be when most disease is seen, but this can vary between years and between rearers. Abnormal patterns in seasonal performance may indicate areas of concern. Some examples of factors to investigate might include the following.

- Inappropriate buildings – poor cover during the colder wetter months, or poor air flow and small outlets during the hotter months might lead to problems.

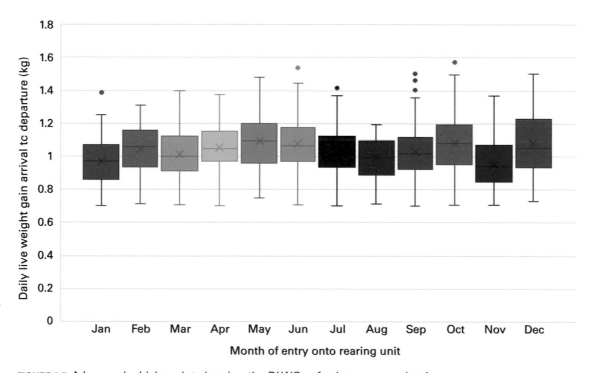

FIGURE 9.7 A box and whisker plot showing the DLWGs of calves on a veal unit.

- Staff – other seasonal work occurring on farm may impact the rearing enterprise.
- Calf quality – different seasonal management procedures on the dairy such as calving environment and colostrum protocols may impact calf performance on the rearing unit.

The veal unit data illustrated in Figure 9.7 showed a decline in weight gains during August due to particularly hot humid weather, which was exacerbated by the buildings having inadequate outlets. The drops in November, January and March were understood to be a stocking issue with different buying patterns leading to an additional 15% of calves being purchased and reared than usual.

When reviewing performance, data are typically grouped within 'calf batch'. This is often the most sensible way of categorising and comparing production in an all-in, all-out system, where each batch is reasonably consistent. Production can be reviewed on a 'per batch' basis as well as a rolling three-batch average which, if farms are continuously rearing, tends to equate to approximately a year of production.

There are a number of key performance indicators that can be assessed on veal units.

- Mortality and rejection rate – the percentage of calves that have died during the rearing period and percentage that have not reached acceptable targets for weight gain and conformation to move onto a finisher, respectively. This may be interpreted as calves that have needed to 'move back a group'. Always consider mortality and rejection rate together as these will often be negatively correlated, relating to culling policies. Alternatively, these figures can be combined to produce a 'percentage of animals that have not been successfully finished' to help with benchmarking.
- Treatments:
  - percentage of animals treated
  - number of treatments per 100 calves
  - retreatment rates – percentage of those treated that required second line treatment, third line treatment etc.

Ideally, treatments should be categorised based on medicine and diagnosis.

- DLWG:
  - overall average
  - spread among the batch (i.e. ± 0.2 kg).
- If weighing facilities are available on farm, then pre-weaning and post-weaning DLWG should be calculated to help with decision making around the milk feed. Appreciating spread of DLWG is also an important feature as average DLWG can be misleading. The percentage of animals that have not met the minimum threshold are often represented as a rejection percentage.
- Total days on farm – arrival to departure. In most cases this will be negatively correlated with DLWG and so is an important reference point to have alongside indicators of performance. In some cases, excessive days on farm may lead to problems if buildings/management are not suitable for larger animals.
- Antimicrobial usage:
  - Mg/PCU – 'Population corrected unit' can be stated as the average weight of animal on farm which is typically ~100 kg on rearing units.
  - Clinical courses – based on average weight of animal treated, standard dose rate and standard number of days for a course of treatment, each antibiotic product dispensed can be expected to treat a certain number of animals.
- Data on medicines prescribed can be used to calculate weight of antimicrobials being dispensed to farm. These data are usually easier to access by the veterinarian but there are issues associated with using this instead of actual treatment records. Veterinary prescribing software contains an accurate record of antimicrobials dispensed to farms but does not tell you what is actually being administered, and to what species and weight of animal it is being used for on farm. Beef farms are often very diverse and

TABLE 9.2 Targets and points of intervention for rearing units.

Key performance indicator	Target	Intervention
Mortality rate (%)	<2	>4
Rejection rate (%)	<1%	>3%
Animals treated (%)	<20	>30
Number of treatments per 100 calves	<25	>35
DLWG from arrival to departure (kg)	>1.1	<1.0
DLWG spread ± variation from the average (kg)	<0.2	>0.3

Note: Rearing units that source from multiple dairy units with mixed infectious disease statuses, have calves arrive at approximately 2 weeks of age, and rear calves for 12–14 weeks before transporting to a finishing unit.

potentially mixed, so it is important to identify which system the medicines are being prescribed for.

The performance indicators discussed above are focusing on information available to the rearer (Table 9.2). Where possible though, information on performance at the finishing unit as well as kill data at slaughter should also be examined. Rearer management and levels of disease will have an impact down the entire chain.

CALVES ENTERING THE REARING UNIT

As with most processes, the quality of a product is affected by the quality of the raw materials you begin with. The same can be said for a beef integrated chain and the calves that it accepts. Having high quality calves enter the rearing unit at the start is crucial for the success of the operation, with unsatisfactory calves having a resonating effect along the entire process.

It is important to understand which calf variables to assess at the point of entry are of interest and how they might affect health and performance going forward. Some 'risk factors' are well described while others still require more investigation – below are some of the better described calf variables that impact future success within the chain.

Bodyweight

Bodyweight (BW) on arrival appears to be one of the best predictors of future disease on the rearing unit. One study found BW at arrival to be associated with the prevalence of respiratory disease within the first 3 weeks, with calves that had a BW >51 kg on entry having the lowest probability of developing respiratory diseases at the rearing unit compared to lighter calves in the study (27). Other studies agree that calves which are lighter on entry, in general have a higher risk of respiratory disease morbidity and early mortality compared to their heavier peers (28, 29).

There are likely to be several factors behind this.

- Heavier animals are typically older, more developed calves with superior immune competence and rumen development.
- As long as calves are of a comparable age, they are more likely to have had improved weight gains prior to purchase, indicative of good management and absence of disease.
- Lower BW may be partly due to losses associated with dehydration and body nutrient mobilisation which has occurred during transportation. In Europe, it has been reported that calves may lose between 3% and 11% of BW during transport to farm, with higher BW losses associated with a reduction in the calf's ability to adapt to its new environment.

TRANSPORT

Young animals are not well adapted to transport, with undeveloped immune systems and an inability to regulate body temperature. Transport is usually a necessary requirement within beef integrated chains with calves being collected from multiple dairy farms, taken to a premise for sorting, and then once grouped transported to a rearing unit. Where transport is necessary, stress should be kept to a minimum. Calves should have sufficient space and bedding to lie down comfortably, with movement on and off the transport as calm as possible. While being transported, efforts should be made to keep calves within their thermo-neutral zone of 15–25°C. Transport duration should be kept as low as possible, with increasing duration linked with increased mortality and BW loss during transport (28, 30, 31).

Infectious disease status

Calves with mixed immune statuses enter the rearing unit and are exposed to a multitude of pathogens. Sourcing from multiple dairies ensures that most pathogens that are of concern will be present, and that not all calves will have previously encountered them or possess the required MDA for protection. Calves that are showing signs of disease at the time of entry have significantly higher mortality and morbidity rates during the rearing period. Interestingly though, calves which on entry have high antibody levels for specific pathogens, are less likely to require treatment during the early rearing phase (20). As a result, it can often be the naïve calves which are sourced from the herds with the best health status which suffer the worst when placed with other calves of mixed unknown health statuses. This further shows the potential benefits of buying from fewer sources with similar health statuses. Unfortunately, this is often not possible when trying to source similar aged animals for a consistent batch. There are obvious advantages to purchasing from sources that provide evidence of controlling certain diseases (e.g. BHV-1-naïve;

BVD monitored and vaccinated; monitoring for *S. enterica* Dublin), but all sources must be of this standard for the rearer to truly benefit. This further promotes the idea of vaccinating calves that are received from mixed sources, in order to 'standardise' a batch's immune status. Vaccination would also be preferably done before movement to the rearing unit, to provide immune-competency when it is most needed.

Immunoglobulin level

When immunoglobulin (Ig) levels were measured in young calves entering veal rearing systems in the Netherlands, Canada and the USA, it was found that on average approximately 40% of animals were found to have immunoglobulin levels below 10 g/L, which was considered to be indicative of a failure in passive transfer from poor colostrum management (18, 19, 20) (see Chapter 3). It is well documented that calves from all types of cattle farming with a failure in passive transfer have a higher risk of disease and mortality. One study found that calves a few weeks of age entering Dutch veal systems with IgG levels below 10 g/L, had an increased likelihood of being treated for pneumonia and a reduced DLWG during the first 3 weeks on farm (20).

Determining whether calves have had a failure in passive transfer at the point of entering rearing units can be a challenge. Testing calves between 2 and 7 days of age is a common procedure performed on the dairy farm and is an important tool when reviewing colostrum management. Most diagnostic tests that are easily accessible and validated for this age of calf look at total protein as an indicator for Ig level rather than the Igs themselves. Total protein levels in older animals above 7-days old do not correlate well with Ig levels, and it is preferable to specifically measure Ig levels when determining whether there has been a failure in passive transfer. Although by 2–3 weeks of age calves have begun to produce their own Igs, which will contribute to a blood measurement of total Ig, a significant proportion of total Ig is still made up of MDA at this point (21). This an important factor when considering whether specifically measuring Igs at the point calves enter will be a viable alternative in the future instead of relying on dairies to review their own colostrum management for calves destined for the beef trade.

Rumen development

When calves enter the rearing unit, they are typically placed on a milk feeding protocol that is aimed at transitioning calves onto hard feed as quickly as possible without the consequences of a growth check or an increase in disease incidence. The desire to wean calves as quickly as possible from a milk feeding regime that is considered more expensive and labour intensive, can mean that calves are weaned abruptly or prematurely with subsequent problems (22). This can be a particular problem where age and weight are the only variables considered before removing the milk feed (see Chapter 6).

Whilst a calf's age and weight is certainly positively correlated with the development of its digestive tract, there are many other factors which influence time taken to becoming a fully functioning ruminant. Providing concentrates, water and forage, as well as ensuring freedom from disease, are all known to help with rumen development. Suboptimal management on the dairy of origin can mean purchased calves have poorly developed rumens despite good weight gains and appearance. An example of this are calves that are fed only whole cow's milk. Removing milk from these animals at 8 weeks of age can often lead to consequences as they struggle with the weaning transition.

Checks in DLWG or peaks in treatment rates can both be signs of a poorly managed weaning process. Concentrate intake is an important measurement for deciding whether calves are fit to wean – more than 2 kg/day is a good threshold to aim for prior to removing milk completely. Some work has looked at validating the measurement of β-hydroxybutyrate as an indicator of concentrate intake and rumen development in pre-ruminant calves. This

has shown promise as a potential screening test for incoming calves to determine intakes on the dairy, but might still be considered impractical due to the validated testing regime requiring daily testing for 3 days to calculate an average result (23).

PRACTICAL ASPECTS OF REARING DAIRY SOURCED BEEF CALVES

Many of the recommendations and known complications discussed within the chapters of this book are relevant to the beef calf sourced from the dairy herd. Whether it is building design, nutrition, cleaning protocols, stocking densities, etc., many of the same principles apply. It could be argued that it is even more vital that these principles are followed to a high standard, due to the nature of the system and the additional detrimental factors that are difficult for the rearer to control. Discussed below are some of the practical areas that are a focus in these systems.

Record keeping

Treatment records can quickly get out of hand with rearers becoming 'blind' to treatments when administered on a frequent basis. Treatments, especially pneumonia treatments, can be an incredibly sensitive detection system for problems. Whether it be lapses in hygiene, deviations in milk feeding or stressful events not being managed correctly, increased pneumonia incidence will often quickly follow as an indicator of overwhelmed immune systems.

It is preferable to record treatment data both in a visual hand-written form that can be reviewed quickly pen-side, as well as in a form that can be analysed using computer software by farmers and advisors. The treatment board in Figure 9.8 is just one example of how you might display a large amount of information easily to multiple members of rotating staff.

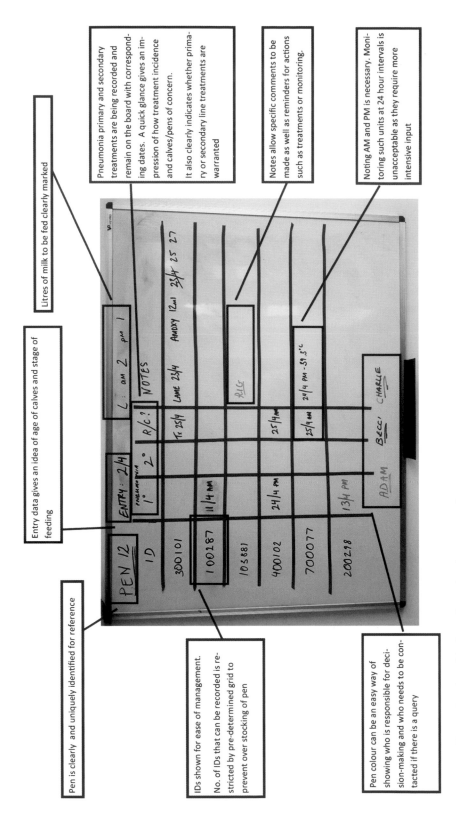

Litres of milk to be fed clearly marked

Pen is clearly and uniquely identified for reference

Entry data gives an idea of age of calves and stage of feeding

Pneumonia primary and secondary treatments are being recorded and remain on the board with corresponding dates. A quick glance gives an impression of how treatment incidence and calves/pens of concern.

It also clearly indicates whether primary or secondary line treatments are warranted

Notes allow specific comments to be made as well as reminders for actions such as treatments or monitoring.

Noting AM and PM is necessary. Monitoring such units at 24 hour intervals is unacceptable as they require more intensive input

IDs shown for ease of management. No. of IDs that can be recorded is restricted by pre-determined grid to prevent over stocking of pen

Pen colour can be an easy way of showing who is responsible for decision-making and who needs to be contacted if there is a query

FIGURE 9.8 Example of a whiteboard used to keep records.

Feeding techniques

There is a huge variety of milk feeding techniques for young calves within the beef rearing unit. The most common examples seen in the UK are discussed below along with their pros and cons.

Teat feeders

Advantages

- Compartments allow a degree of individual feeding to ensure milk is shared out equally.
- Requirement of stockperson to stand by feeder ensures that calves are individually inspected.
- Believed to stimulate an improved oesophageal groove closure though evidence is lacking.

Disadvantages

- Difficult to clean compared to troughs.
- Can be labour intensive and time consuming as there is a requirement to stand by the feeders until all milk has been finished.

Things to consider

Teat feeders are often considered to be the most 'natural' form of feeding (Figure 9.9). The method promotes good saliva production and improved oesophageal groove closure. Studies have been equivocal though with little difference documented between teat feeding and open bucket or trough feeding.

Consequences arise when teat feeders are not kept clean and well maintained. Teat openings need to have good tight seals to prevent excessive milk flow, and the teat surface needs to show no signs of perishing or wear with cracks allowing pathogens to persist. Teats should be replaced frequently with a calf batch change often providing a good opportunity. When cleaning it is important that all surfaces of the feeder are checked, and

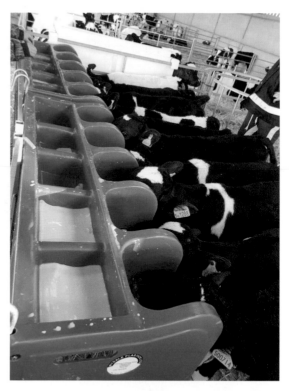

FIGURE 9.9 Wydale teat feeders with an individual compartment for each calf to drink from. It can be seen that the calves are drinking at different speeds, something which requires constant monitoring by staff.

that teats are frequently removed and cleaned as build up between the feeder's parts is common (Figure 9.10).

The gold standard would be to have a teat feeder specific for each pen, but cost often prohibits this. An advised compromise is to have a specific teat feeder for each 'row' of pens that may have physical contact. Feeding equipment is then not shared between rows or buildings to limit potential spread of disease pathogens (Figure 9.11).

Trough feeding

Advantages

- Cheapest to install.
- Easiest to clean.
- Least labour intensive when feeding.

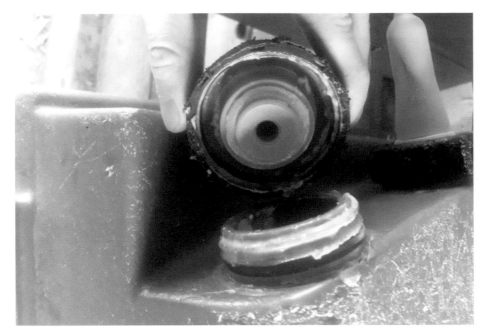

FIGURE 9.10 Congealed milk deposits between the threads when teats are not removed and cleaned thoroughly.

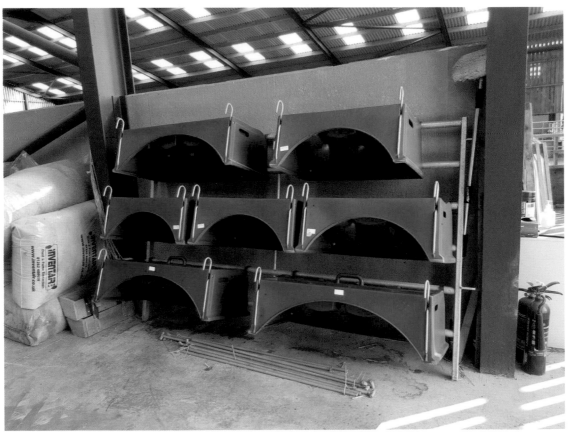

FIGURE 9.11 Example of excellent storage of feeders between feeding sessions.

Disadvantages

- No way of assessing volume of milk consumed by individuals. Different milking speeds can lead to a large variation within a group.
- Difficult to measure volumes fed 'by eye'. Requires flow meter or feeds to be individually measured out and poured.
- Concerns about lack of stimulation for oesophageal groove closure leading to increased ruminal problems (24).

Things to consider

Milk troughs are potentially the quickest and least labour-intensive form of feeding milk calves (Figure 9.12). Unfortunately, they lack the ability to ensure individual calves receive an adequate volume each feed. The 'race' by all calves to finish the feed inevitably leads to some calves receiving more than planned and others much less. This can lead to serious issues if smaller weaker calves are not prioritised by moving to less competitive groups or individually fed from bottles or buckets. Systems that utilise milk troughs poorly will typically have a larger range in weight gains with the highest risk calves towards the bottom of this range.

The total volume of milk fed to the group can also be difficult to quantify – if using a milk bowser with pump, a flow meter needs to be installed.

Troughs are usually cheap to install with one potentially being purchased for every individual pen. A positive knock-on effect of this can be reduced disease spread between pens by removing the need to share feeding equipment. This

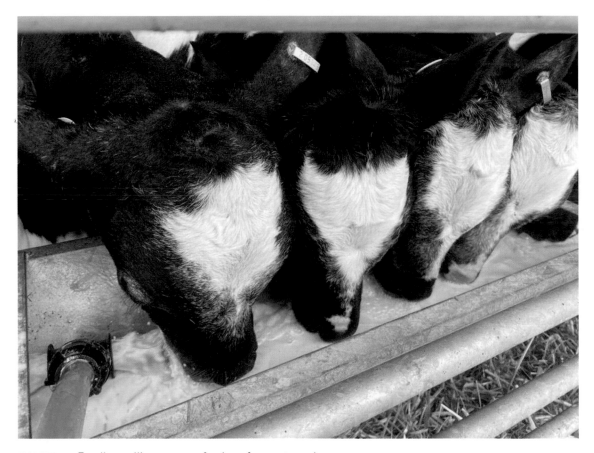

FIGURE 9.12 Feeding milk to a pen of calves from a trough.

though is often countered by a requirement to frequently swap calves between pens based on drinking speed.

Individual pens with bucket feeding

Advantages

- Good for disease control.
- Ensures correct volume of milk drunk by each calf.
- Ideal for monitoring.
- Dividers can be taken out after calves are drinking adequately with no initial signs of disease.

Disadvantages

- Additional cost of separating structures which may be used for only a short time in the rearing period.
- Labour intensive when penned individually.
- Concerns about lack of social interaction and exhibiting normal behaviour when separated.
- Concerns about lack of stimulation for oesophageal groove closure if using buckets – individual bottles with a teat though are an alternative option, seen less commonly in the UK.

Things to consider

The act of separating calves into individual pens on entry, regardless of feeding method, has significant advantages when it comes to controlling the spread of disease and monitoring feed intake and health parameters. Though there is no set time, units which employ this method tend to remove the dividers 10–14 days after entry, when calves are fully competent at drinking and the incidence of disease has begun to plateau. An alternative form of separating calves during the early rearing stages is to use hutches outdoors, with calves then being moved to a large group pen later.

Though the separation is only for a short time, there can be concerns about limiting social contact and the public perception of this. Separation of calves, whether it be by dividers or hutches, inevitably leads to increased labour with additional time needed to feed, bed up and clean the environment.

Automatic calf feeders (ACFs)

Advantages

- Easiest for time management.
- Increased number of feeds per day allows increased total volume fed with the potential for improved growth rates.
- Feed data generated and alert systems for when calves are not feeding.

Disadvantages

- Considerable initial investment.
- High cleaning requirements.
- Consideration about placement and drainage needed.
- Potential for increased risk of disease spread.
- Most difficult to repair if malfunctions occur.
- Calves need to be 'taught' on entry.
- Can lead to reduced monitoring.

Things to consider

Automatic milk feeders have the potential to produce superior growth rates with additional quantities of consistently mixed milk being fed over an increased number of feeds per day. They also require the most planning and greatest expertise, leading to a greater potential for problems.

There needs to be a great amount of consideration when installing the feeder. Adequate drainage that ensures effluent around the feeder is removed quickly from the building is vital, as excessive amounts of milk, cleaning fluid and urine is deposited in a very small area.

While the feeder performs regular internal cleaning, the single teat will not be adequately

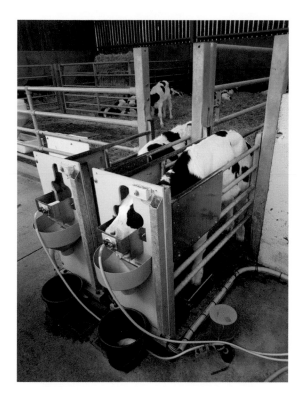

FIGURE 9.13 ACF stations set up outside of the pen with specially placed drainage directly below the feed areas to improve effluent flow.

cleaned externally and acts as an incredibly effective spreader of disease. The teat should be removed and cleaned at least twice a day. Soaking in hypochlorite solution in between changes is a common method of cleaning. The machine and internal workings should also be hand cleaned and calibrated on a regular basis, preferably weekly. Similar to teat feeders, teats need to be regularly checked and replaced when there are signs of wear.

Stocking density should also be favourable. While many may have up to 25 calves on one teat, less than 15 is advised to limit pressure on the teat, feeder area and environment. The automatic milk feeder allows flexibility with time management but should not be used as an excuse to not check stock regularly. Although the alert system is a helpful tool to monitor calf drinking, do not solely rely on it for disease detection.

Ruminal drinking

The oesophageal groove is a muscular channel that runs from the distal end of the oesophagus to the omasal orifice. The closure of this channel results in an enclosed pipe that directs ingested milk past the rumen and reticulum, straight into the abomasum. Closure of the oesophageal groove is a reflex triggered by nerve stimulation which is in turn aroused by the anticipation of the milk feed (25). It is important that the calf is aware of what is to come, with a consistent stress-free approach to the milk feed if it is expected to respond in the desired way.

When there is a failure of the oesophageal groove to close due to a stressful situation, the milk feed spills into the rumen instead of taking its normal route. Milk then begins to go through bacterial fermentation, producing high levels of lactic acid with a subsequent drop in pH level. The immediate consequence of a pH drop within the rumen can be ruminal bloat, depression, discomfort and inevitable poor performance. The longer term pathology associated with ruminal drinking can include hyperkeratosis of the rumen mucosa, poor rumen motility, and a chronic recurring bloat (26). It is good to note that the condition described is also seen when oesophageal feeders are used on calves to forcibly feed milk. The feeder prevents closure of the oesophageal groove and is the reason that calves should never be fed milk feeds in this manner – the exception being the first colostrum feed.

It is maybe unsurprising that beef units rearing calves from multiple dairy sources can sometimes see a higher incidence of this condition than other calf rearing systems and is the reason it is specifically mentioned within this chapter. Calves that have been stressed, transported, and had multiple management and environmental changes forced upon them in a short period of time are particularly susceptible.

While some of the risk factors for this condition are unavoidable in this type of system, if a high incidence of ruminal drinking is detected (>1%), management on the rearing unit should be reviewed to see if any corrections need to be made. When reviewing whether management may be contributing to ruminal drinking, remember that consistency is key.

- **Time of day** – calves need to expect the feed. Preparation in front of them following a set regime is ideal.
- **Method of feeding** – switching between methods of feeding, for example, bucket feeding to teat feeding or vice versa, is likely to be disastrous. Some believe feeding from a teat compared to an open bucket or trough promotes an improved oesophageal groove closure with a reduction in diseases associated with poor oesophageal groove closure and as a result improved performance (24, 25). The author anecdotally sees more digestive problems associated with open bucket feeding in comparison to teat feeding but this may be more related to the change in method from the dairy source – where calves have become accustomed to teat feeders or were still suckling from the cow – rather than the method itself.
- **Drinking speeds** – continuing to use old, perished teats with worn, open endings will result in excessive and/or inconsistent milk flow when calves are feeding.
- **Volume** – the volume of milk will need to be reduced during the weaning process but make sure it is done in a controlled manner, preferably over 2 weeks while monitoring concentrate intake and performance.
- **Temperature** – the milk feed should be consistently reaching the calves at approximately body temperature (39–40°C). When mixing make sure that the powder does not reach temperatures unsuitably high (>55°C) as this may damage proteins reducing the powder's digestibility. Measuring temperatures accurately requires a thermometer.
- **Mixing** – well mixed homogenous milk ensures all calves receive a consistent digestible feed. Concentrations should not be changed dramatically or be excessively high. Most calf milk

replacer (CMR) product guidelines advise 125–150 g/L.
- **Cleanliness** – strict cleaning protocols that incorporate a detergent ensure that hygiene is adequate. Performing coliform counts on the milk feed at different intervals during the feeding routine can be a useful objective measure of cleanliness – target is <1000 cfu/mL.
- **Calf milk replacer** – the quality of CMR products can be variable with poorly processed milk proteins and plant proteins leading to poor digestibility. Rapidly changing between different products, as well as sticking with a poor quality one, can both be detrimental.

In addition to ruminal drinking, poorly managing any of the above variables can lead to diarrhoea caused by nutrition, as well as unsatisfactory performance in general. Assessing the milk feeding procedure is a critical part of any calf rearer review.

THE FUTURE OF DAIRY SOURCED BEEF

As it stands, there are distinct veterinary health challenges that face the beef integration chain sourcing from multiple dairies. Nevertheless, there are indications that this form of farming will continue to become more widespread in the UK. Although the UK sector is well placed compared to similar sectors across the world with regards to its antimicrobial usage; specified levels of welfare and transparency with industry partners and veterinary health advisors is needed in order to confront the barriers to its climbing sustainability.

Disease status

As discussed previously, the varying infectious disease status of different dairy herds providing calves to produce one batch is a serious issue. Ideally calves would be consistent in their infectious disease status on arrival. Vaccination acts as a

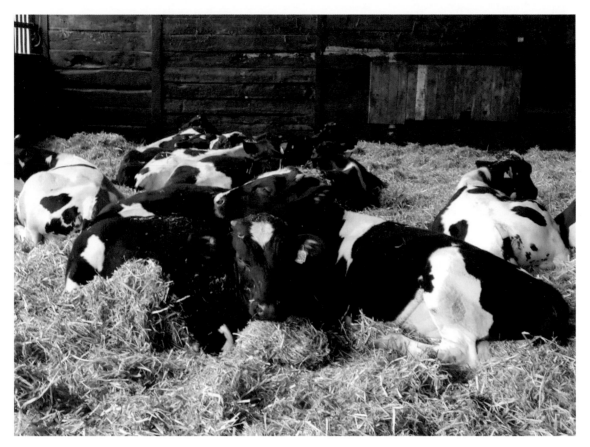

FIGURE 9.14 Consumer perception needs to change to allow veal to be accepted as a high value product.

means of 'forcing' a consistent status of immunity across an entire batch of calves, reducing the potential for pathogen spread. The dairy farms providing calves to the integration chain remain a weak link in controlling management. It might be hoped that perhaps with improved relationships, contractual agreements and premiums on measurable outcomes, source dairies may be tasked with ascertaining a certain disease status or vaccination status prior to movement to the rearing unit. Currently though, logistical issues and concerns about compliance remain a barrier to requesting this.

Calf value

Veal is a high quality product. It is important for Holstein-Friesian bull calves not to be seen purely as a worthless by-product of the dairy industry. Increasing the Holstein-Friesian bull calf's worth to the integrated chain through proactive changes by the dairy farm would be expected to produce an animal with improved performance that also has an increased sale value for the dairy farm. Potential areas for adding value might include the following.

- Genetics – considering traits that are worthwhile to the beef industry (e.g. weight gains, carcase quality, feed efficiency) when constructing breeding strategies with conventional dairy semen. Breeding decisions continue to be one of the most cost-effective points of intervention regardless of livestock sector.
- Evidence of successful passive transfer – Good colostrum management is vital to the success of calves entering the rearing unit. Current

commercial tests are focused on detecting Ig levels in calves aged 2–7-days old. Further work is needed to develop commercial tests that accurately measure Ig levels in calves a few weeks old so that they can be used at the point of calves entering rearing units via the collection centre. Until this is available though, evidence by the dairy farm of successful passive transfer could add value.

- Ensuring certified disease status or pre-vaccination to set specifications.

Big data – getting smarter

There are multiple factors determining whether calves succumb to disease or experience poor performance during their time on the rearing unit and understanding these factors will help us to make more informed decisions at all stages of the supply chain. The largest beef integration chains in the UK will be accepting thousands of calves every week and taking them through from start to slaughter. During this process, a vast amount of information is available for capture at all stages. A large array of calf information on entry – dates, dairy source, travel times, age, weight on entry, sire – is being recorded. Performance data are also recorded throughout the process including mortalities, treatment data, weight recordings, rejections, and kill data. Although we are aware of many of the risk factors for poor performance in animals that enter the chain, considering these factors and then individually responding to every animal can be an immense challenge. Data sets are becoming too large and complex to interpret and react on. The consequence of this is for integration chains to use advanced analytical techniques to extract and analyse the data sets available, revealing relationships and dependencies that lead to insights and the prediction of outcomes. By understanding factors that contribute to calves being at a high risk of poor performance, algorithms that employ specific management can be arranged. Practically, interventions would include grouping and allocating calves by

disease risk, specialised feeding and management plans, focused treatments in the event of disease outbreaks, and the ability to review and feedback to the source dairies that supply the chain. The result is a system that promotes continual improvement in its management and decision making.

REFERENCES

1. Hyde RM, Green MJ, Sherwin VE, Hudson C, Gibbons J, Forshaw T, et al. Quantitative analysis of calf mortality in Great Britain. J Dairy Sci 2020 Mar 1;103(3):2615–23.

2. Rell J, Wunsch N, Home R, Kaske M, Walkenhorst M, Vaarst M. Stakeholders' perceptions of the challenges to improving calf health and reducing antimicrobial use in Swiss veal production. Prev Vet Med 2020 Jun 1;179. Available from: https://pubmed.ncbi.nlm.nih.gov/32407997/:104970.

3. Ayling RD, Rosales RS, Barden G, Gosney FL. Changes in antimicrobial susceptibility of Mycoplasma bovis isolates from Great Britain. Vet Rec 2014 Nov 14;175(19):486. Available from: https://veterinaryrecord.bmj.com/content/175/19/486.1.

4. Bokma J, Boone R, Deprez P, Pardon B. Short communication: Herd-level analysis of antimicrobial use and mortality in veal calves: Do herds with low usage face higher mortality? J Dairy Sci 2020 Jan 1;103(1):909–14.

5. Jarrige N, Cazeau G, Morignat E, Chanteperdrix M, Gay E. Quantitative and qualitative analysis of antimicrobial usage in white veal calves in France. Prev Vet Med 2017 Sep 1;144:158–66.

6. SDa. Usage of antibiotics in agricultural livestock in the Netherlands in 2018: Trends and benchmarking of livestock farms and veterinarians; 2019.

7. Lava M, Pardon B, Schüpbach-Regula G, Keckeis K, Deprez P, Steiner A, Meylan M. Effect of calf purchase and other herd-level risk factors on mortality, unwanted early slaughter, and use of antimicrobial group treatments in Swiss veal calf operations. Prev Vet Med 2016 Apr 1;126:81–8.

8. Graveland H, Wagenaar JA, Heesterbeek H, Mevius D, van Duijkeren E, Heederik D. Methicillin resistant Staphylococcus aureus ST398 in veal calf farming: Human MRSA carriage related with animal antimicrobial usage and farm hygiene. PLOS ONE

2010;5(6):e10990. Available from: /pmc/articles/PMC2882326/?report=abstract.

9. RUMA. Targets task force: Two years on; 2017.

10. Pardon B, De Bleecker K, Hostens M, Callens J, Dewulf J, Deprez P. Longitudinal study on morbidity and mortality in white veal calves in Belgium. BMC Vet Res 2012 Mar 14;8:26. Available from: /pmc/articles/PMC3366893/?report=abstract.

11. Pardon B, De Bleecker K, Dewulf J, Callens J, Boyen F, Catry B, Deprez P. Prevalence of respiratory pathogens in diseased, non-vaccinated, routinely medicated veal calves. Vet Rec 2011 Sep 10;169(11): 278.

12. Williams P, Green L. Associations between lung lesions and grade and estimated daily live weight gain in bull beef at slaughter. Cattle Pract 2007;15(3):244–9. Available from: https://www.researchgate.net/publication/289841711_Associations_between_lung_lesions_and_grade_and_estimated_daily_live_weight_gain_in_bull_beef_at_slaughter.

13. Godinho KS, Sarasola P, Renoult E, Tilt N, Keane S, Windsor GD, et al. Use of deep nasopharyngeal swabs as a predictive diagnostic method for natural respiratory infections in calves. Vet Rec 2007 Jan 6;160(1):22–5.

14. Perez-Casal J, Prysliak T, Maina T, Suleman M, Jimbo S. Status of the development of a vaccine against Mycoplasma bovis. Vaccine 2017;35(22):2902–7.

15. Davison HC, Smith RP, Pascoe SJS, Sayers AR, Davies RH, Weaver JP, et al. Prevalence, incidence and geographical distribution of serovars of Salmonella on dairy farms in England and Wales. Vet Rec 2005 Nov 26;157(22):703–11. Available from: https://pubmed.ncbi.nlm.nih.gov/16311384/.

16. Nielsen LR. Review of pathogenesis and diagnostic methods of immediate relevance for epidemiology and control of Salmonella Dublin in cattle [Internet]. Vet Microbiol 2013;162(1):1–9. Available from: https://pubmed.ncbi.nlm.nih.gov/22925272/.

17. Bosman AB, Wagenaar JA, Stegeman JA, Vernooij JCM, Mevius DJ. Antimicrobial resistance in commensal Escherichia coli in veal calves is associated with antimicrobial drug use. Epidemiol Infect 2014;142(9):1893–904. https://doi.org/10.1017/S0950268813002665.

18. Stilwell G, Carvalho RC. Clinical outcome of calves with failure of passive transfer as diagnosed by a commercially available IgG quick test kit. Can Vet J

2011 May;52(5):524–6. Available from: http://www.midlandbio.com/.

19. McDonough SP, Stull CL, Osburn BI. Enteric pathogens in intensively reared veal calves. Am J Vet Res 1994;55(11):1516–20.

20. Pardon B, Alliët J, Boone R, Roelandt S, Valgaeren B, Deprez P. Prediction of respiratory disease and diarrhea in veal calves based on immunoglobulin levels and the serostatus for respiratory pathogens measured at arrival. Prev Vet Med 2015 Jun 15;120(2):169–76.

21. Hassig M, Stadler T, Lutz H. Transition from maternal to endogenous antibodies in newborn calves. Vet Rec 2007 Feb 17;160(7):234–5.

22. Khan MA, Bach A, Weary DM, von Keyserlingk MAG. Invited review: Transitioning from milk to solid feed in dairy heifers. J Dairy Sci 2016 Feb 1;99(2):885–902.

23. Deelen SM, Leslie KE, Steele MA, Eckert E, Brown HE, DeVries TJ. Validation of a calf-side β-hydroxybutyrate test and its utility for estimation of starter intake in dairy calves around weaning. J Dairy Sci 2016 Sep 1;99(9):7624–33.

24. Abe M, Iriki T, Kondoh K, Shibui H. Effects of nipple or bucket feeding of milk-substitute on rumen by-pass and on rate of passage in calves. Br J Nutr 1979 Jan;41(1):175–81. Available from: https://pubmed.ncbi.nlm.nih.gov/420750/.

25. Wise GH, Anderson GW. Factors affecting the passage of liquids into the rumen of the dairy calf. I. Method of administering liquids: Drinking from Open Pail versus sucking through a rubber nipple. J Dairy Sci 1939 Sep 1;22(9):697–705.

26. Breukink HJ, Wensing T, van Weeren-Keverling Buisman A, van Bruinessen-Kapsenberg EG, de Visser NA. Consequences of failure of the reticular groove reflex in veal calves fed milk replacer. Vet Q 1988;10(2):126–35. Available from: https://pubmed.ncbi.nlm.nih.gov/3413970/.

27. Brscic M, Leruste H, Heutinck LF, Bokkers EA, Wolthuis-Fillerup M, Stockhofe N, et al. Prevalence of respiratory disorders in veal calves and potential risk factors. J Dairy Sci 2012;95(5):2753–64.

28. Renaud DL, Duffield TF, LeBlanc SJ, Ferguson S, Haley DB, Kelton DF. Risk factors associated with mortality at a milk-fed veal calf facility: A prospective cohort study. J Dairy Sci 2018;101(3):2659–68.

29. Winder CB, Kelton DF, Duffield TF. Mortality risk factors for calves entering a multi-location white veal farm in Ontario, Canada. J Dairy Sci 2016;99(12):10174–81.

30. Cernicchiaro N, White BJ, Renter DG, Babcock AH, Kelly L, Slattery R. Associations between the distance traveled from sale barns to commercial feedlots in the United States and overall performance, risk of respiratory disease, and cumulative mortality in feeder cattle during 1997 to 2009. J Anim Sci 2012;90(6):1929–39.

31. Jongman EC, Butler KL. The effect of age, stocking density and flooring during transport on welfare of young dairy calves in Australia. Animals (Basel) 2014 Apr 11;4(2):184–99.

Chapter 10

Economics of calf rearing

Peter Plate

CHAPTER CONTENTS

The rearing of calves, and particularly dairy replacements, is a long-term investment. This often means that the rearing period is seen as an expense to the farm and the costs of which should be reduced as far as possible. However, this is the wrong perspective to take, as the rearing period should be seen as a time of investment through which the farm can produce a healthy and productive animal, while still being efficient with both time, resources and money.

THE BASICS OF FARM ECONOMICS

There are many definitions of economics, but one often quoted describes economics as the 'science which studies human behaviour as a relationship between ends and scarce means which have alternative uses' (1).

On farms not every investment with a positive cost–benefit ratio can be justified. For example, capital (or the willingness of the banks to lend) is a limited resource, and on a purely cost–benefit ratio it is tempting for a mastitis consultant to justify a new parlour, an agronomist to justify a new piece of machinery and a calf consultant to justify investments in calf housing. They may all give a multiple return on the money invested, but are competing for limited resources, and there will be an opportunity cost to installing a new parlour by forgoing the benefits from improving the calf housing and vice versa. Farmers receiving advice from various 'specialists' may feel drawn in conflicting directions; in practice it is often a sensible approach to start with the weakest link – improving or replacing equipment or procedures that are in the poorest state is likely to give better returns than improving something which is 'bearable' and further down the wish list.

Key economic terminology

- Economics is a science that studies human behaviour, therefore outcomes are less predictable compared to natural sciences. 'Laws of economics' are less static than 'laws of nature'.
- The 'ends' or outputs are sought to satisfy people's wants, and wants are often unlimited (as opposed to needs). If one want is satisfied, other wants may arise. If wants were limited there would be no economic pressure.
- 'Means' or resources are scarce and have to be used to maximum effect. In an agricultural context these means are, for example, land, time, capital, labour, etc.
- Alternative uses of limited means results in choices being made on how to 'invest' these resources to maximise the desired outcomes. In business this is often done following a cost–benefit analysis, calculating the different expected outcomes of different 'investments', maximising the return for every unit invested.
- In a further step, 'opportunity costs' are taken into account – the cost of forgoing the benefit of an alternative choice.

Another common example of opportunity cost is that too many calves are kept on farms, for example, dairy farms keeping more heifers than needed or beef calves. This can lead to opportunity costs such as reduced space and increased labour hours. While the selling of excess heifers or beef animals may be cost effective in itself and bring in immediate revenue, further rewards may be reaped from the redirection of resources to other areas.

WHAT ARE THE LIMITED RESOURCES IN CALF REARING?

Time

Time is often the biggest constraint on many farms. Competing uses include milking and feeding cows, harvesting, maintaining machinery, catching up with accounts and paperwork, or taking time off, rather than spending additional time with a calf unwilling to suck.

Money

Capital can be spent or invested in different ways, and it is not always obvious what the return in investment will be compared to spending it in other areas (e.g. machinery, parlour upgrade, a pay rise for employees). These choices are harder to make at times of low milk or meat prices.

The calf itself

Decisions have to be made whether to rear a calf at all, sell it early or even euthanase it at birth. These decisions will be driven by factors such as available space (rear fewer calves with more space, or more calves with less space), regulations, and increasingly by public opinion and the constraints put in place by milk buyers and their contracts.

WHAT ARE THE ENDS (OUTPUTS)?

These may be different to different people, but most stakeholders agree with a combination of the following ends:

- a healthy, productive animal
- high welfare – Five Freedoms for the animals

- environmental sustainability and optimum use of limited resources
- quality of life for the people involved in the work.

Some of these ends are directly measurable and quantifiable (e.g. profit), but some are less so (e.g. well-being of people, animal welfare) but are just as real. This also includes indirect outcomes like staff morale, which may be severely affected if many calves get sick or die. Ignoring those aspects purely because they are difficult to quantify would lead to a reductionist view and as a consequence suboptimal decisions.

Furthermore, the efficiency with which inputs are transformed into outputs can be reduced by factors such as disease, poor nutrition, poor climate, stress and poor stockpersonship.

There are other aspects to consider when talking about investment (input of limited resources) and return (output of desirable ends). Cattle are 'slow' animals in economic terms – while a pig starts reproducing at less than 1-year old and can then produce over 30 piglets per year, a cow calves at around 2 years and produces 0.9 calves a year. In dairy farming the rearing costs are paid back on average halfway through the second lactation, 530 days after the first calving (2), which is at nearly 3.5 years of age.

Farming is a high risk business – investments made can fail to give returns due to circumstances beyond a farmer's control (e.g. price fluctuations, abnormal weather conditions, bovine tuberculosis breakdowns and other diseases, political changes and consumer attitude). On average 58% of heifer calves fail to reach their third lactation in the UK (3), therefore failing to achieve optimum economic potential.

The fact that returns are slow and uncertain (as opposed to, for example, contractually guaranteed subsidy payments for renewable energy projects) require a highly positive cost–benefit ratio in livestock to make investments worthwhile. If the calculated benefits only marginally outweigh the costs, and this benefits accrue with time delay and with uncertainty, farmers are wise not to invest.

As mentioned above, investment in improved calf rearing competes with other investment opportunities, and while promoting optimisation of calf rearing the author is aware that other priorities may exist on many farms. However, some investments in calf rearing require very little additional resources and give a quick return, namely colostrum management, optimised nutrition and preventative healthcare measures, such as respiratory vaccines or bovine viral diarrhoea (BVD) control. While a new barn or major building alteration has to be costed against other investment opportunities, measures like increasing the daily milk allowance from 4 to 8 L, ensuring adequate colostrum intake, eradicating BVD or vaccinating against respiratory diseases are minor ongoing costs with frequently quick returns in reduced mortality and improved feed conversion efficiency. These therefore have very little opportunity costs attached to them.

THE CALF – A FELLOW BEING OR A MEANS OF PRODUCTION?

It is beyond the scope of this book to discuss in depth the ethics of keeping, using and killing animals for human food production and economic purposes per se. While this question is a purely ethical/philosophical one, science can aid the argument. The question of whether livestock farming, including dairy and beef production, is a justified use of limited resources and sustainable in environmental terms can (and should) be approached scientifically and through the use of available data.

Available agricultural land per person worldwide is diminishing (Figure 10.1), and considering the opportunity cost of using land to produce human edible protein, beef suckler production uses considerably more land than other livestock systems, such as pig and poultry rearing. However, cattle conversion of human non-edible resources into human edible protein is superior

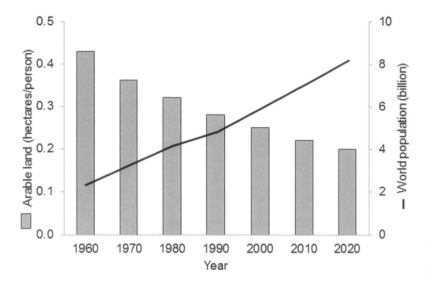

FIGURE 10.1 World population compared to arable land per inhabitant between 1960 and 2020 (5).

to monogastric animals, and many extensive beef systems can also form part of conservation projects enhancing biodiversity and building up soil fertility in rotations, so allocating this land purely to the most efficient protein production may be incorrect. Dairy production favours well in both land use and protein conversion, except for the latter in very high yielding cows. Flachowsky et al. in 2017 produced a detailed review of the efficiency of various animal production systems with regards to protein conversion and land use (4).

In ethical terms the views on animal husbandry are as variable as are views on human to human relationships. The animal can be seen as a pure means of production without any rights and lacking the ability to suffer (or if this ability is recognised it is not seen as relevant) – the human equivalent to slavery. At the other end of the spectrum, the animal may be seen as equal to humans in terms of its value and rights. The idea of positioning humans above animals has been labelled as 'speciesism' by some thinkers, analogous to the view embodied in racism and sexism. One protagonist of this idea, Peter Singer, found it morally acceptable to euthanase newborn babies with severe disabilities, as the boundary between humans and animals is seen as 'artificial'. The equivalent of human structures would be that of a non-hierarchical one, like anarchy.

Most people's attitude to human–animal relationships are somewhere between these extremes. The Five Freedoms can be seen as an equivalent to a human rights declaration. Using employees for economic benefit, but treating them well and paying them fairly. Using animals for economic benefit but meeting their needs in a wider sense (including psychological and behavioural needs) is the most common consensus of a 'fair play'. Many authors confirm that businesses are more successful if they know their employees and deal with them with empathy, meeting their needs. Similarly, in farming it is a common observation that those farmers who 'know' their animals, meet their needs and assure high welfare, are economically more successful.

ECONOMICS OF COLOSTRUM MANAGEMENT

Colostrum is vital for the successful protection of the newborn calf due to the lack of circulating antibodies (see Chapter 3). The main input for colostrum management is time. Colostrum is 'free' (unless bought as a substitute), although there are some fixed costs involved with good management (e.g. clean equipment, a colostrometer or

The Five Freedoms – Farm Animal Welfare Council, 1979

1 **Freedom from hunger and thirst** – ready access to fresh water and a diet to maintain full vigour and health.
2 **Freedom from discomfort** – provision of an appropriate environment including shelter and a comfortable resting area.
3 **Freedom from pain, injury or disease** – prevention or rapid diagnosis and treatment.
4 **Freedom to express normal behaviour** – provision of sufficient space, proper facilities and company of the animal's own species.
5 **Freedom from fear and distress** – ensuring conditions and treatment which avoid mental suffering.

Example case 1

On a dairy unit with 200 calves per year additional time is spent to reduce the rate of FPT modestly from 30% to 20%. This will prevent FTP in 20 calves, and at a cost of about £50 each this will save the farmer £1000. At £10 per hour labour costs, this would justify an additional 100 hours as a break-even point to achieve this goal. However, due to other risks and the time delay in cattle farming, working near the break-even point is not sufficient, and higher returns of investments are required.

However, the economic benefit can be illustrated in a different way – it can be argued that if these measures require an additional 20 hours of time as the sole investment (on average 6 additional minutes per calf), these hours would be 'paid' at a rate of £50 per hour. It appears obvious that there are not many areas in farming giving this return, so even when looking at the opportunity costs of investing this time into colostrum management, it is worthwhile.

refractometer to assess the quality and, potentially, a pasteuriser).

From the animal's point of view colostrum feeding is a once in a lifetime event. The clinical benefits are explained in Chapter 3, but reduced antibody uptake from colostrum (failure of passive transfer (FTP)) leads to an increase in risks by factors of 2.16 for mortality, 1.75 for respiratory disease and 1.51 for diarrhoea (6). Calves with FTP on average have a reduction in daily liveweight gain (DLWG) of 81 g, with an estimated mean total cost of FTP of £52 and £69 per affected calf for dairy and beef calves, respectively.

ECONOMICS AND NUTRITION

Many farmers try to save money by restricting expensive milk or milk replacer feeding to pre-weaned calves. The cost of milk replacer is about six times that of calf concentrates (7), and the initial reaction of many farmers is to restrict the former, which is also still reflected on label instructions for many milk replacers. Milk accounts for 40%

of the pre-weaning rearing costs, the most expensive phase of calf rearing (2). However, restricting milk and effectively starving the newborn is false economy – a recent study from the USA showed that higher amounts of milk/milk replacer lead to higher feed costs in total, but a decrease in feed costs per kilogram of weight gain (8).

With calf milk feeding, there are two principal approaches in terms of economics.

• Rearing a calf as *cheaply* as possible – spending as little as possible.
• Setting a target and achieving this in the most *cost-effective* way – spending money/resources in a way that it gives the highest returns.

The argument is similar to comparing cars and buses – cars need less fuel and emit less than

TABLE 10.1 The feed cost per kilogram of DLWG for pre-weaned calves fed different types of milk.

Milk source	Milk allotment (L)			
	6	8	10	12
Average daily weight gain (kg)	0.3	0.3–0.6	0.6–0.9	0.9–1.2
Milk replacer	£2.67	£2.10	£2.04	£1.99
Whole milk	£2.27	£2.26	£2.23	£1.98
Pasteurised whole milk	£2.74	£2.63	£2.52	£2.21

Source: Adapted from Hawkins et al. (8).

buses, but they emit more by passenger kilometre travelled.

Farmers adopting the first approach (rearing as cheaply as possible) actually end up spending more in the long term in an attempt to save money in the short term. The reason for this is that if calves grow slower, overall they will need more days of being fed (maintenance + growth), which results in a larger amount of food overall. The feed conversion efficiency is highest in calves, and declines quickly when they become ruminants, therefore an additional unit of energy will give higher growth rates in early life compared to when fed in later life. This is why the age at first calving (AFC) is the biggest determinate for the total rearing costs, accounting for 44% of its variation (2). It has also been shown that calves with higher milk intakes pre-weaning will achieve higher yields in their first lactation due to metabolic programming (epigenetics). As a result, farmers who feed their calves 'natural' amounts of milk (8–10 L or 20% of bodyweight, (9)) will generate a higher quality 'product' at a lower cost.

It is surprising that while a simple cost–benefit analysis will expose the error associated with a 'cheap as possible' approach, it is still widespread on farms. Often the reasons behind decision making for calf feeding practices are based on farmers' attitudes regarding the ease of management and well-being of their calves, only making alterations in response to perceived problems with calf health or growth rates even though many farmers struggle to accurately assess calf performance due to a lack of calf monitoring data (10).

An added difficulty in assessing the cost effectiveness of a higher calf milk replacer (CMR) feed rates is that there is a direct benefit in higher growth rates and increased feed conversion efficiency (which is fairly consistent), but also an indirect effect of improvement in immune function and a reduction in disease, which is more variable and dependent on other environmental factors. As a result some of the increased DLWG seen with higher feeding rates is directly attributed to the nutrition, and some of it is indirect due to decreased rates of diseases like BRD (11).

ECONOMICS OF DISEASES

There are several published comprehensive approaches on how to evaluate disease costs (12, 13), with seven main economic impacts of disease being assessed:

1. reduction in the quantity of outputs (a direct cost)
2. reduction in quality (actual or perceived) of the outputs (a direct cost)
3. waste or higher level of inputs (a direct cost)
4. prevention and control costs (a direct cost)
5. human health costs either due to zoonotic potential or certain control measures (e.g. organophosphate sheep dips)
6. negative animal welfare impacts
7. international trade restrictions.

While economics is defined in a wider sense, including animal welfare, the indirect effect of staff

Example case 2: Milk yield in the first lactation

Soberon et al. (11) found an increase in first lactation milk yield of 850 kg to 1113 kg for every kilogram of pre-weaning DLWG. Pre-weaning DLWG accounted for 22% of the variation in first lactation milk yield.

In simpler and practical terms, it is reasonable to expect an additional 100 L of milk for every additional 0.1 kg per day pre-weaning growth rate. Looking at the return in investment of increasing the pre-weaning DLWG moderately from 0.4 kg to 0.6 kg, this requires an additional intake of about 3 MJ per day which is the equivalent of about an additional 1.2 L of whole milk per day. Over an 8-week pre-weaning period this would require an additional 67 L of whole milk. If this leads to an additional 200 L of additional milk in the first lactation the return in investment is 1 : 3.

The obvious opportunity cost would be selling the milk (provided it is not waste milk). This is especially tempting in high milk price scenarios like direct supermarket contracts or organic milk production. However, the cost–benefit ratio will be the same in any price scenario. Most investors would choose to invest money with a 3 : 1 return after 3 years, this return is superior to most other investment opportunities including subsidised renewable energy schemes, even after taking account of time and risk. This simple calculation does not take into account the lower production cost due to a faster growing calf with improved disease resistance, the continued positive effect into the second lactation, or any losses that may occur if an animal does not complete its first lactation (11).

Example case 3: Reducing the AFC

Boulton et al. confirmed the optimum AFC with regards to rearing costs at 23 to 24 months (2). They calculated the cost of an additional day over 24 months at £2.87. This is a higher figure than most sources quote for an increase in the calving interval of lactating cows, as delaying the AFC means heifers spend more of their time producing no milk at all!

This figure is useful when considering the cost of lower growth rates, either due to poor nutrition or due to disease. Assuming a birth weight of 40 kg and a target weight after first calving of 600 kg (85% of mature BW of 700 kg for a Holstein heifer), 767 g DLWG is required to achieve this. Any reduction in DLWG can be translated into additional days till first calving and costed accordingly. Therefore, a reduced feed rate reducing DLWG mildly to 0.7 kg per day will increase the AFC to 800 days – the additional 70 days cost £200!

This does not take into account the economic benefits of earlier calving heifers with regards to productivity, fertility and longevity.

Neonatal diarrhoea

In the UK 48.2% of calves are diagnosed with diarrhoea during the whole pre-weaning period, with an incidence of 7.8 cases per 100 calf weeks at risk (14). This would give an estimated 203,000 animals being affected by enteric disease, at a total cost of £11 million, which results in costs of £54 per affected animal (13). The biggest cost factors are treatment and control, followed by mortality and liveweight loss. Again, the difficulty in quantifying control costs is that certain measures have other beneficial effects, for example, calving and colostrum hygiene and prompt removal of calves will also reduce the transmission of Johne's disease, and high colostrum intake will also reduce respiratory disease.

motivation is not considered here, although the increased labour required is part of the higher level of inputs.

While mortality is seen as the biggest cost factor, reduced growth rates are also important (15). Specifically, for cryptosporidiosis, one study followed calves in the UK over 6 months and scored their severity of clinical signs for cryptosporidiosis – the high scoring calves had significantly lower weights at 6 months than the low scoring ones, being on average 34 kg lighter (16).

Coccidiosis

While high doses of pathogenic *Eimeria* species can cause severe clinical disease, followed by a protective immunity if animals survive, the more common picture is that of a lower degree 'trickle infection'. In an economic simulation model based on a 100-cow herd, a delay to first service was identified as the main economic loss of low grade coccidiosis, followed by calf mortality – the opposite picture of neonatal calf diarrhoea (17).

Respiratory disease

The most comprehensive study on the cost of calf pneumonia in the UK looked at short-term costs which averaged £43.26 per ill dairy and £82.10 per ill beef calf (18). Even with several limitations to the model, reduced DLWG was identified as the biggest cost factor, contributing 26% of the total cost without considering longer term factors like first lactation yield, which has now been identified to be reduced in affected and treated calves (11). One study demonstrated a reduced growth rate of 66 g/day which can have a significant impact on reaching growth targets (19).

Costs of calf pneumonia can vary very widely, with a large impact being made by the speed with which disease is detected and treated. The reduction in DLWG is minimal if respiratory disease is detected early and treatment given promptly, with chronicity and severity increasing the overall cost. One study demonstrated that calves that are treated only once for respiratory disease performed similarly to unaffected animals, whereas animals with severe lung and pleural lesions or animals treated more than twice performed poorly, with an estimated cost of £279 (20). Similarly, when calves' lungs were assessed at weaning using ultrasound, heifers with lung consolidation were less likely to get pregnant and more likely to be culled before their first lactation, although in this study there was no difference in milk yield for the first lactation (21).

Practically, on farm calf pneumonia costs are extremely difficult to quantify and are highly variable depending on infectious agent, immune status of the calves, mortality and treatment regimes. For example, the real costs of mortality may be

---

Example 4: Instigating a vaccination programme against calf respiratory disease

A dairy herd with 200 calves has an annual pneumonia incidence of 40%. Cases are generally detected early by well trained staff, who also weigh the calves regularly, but those who had pneumonia were growing on average 30 g per day less and as a consequence calved 30 days later (25 instead of 24 months).

The vaccine cost is £7 per calf (single intra-nasal vaccine given at ≥10 days of age) and as the agent has been identified and is part of the vaccine, it is expected to reduce pneumonia incidence from 40% to 30%.

> Cost per case, based purely on growth rate:
> 30 days × £2.87 = £86.10
> 20 cases prevented = cost saving is £1722
> Cost of vaccinating 200 calves: £1400

Although this is close to the break-even point (123% return in investment), other important but variable factors, such as mortality, treatment costs, staff time, frustration and, above all, welfare, have not been included in the calculation, and higher reductions are achieved on many farms.

the value of a calf plus disposal costs, but in closed herds with marginal replacement heifer numbers the losses may mean empty spaces in the milking herd. For this reason, a very conservative approach has been taken in the herd example, taking into account mainly the reduced growth rates and the resulting increased rearing costs:

REFERENCES

1. Shizgal P. Scarce means with alternative uses: Robbins' definition of economics and its extension to the behavioral and neurobiological study of animal decision making. Front Neurosci 2012; 6:20.
2. Boulton AC, Rushton J, Wathes DC. An empirical analysis of the cost of rearing dairy heifers from birth to first calving and the time taken to repay these costs. Animal 2017;11(8):1372–80.
3. Brickell JS, McGowan MM, Wathes DC. Effect of management factors and blood metabolites during the rearing period on growth in dairy heifers on UK farms. Domest Anim Endocrinol 2009 Feb;36(2):67–81.
4. Flachowsky G, Meyer U, Südekum KH. Land use for edible protein of animal origin—A review. Animals (Basel) 2017;7(3):1–19.
5. FAO. Dietary protein quality evaluation in human nutrition; 2013.
6. Raboisson D, Trillat P, Cahuzac C. Failure of passive immune transfer in calves: A meta-analysis on the consequences and assessment of the economic impact. PLOS ONE 2016;11(3):e0150452.
7. Redman G. John Nix farm management pocketbook. 48th ed. 2017.
8. Hawkins A, Burdine K, Amaral-Phillips D, Costa JHC. An economic analysis of the costs associated with pre-weaning management strategies for dairy heifers. Animals (Basel) 2019;9(7):1–11.
9. Khan MA, Weary DM, von Keyserlingk MA. Invited review: Effects of milk ration on solid feed intake, weaning, and performance in dairy heifers. J Dairy Sci 2011;94(3):1071–81.
10. Palczynski LJ, Bleach ECL, Brennan ML, Robinson PA. Appropriate dairy calf feeding from birth to weaning: 'It's an investment for the future'. Animals

2020 Jan 10;10(1):116. Available from: https://www.mdpi.com/2076–2615/10/1/116.
11. Soberon F, Raffrenato E, Everett RW, Van Amburgh ME. Preweaning milk replacer intake and effects on long-term productivity of dairy calves. J Dairy Sci 2012 Feb;95(2):783–93. Available from: http://www.ncbi.nlm.nih.gov/pubmed/22281343.
12. Bennett R. The "direct costs" of livestock disease: The development of a system of models for the analysis of 30 endemic livestock diseases in Great Britain. J Agricultural Economics 2003;54(1):55–71.
13. Bennett R, Ijpelaar J. Updated estimates of the costs associated with thirty four endemic livestock diseases in Great Britain: A note. J Agricultural Economics 2005;56(1):135–44.
14. Johnson KF, Chancellor N, Burn CC, Wathes DC. Prospective cohort study to assess rates of contagious disease in pre-weaned UK dairy heifers: Management practices, passive transfer of immunity and associated calf health. Vet Rec Open 2017 Apr 1;4(1). Available from: https://pubmed.ncbi.nlm.nih.gov/29259784/:e000226.
15. Pardon B, Hostens M, Duchateau L, Dewulf J, De Bleecker K, Deprez P. Impact of respiratory disease, diarrhea, otitis and arthritis on mortality and carcass traits in white veal calves. BMC Vet Res 2013;9:79.
16. Shaw HJ, Innes EA, Morrison LJ, Katzer F, Wells B. Long-term production effects of clinical cryptosporidiosis in neonatal calves. Int J Parasitol 2020;50(5):371–6.
17. Lassen B, Østergaard S. Estimation of the economical effects of Eimeria infections in Estonian dairy herds using a stochastic model. Prev Vet Med 2012;106(3–4):258–65.
18. Andrews A. Calf pneumonia costs! Cattle Pract 2000;8(2):109–14.
19. Magnier S. The impact of early calf hood disease. Vet Irel J 2014;4(5):267–9.
20. Blakebrough-Hall C, Dona A, D'occhio MJ, McMeniman J, González LA. Diagnosis of Bovine Respiratory Disease in feedlot cattle using blood 1H N.M.R. metabolomics. Sci Rep 2020;10(1):115.
21. Teixeira AGV, McArt JAA, Bicalho RC. Thoracic ultrasound assessment of lung consolidation at weaning in Holstein dairy heifers: Reproductive performance and survival. J Dairy Sci 2017 Apr;100(4):2985–91. Available from: https://linkinghub.elsevier.com/retrieve/pii/S0022030217301510.

Appendix I

P00222BG VitaMilk Hipro Heifer
Complementary milk replacer for rearing calves up to 4 months

Analytical constituents:

Crude protein	26.0%
Crude fat	17.0%
Crude fiber	0.0%
Crude ash	8.5%
Calcium (Ca)	0.80%
Phosphorus (P)	0.67%
Sodium (Na)	0.74%

Additives per kg
Nutritional:

3a672a Vitamin A	25.000 IU
3a671 Vitamin D3	5.000 IU
3a700 Vitamin E (all-rac-alpha-tocopheryl-acetate)	350 mg
3b103 Iron (II) sulphate monohydrate	100 mg
3b405 Cupric (II) sulphate pentahydrate	8 mg
3b503 Manganous sulphate monohydrate	55 mg
3b605 Zinc sulphate monohydrate	70 mg
3b201 Iodine, potassium iodide	1 mg
3b801 Sodium selenite	0.3 mg

Technologial:

E310 Propyl gallate	3 mg
E320 BHA	3 mg

Composition:
Whey powder; Vegetable oil (Palm, Coco, Rape); Wheat protein, hydrolised;
Wheat flour Calcium carbonate; Yeast; Magnesium sulfate anhydrous.

Directions for use:
Complementary feed for calves. Use for target animals only.
Feed as directed - Do not feed to sheep.
For expiry date and batch number, see below.
Store in dark, cook and dry conditions.

UFAS No. 794
Creditation number: α-NL09882

For Farmers, Horizon House, Fred Castle Way,
Rougham Industrial Estate
Rougham, Bury St. Edmunds, IP30 9ND

	Best befor:	01-01-2015
PO 1103191252		
Batch 1234567	11506705	Net Weight: 20kg

FIGURE 5.6 A list of constituents on a CMR bag.

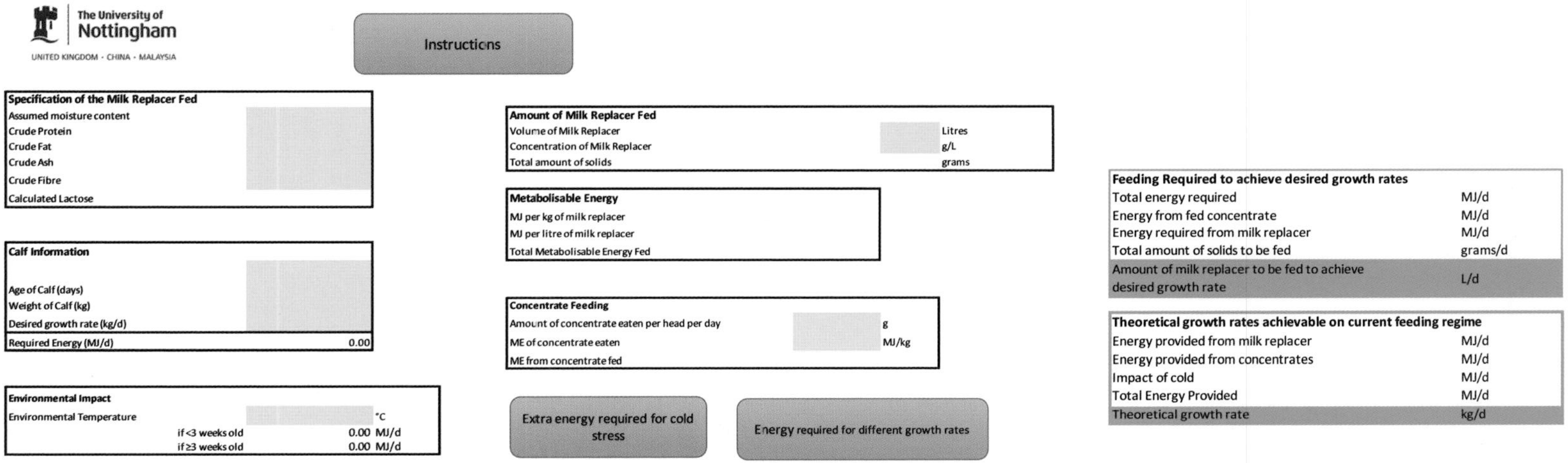

FIGURE 5.5 A screenshot of the AHDB CMR energy calculator that was designed in conjunction with the University of Nottingham.

Index